W9-BKI-007

THE PROBLEM OF
ALZHEIMER'S

ALSO BY JASON KARLAWISH

Open Wound: The Tragic Obsession of Dr. William Beaumont

THE PROBLEM OF ALZHEIMER'S

· · · · · · · · · · · · · ·

HOW SCIENCE, CULTURE, AND POLITICS TURNED A RARE DISEASE INTO A CRISIS AND WHAT WE CAN DO ABOUT IT

JASON KARLAWISH

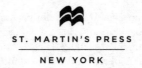

ST. MARTIN'S PRESS

NEW YORK

First published in the United States by St. Martin's Press, an imprint
of St. Martin's Publishing Group

THE PROBLEM OF ALZHEIMER'S. Copyright © 2021 by Jason Karlawish. All rights
reserved. Printed in the United States of America. For information, address St. Martin's
Publishing Group, 120 Broadway, New York, NY 10271.

www.stmartins.com

Library of Congress Cataloging-in-Publication Data

Names: Karlawish, Jason, author.
Title: The problem of Alzheimer's : how science, culture, and politics turned a
rare disease into a crisis and what we can do about it / Jason Karlawish.
Description: First edition. | New York : St. Martin's Press, 2021. | Includes
bibliographical references and index.
Identifiers: LCCN 2020026249 | ISBN 9781250218735 (hardcover) |
ISBN 9781250218742 (ebook)
Subjects: MESH: Alzheimer Disease | Delivery of Health Care | Caregivers |
Bioethical Issues | Psychosocial Support Systems | Case Reports
Classification: LCC RC523 | NLM WT 155 | DDC 616.8/311—dc23
LC record available at https://lccn.loc.gov/2020026249

Our books may be purchased in bulk for promotional, educational, or
business use. Please contact your local bookseller or the Macmillan Corporate
and Premium Sales Department at 1-800-221-7945, extension 5442, or by email at
MacmillanSpecialMarkets@macmillan.com.

First Edition: 2021

10   9   8   7   6   5   4   3   2   1

FOR JOHN

CONTENTS

THE PROBLEM OF ALZHEIMER'S

INTRODUCTION:
THE DISEASE OF THE CENTURY

It is the worst of all diseases, not just for what it does to the patient, but for
its devastating effects on families and friends.
—Lewis Thomas, "The Problem of Dementia," 1981

BY THE COLD Friday afternoon in January 2010 when I met Edith Harrison for a new patient appointment at the Penn Memory Center, her memory
problems had been going on for at least four, maybe five years. Her husband,
Ed, struggled to pinpoint exactly when they started.

At first, the problems were subtle. She was making more lists.

She snapped, "You do too," when he pointed this out to her.

"But I've always made them. You've just started."

She turned on her heel and strode smartly out of the kitchen. A door
slammed.

Maybe it is just aging, he decided. And so he let it go.

In the months that followed, her memory trickled away. She'd forget an
item from the grocery store and repeat a story she'd told him earlier in the
day. Otherwise, though, she seemed fine.

It was the call from the home owners' association that caused him to
worry. "Is there something wrong, Mr. Harrison?" asked the officious dep-
uty director. "You haven't paid your fee in three months." For the first time
since they married, he looked at their joint checking account. Her handwrit-
ing, like her, was still elegant, but the balance was in disarray.

Maybe this isn't aging.

A visit to her primary care doctor for help was too quick and essentially
useless. It ended not with a diagnosis but instead with an antibiotic. The

nurse who telephoned with the results of the MRI of her brain reported there was no tumor or stroke, but there was sinusitis. The prescribed antibiotic caused two weeks of diarrhea.

That was in 2008. There were more doctors and more medications—for low thyroid, high anxiety, and chronic fatigue—but no clear diagnosis. In time, they settled into a new normal. He did the bills. They shopped and cooked together, and she watched a lot of TV. Diagnosis didn't seem to matter.

It was their daughter who sounded the alarm. She was back from an extended tour of duty with the army in the Middle East. "Dad, something's really wrong with Mom." She held her hands out before her father like she intended to shake him.

They waited six months for a new patient appointment at the Memory Center.

"This seems more than memory," Ed anxiously explained to me. He worried she was depressed. Her once-inspiring initiative and conscientiousness were fading away. She'd ceased going to her book club and choir. "Not interested," she explained as she sat before the TV. The day of the week was becoming unmoored from ordered time. The repetitious questions—"Is today Monday?"—were increasing, and they were profoundly annoying, a kind of slow verbal tennis match. She'd ask, he'd answer, and then fifteen minutes later, she'd ask again. Back and forth until she seemed to finally get it.

Or he blew up at her.

My examination of Mrs. Harrison displayed her cognitive impairments. Her struggle to learn the five items of a street address and after a five-minute delay to recall only one of those items—"Chicago"—showed not only problems with memory (her recall of the address) but also with attention and concentration (her struggle to learn the address). In those minutes between learning and recalling the address, I put her through other tests. Counting down from one hundred by sevens. Calculating the change on a purchase. I handed her a pencil and a clipboard with a sheet of plain white paper.

"Please draw me the face of a clock, fill in all the numbers, and show the time as five minutes to one."

Explanations for all the notes about the house, the double-paid bills, and the disordered checkbook were clarifying. She had a problem with memory—the ability to recall new information. And she had problems with the ability to plan, sequence, and organize a task, what psychologists call executive function, a term that describes the adult brain's capacity to conduct itself, to orchestrate its myriad of cognitive abilities—such as memory, language, and attention—into a song of yourself.

This test—we call it the clock draw test—is just one among many tests to measure executive function, but it is the one I favor. Its results are so evident. Truly, this one picture displays what I sometimes struggle to explain. Your cognition isn't normal anymore.

This one picture also displayed her quiet sufferings.

"Not too good," she murmured as she returned to me the clipboard and pencil. She folded her hands in her lap. She wouldn't look at me. This seventy-one-year-old retired art teacher was plainly embarrassed over her drawing, a surreal jumble of lines and misplaced numbers.

In 1981, the physician and National Book Award–winning essayist Lewis Thomas published "The Problem of Dementia" in the popular science magazine *Discover*.[1] Thomas, a prominent cancer researcher, began his essay with a stern admonition to the American public: do not let the government intrude into the work of scientists like him. The esteemed and accomplished sixty-eight-year-old former dean of New York University's and Yale University's medical schools and, at the time of this essay, president of Memorial Sloan Kettering Cancer Center, argued that the right way to discover treatments for common and devastating diseases such as cancer was to follow a "nontargeting rule."

"Nontargeting" meant studying normal biological processes at a pace set by scientists, not by politicians. He dismissed politicians directing scientists to mount "frontal, targeted assaults on one disease after another." He disparaged this approach as "the 'disease-of-the-month' syndrome."

Congress agreed. Leaving to scientists the decisions over how much research funding they needed and how best to spend it dodged the difficult politics of yet another desperate constituent's plaintive and unceasing plea for a moonshot effort to cure their disease.

But then, in that same article, Thomas argued for an exception to his rule. He urged "special consideration and high priority for one particular disease, not a disease of the month," he wrote, "but a disease-of-the-century, the brain disease that affects increasing numbers of our population because of the increasing population of older people in the society—senility, or, as it is now termed, senile dementia. The major form of the disorder, Alzheimer's disease, affects more than 500,000 people over the age of fifty, most of them in their seventies and eighties. It is responsible for most of the beds in the country's nursing homes, at a cost exceeding $10 billion now and scheduled to rise to $40 billion or more within the next few years."

"It is," he concluded, "the worst of all diseases, not just for what it does to the patient, but for its devastating effects on families and friends."

Thomas was writing at the dawn of a new age. Just five years earlier, in a short essay in the *Archives of Neurology* (now called *JAMA Neurology*), the neurologist Robert Katzman argued for a new disease. Medicine and society should cast aside the label of senility and replace it with Alzheimer's disease.[2] He warned America: this disease is common, and it is "a major killer."

Katzman's "The Prevalence and Malignancy of Alzheimer Disease" was a call to action. He argued that the multiplicity of older adults with dementia were no longer victims of senility, an extreme and unfortunate stage of normal aging. They were patients with a disease. We must therefore cease hiding them away in families' homes or asylums. They needed doctors and researchers dedicated to accurate diagnosis, treatment, and, ultimately, a cure.

America listened.

On December 4, 1979, seven desperate and determined families met at the Hilton Chicago O'Hare Airport Hotel and passed a resolution to form a national patient advocacy and self-help group that came to be branded the Alzheimer's Association. They set to work advocating for better care and research so that other families did not suffer as they did. Things began to change.

The National Institutes of Health's newly created National Institute on Aging took on Alzheimer's disease as its charge, devoting as much as half of its research budget to the disease. Congress held numerous hearings and authorized funding for a national network of Alzheimer's disease research centers. By 1988, the association joined with the American Association of Retired Persons (AARP) and other advocacy groups to campaign on behalf of the millions of families threatened with bankruptcy by the staggering yearslong, daily costs of caring for a patient at home or in a nursing home. They persuaded the presidential candidates, Republican and Democrat, to sign on to a national long-term care social insurance program modeled after Medicare. In 1993, the Food and Drug Administration (FDA) approved the first pharmaceutical treatment for Alzheimer's disease.

The dark ages were ending.

Some thirty-five years after Katzman's call to action, Congress asked a bipartisan study group to take stock of the nation's progress against Alzheimer's disease. The 2009 report, *A National Alzheimer's Strategic Plan: The Report of the Alzheimer's Study Group*, was a breathtaking, unqualified, even apocalyptic assessment of America's failed progress, an indictment of both the national research effort and the health care system.[3]

The report began: "Alzheimer's disease poses a grave and growing challenge to our Nation." The numbers of persons affected (10 million caregivers providing 94 billion hours of care for 5 million patients) and the costs of their care ($100 billion per year) were arresting multiples of the facts and figures Thomas cited in his 1981 essay. The word "crisis" appeared twenty-four times.

At the time of the Alzheimer's Study Group report, I was moving along in my career as a physician and researcher. My focus was Alzheimer's disease. My research examined issues at the intersections of care, ethics, and policy. It was work dedicated to improving the dignity and respect for the personhood of people living with dementia. Our discoveries included methods to assess a patient's ability to make risky decisions and policies to protect the voting rights of persons living in long-term care facilities. Once a week on a Friday, I saw patients for diagnosis and treatment at the Penn Memory Center.

The report, I was quite certain, was correct. This was a crisis. The Harrisons were yet one more casualty.

The glass-and-steel tower where I saw them housed state-of-the-science cancer and cardiovascular centers where colleagues administered astonishingly accurate diagnostic tests and spectacularly effective treatments. I, on the other hand, was still performing a diagnostic assessment that had changed little since the work-up Dr. Alois Alzheimer and his colleagues performed in the first two decades of the twentieth century.

The story of Mr. Harrison's efforts to obtain a diagnosis and care for his wife was all too typical. In addition to her internist, they'd sought answers from a neurologist who'd mentioned dementia, never said "Alzheimer's disease," and then quickly focused the visit on a medication to treat memory problems and scheduled follow-up in one year.

They were frustrated and so was I. Our new patient visits were booked out months in advance. The medications the neurologist and I prescribed were largely ineffective. The treatments that could help the Harrisons—social, environmental, and psychological interventions—Medicare wouldn't pay for, and even if it did, they weren't routinely available.

Why, in the twenty-eight years between Dr. Thomas's essay and the Harrisons' visit with me, had nothing really changed? Why did the richest and most powerful nation—the beacon of can-do, go-ahead innovation—fail to listen to revolutionaries like Robert Katzman, Lewis Thomas, and the seven families?

This book recounts the answers to these questions. It is the story of how once upon a time, Alzheimer's disease was a rare disease, and then it became common, and then it turned into a crisis. By the middle of the twentieth century, after the catastrophes of two world wars, much of the story of Alzheimer's crosses the Atlantic from Germany to America. What follows may seem, therefore, to be an American view taken by an American writer on an American problem. And yet a story of a disease as vast and all encompassing as Alzheimer's must focus on one nation's response.

The focus is national, but the crisis is international. Readers from other nations will recognize unfortunate similarities with their nations' uneven responses to Alzheimer's. Undoubtedly, they'll nod with understanding and empathy over the plight of people like the Harrisons.

Part 1 explains the changing meanings of what Alzheimer's disease is and the enduring challenges of translating this complicated and nuanced diagnosis to patients, their families, and health care systems. Part 2 looks back over the course of the twentieth century to show a tragedy of science and medicine colliding with politics and culture in ways that kept the disease largely hidden and untreated and then—once recognized as common—underdiagnosed, leaving patients and families neglected. Part 3 shows the opportunities to address this crisis. Scientific advances have discovered ways to improve care in the physician's office, home and community, and hospital and nursing home. There are also astonishingly promising advances in the ability to diagnose and treat the disease before a person has dementia. The problem isn't science. Part 4 explains why and what we have to do.

Alzheimer's disease starts out in individuals, people like Mrs. Harrison. Soon it spreads to other people, men and women like her husband and their daughter, who switched from full- to part-time work to help her father care for her mother for five years. Together, millions of patients and caregivers experience physical, psychological, financial, and moral suffering. Their awesome tally adds up to a humanitarian problem. The solution isn't simply better medical care. To overcome this crisis, we must mobilize our cultural, civic, and social systems.

PART 1

. . . .

ALZHEIMER'S UNBOUND

Considering everything, it seems we are dealing here with a peculiar
illness.
> —Alois Alzheimer, "An Unusual Disease of the Cerebral Cortex," 1907

1

A PECULIAR DISEASE
OF THE CEREBRAL CORTEX

The dementia of Alzheimer's disease is typically gradual in onset, so insidious that families and afflicted individuals may not recognize the disease until glaring deficits have appeared.

—Valerie Denisse Perel, "Psychosocial Impact of Alzheimer Disease," *JAMA*, 1998

"WHAT'S THE DIFFERENCE between dementia and Alzheimer's disease?"

That was the Harrisons' first question to me after I told them Mrs. Harrison had dementia and the most likely cause was Alzheimer's disease. He asked. She nodded. She was characteristically silent for much of the visit.

This question is the most common question patients and their family members have. It's as if this disease that causes a person to repeat questions because she forgets the answers were having fun with us.

Dementia, I explained, describes progressive impairments in cognition that cause problems with day-to-day function. Alzheimer's disease is one of several diseases that cause dementia. When I saw the Harrisons in 2010, I was following a strict rule set forth in diagnostic criteria written in 1984 by an expert panel of neurologists.[1]

No dementia. No Alzheimer's disease.

"And how's dementia different from aging?" he asked.

Cognition does change with aging, I explained. Quite slowly. Much of the change is in the speed of thinking and deciding, annoying to be sure and sometimes the cause of mistakes, but not disabling. A person with dementia, in contrast, has months to years of progressive declines in multiple cognitive abilities. These declines cause them to have troubles performing their usual and everyday activities. "Cognitive abilities" describes the workings of our brain, such as recalling new information (memory), naming things (language), and switching between activities (multitasking). Usual and everyday activities are the stuff of life, such as logging on to the computer, ordering a gift, and, later, traveling to a restaurant to present it to a friend.

Much of what I needed to diagnose whether Mrs. Harrison had dementia came from the history of her day-to-day life. Her repetitious questions were an example of problems with short-term memory. Her problems balancing the checkbook were an example of problems with executive function and calculations.

To be sure, the cognitive tests were valuable. They helped to firm up the diagnosis and identify the particular disease that was causing her dementia. The history, though, is key. I tell trainees: "Nine-tenths of the work-up is the history." I organize this history along three themes.

The first is difficulties performing the usual, everyday tasks the person once performed effortlessly, such as taking medications or traveling outside the home, and difficulties in making decisions, such as whether to take a medication. In Mrs. Harrison's story, what stood out to me was problems with finances and baking Thanksgiving pies she was so noted for. These are cognitively demanding activities.

The second is changes in behavior and mood. Among the earliest and most common of these symptoms is apathy, a term describing fading initiative and conscientiousness. Many days, Mrs. Harrison seemed content to sit and do little. Other common changes are anxiety, depression, and false beliefs, or delusions. These symptoms vary in their frequency and intensity and, if they occur, like the moon, they wax and wane over the course of the disease.

The third theme is the loss of remote memory, or autobiography, the knowledge about one's self, your story, such as where you grew up, your first love, the birth dates of your children. This occurs in the later stages of the disease.

These themes are conveyed through histories that are typically quite vivid, routinely deeply personal, and sometimes very tragic (I once diagnosed a woman whose grandchildren scammed her of tens of thousands of dollars). Together, the histories form a kind of literature of the decline of a person's ability to self-determine her life. There is a word for this ability: "autonomy," meaning self-rule, from the Greek *autonomos* (having its own laws). Dementia in a sense is a disease of autonomy, and the lives of persons with it are an extended conversation over a question: "What's a good life when you're losing your ability to determine that life for yourself?"[2]

As a physician at a memory center, I write histories about the slow abridgement of the self. I begin this with the questions: "What's the problem? How can I help you?" Mr. Harrison's answers were all too common. "Memory problems" and then he launched into a plaintive story of their years of searching for answers.

Questions are my diagnostic tools. All I need is a clipboard, paper and pen, and the time to listen. Among my most powerful tools is a four-word question: "What's a typical day?" Upon administration, it elicits the story of a brain interacting with its world. Mrs. Harrison's day seemed normal, but it wasn't like it used to be. She was reading magazines not books. She was still cooking but not as well as she used to. Mr. Harrison had taken over the finances. This vivid account was the disease talking through her, a kind of slow entropy of her consciousness.

I used her history not only to diagnose her with dementia and determine that the cause was Alzheimer's disease but also to stage the dementia. When I met Mrs. Harrison, she was in the mild stage because her problems were largely confined to troubles performing the activities we undertake to maintain our house and home and to live well in it, such as cleaning and cooking, managing money and medications, using technologies like the computer or television remote control, and using transportation such as the bus. These are what we elect to do to flourish and live life as we choose. She was experiencing troubles with some of these, but she was still performing as usual on others. In a casual conversation, she seemed fine.

The moderate stage of dementia is characterized by consistent troubles with most of these activities. At this stage, the person had transformed from an adult who managed more or less on her own to a person whose survival now depends on others. In the years to follow their new patient visit with me, Mr. Harrison told me of the progressive exchange of activities from her to him. She was less conversational. And, notably, she was increasingly unaware of her problems with memory and performing day-to-day tasks. As the moderate stage worsened, she began to need some help with what are called basic activities of daily living, what we do to begin and end a day, namely walking to the bathroom to use the toilet, washing and dressing, and then walking to the kitchen for breakfast. The first sign is often the need for reminders to change clothes.

Mrs. Harrison was in the severe stage when she needed more assistance with basic activities. She lost these in a stereotypical pattern. Her dressing became disorganized. She needed reminders to bathe and then help to bathe. Then her walking became slow and unsteady and she needed help with the toilet. In time, if Mr. Harrison didn't spoon-feed her, the meal would be left cold and untouched.

Mr. Harrison pushed back when I labeled his wife as mild stage. "Her anger . . . it's so disruptive. This has to be severe," he countered. The count or severity of the emotional and behavioral problems is not factored in to staging, I explained. The focus is function and cognition because they best predict what to expect in the future and the time that will pass between diagnosis and death.

The most common word people use when they talk about Alzheimer's disease is "memory" or variations on it, like "memory loss" and "forgetfulness." This is sensible. Alzheimer's disease most commonly presents like Mrs. Harrison's did, with bothersome problems with memory. She'd forget new information. If Mr. Harrison didn't remind her of appointments, she'd miss them.

Memory is the earliest symptom because the hippocampus is often affected earliest by the disease. This region of the brain, so named for its resemblance to the mythical fishtailed horses that pulled Poseidon's chariot through the seas, has a critical role in our ability to learn and remember new information. When Alzheimer's begins here, it causes what my colleagues and I call the amnestic presentation of the disease.

Alzheimer's disease can start in other places in the brain. The result is a history of dementia that begins not with forgetfulness but other cognitive problems. In addition to the common amnestic presentation, three other presentations of Alzheimer's disease have been described.

One begins with vision problems. The patient describes frustrating months running through multiple eyeglass prescriptions in a vain effort to address troubles judging distances and reading. Another begins with problems with speech. The patient struggles to find words and uses more general terms, such as "thing" instead of the specific name for a familiar object. Finally, some stories begin with problems with attention, concentration, and problem solving. A patient will make mistakes paying bills. Early on, this presentation is perhaps the most difficult to diagnose because these symptoms are so similar to the age-related changes in cognition, that feeling of not being as sharp as one once was. Often, I have these patients return months later for a reassessment. Time tells whether the problem is the slow change due to aging or the fury of a disease.

Alzheimer's disease is one cause of dementia, and because it is thought to be the most common cause, it has attained eminence over the other diseases that also cause dementia. In Lewy body disease, for example, the patient has vivid hallucinations, typically of animals or people, such as seeing a cat in the fireplace. A person with frontotemporal lobar degeneration—so named for the particular regions of the brain affected—has marked changes in personality.

These diseases are collectively called neurodegenerative diseases. This term describes their common feature. The brain's complicated and elegant network of cells, called neurons, is dying, or degenerating. Pathologists describe the visibly shrunken brain they autopsy as "atrophied." They'll run their gloved finger over the brain's surface and remark how much more space there is between the folds of tissue that make up the walnut-shaped organ. Next, they'll slice up the tissue and, using a microscope, see missing neurons and the pathologies characteristic of the different diseases.

Not all dementias are caused by a neurodegenerative disease. Infections can cause dementia. In the nineteenth century, one of the most common causes of dementia was infection with syphilis. In addition to notable changes in mood and cognition, patients often developed trouble walking.

A careful history, tests of her memory and other thinking skills—or in a word her "cognition"—and a neurological exam provided me with most of the data I needed to diagnose Mrs. Harrison with dementia and that the cause was Alzheimer's disease.

My confidence in her diagnosis was, however, only "probable." The preamble to the section "Laboratory Assessments" in the 1984 Alzheimer's disease diagnostic criteria advised me: "At present, there are no specific diagnostic laboratory tests for Alzheimer's disease." I could only make a diagnosis of "definite Alzheimer's disease" when she died. Then, in addition to her history and exam, I would order a brain autopsy to look for the characteristic pathologies.

These diagnostic criteria—probable in life, definite in death—reinforce lurid metaphors of the disease as a mysterious, gothic horror story. Mrs. Harrison would have to die before I could tell her husband the cause of her dementia.

A PECULIAR DISEASE, DIAGNOSED IN A PECULIAR PLACE, AND IN A PECULIAR WAY

The memory center where I diagnosed Mrs. Harrison is, like the disease she had, strange. The physicians might be neurologists, psychiatrists, or geriatricians (a doctor who specializes in the care of older adults). There are psychologists and technicians who administer cognitive testing, nurses to review health history and medications and answer calls from the family, and social workers who educate patients and families and lead education and support groups for each.

Our space is unusual. The waiting and exam rooms have extra chairs to accommodate the patient and their family. There are windowless, austere rooms, minimalist spaces where, free of distractions, the technicians perform cognitive testing.

After I introduced myself to the Harrisons in the waiting room, I sent Mrs. Harrison off to that windowless room with the promise that I'd meet her later. Then I asked her husband to follow me to my exam room. We took our catty-corner seats at the small exam room desk. I pushed the computer screen out of the way, took up my clipboard and pen, and began her new patient visit.

"What's the problem?" I asked him. "How can I help you?"

I don't start with the patient. I start with the family.

My patients are adults, but to deliver the standard of care, my colleagues and I routinely violate their privacy and authority. To obtain a detailed and accurate history, we require patients to bring a close friend or family member. We instruct this person—not the patient—to fill out the details on the new patient assessment form. At the start of the visit, I routinely separate the patient from her family.

I do this because patients often minimize or even don't recognize their disabilities. If I relied on Mrs. Harrison for her history, I might miss her diagnosis. In fact, she might not even come to a memory center, insisting that all is well.

Awareness of how cognitive problems impact daily life is often nuanced. This tends to mitigate the patient's distress. One of my patients explained her emotions after the diagnosis. "In the beginning, I was very sad about this, but right now I'm just going with it. I'm doing the best I can. I'm going to have a positive attitude, but I'm not going to be a crybaby. I don't want to go away. I want to do as best as I can." Her experience wasn't a denial of but rather living with the diagnosis.

Some patients interpret their problems not as a disease but instead as a disability. A patient told me: "I'm totally healthy from the neck down. I don't feel like I have an illness. I feel like I have a disability. I don't see myself as sick. I think I have a condition like a bum foot." Her turning away from illness and disease and toward disability was a reframing. It allowed her to once again feel normal. I find her analogy to a physical disability fascinating. A person with quadriplegia, for example, needs devices such as a scooter or a wheelchair. A person with dementia also needs a device. We call it the caregiver.

Some family members new to this role gesture to the empty chair where their relative might sit beside them and confess they feel I'm turning them into spies. But I reassure them. This is the standard of care. What's considered extraordinary practice elsewhere is, at a memory center, not peculiar but rather usual and ordinary practice.

The empty chair signifies endings and beginnings. For Mrs. Harrison, it was the end of being an older adult with a memory problem and the beginning of becoming a patient with dementia caused by Alzheimer's disease. For Mr. Harrison, the empty chair marked the end of simply being her husband and the beginning of being her husband and her caregiver.

Some patients and caregivers complain about our practice. A caregiver once snapped at me: "Isn't there some test you can do to figure out what *exactly* is going on? All we seem to do at a memory center is tell each other stories." He might have added: "And wait until my wife dies to tell me what killed her."

I understand his anger.

He and his wife came to me seeking a simple answer to a simple question: "Doctor, am I still normal?" Two hours later, I had subjected them to an unusual and invasive work-up. I intruded into their privacy, upended her authority, and challenged their identity and sense of being normal. My answer was definitive—you have dementia and you are her caregiver—but it was also uncertain. The cause is *probably* Alzheimer's disease. Moreover, all my efforts in diagnosis led to comparatively meager treatments. The only medications I could prescribe were minimally effective drugs to palliate the symptoms. I possessed no treatment to slow the relentless losses in day-to-day function.

NOT ONE BUT TWO PATIENTS

In 2000, Dr. Arthur Kleinman's professional and personal lives collided. The cause of his wife Joan's bothersome problems with reading and a frightening, near catastrophic accident while running were not problems with her aging eyes. Kleinman, a psychiatrist and anthropologist at Harvard University, was renowned for his studies of how patients make sense of disease, how culture shapes those experiences, and the role clinicians have in eliciting these experiences. He was now turning his academic skills on his life and its new and disturbing roles. Joan had Alzheimer's disease and he was her caregiver (hers was the visual form; the earliest symptoms are troubles organizing visual images).

He started publishing essays about his experiences caring for her. In time, he wrote a book, *The Soul of Care*.[3] He came to see how the person with the disease and the person who cares for her essentially exchange roles. He concluded, "She is happy much of the time. It is me, the caregiver, who, more often, is sad and despairing."[4]

Studies reinforce this. Patients consistently rate their quality of life and functional abilities better than caregivers rate the quality of life and functional abilities of the person they care for,[5] and caregivers experience notable symptoms of anxiety and depression.[6] The caregiver's anxiety is a distinct and persistent preoccupation with the future. A wife explained to me: "If things could stay the way they are, that would be fine. I'm scared. I worry. I worry about the future and how to handle it physically." Her words describe two other aspects of the caregiver's illness experience: tasks and time.

The tasks of caregiving involve taking on the activities the patient leaves off. As the patient loses the ability to manage day-to-day activities and make decisions, the caregiver takes these up.

One of the most widely read books to educate and train caregivers is *The 36-Hour Day*.[7] The title is sadly brilliant. Assisting or entirely performing either instrumental or basic activities of daily living, or both, encumbers a caregiver's time. "Pills and bills," a caregiver once lamented to me. The tally of hours spent providing this care (instead of other activities such as working, going to the gym, or being with friends) is estimated to be as much as 171 hours a month.[8]

One of the greatest advances in assessing the totality of the harms of Alzheimer's disease occurred not in medicine coming up with some novel way to measure the suffering of patients or more nuanced ways to measure their impairments in cognition or day-to-day function but rather in economics and related social sciences. These outsider fields began to explore novel ways to think about, measure, and so talk about the experience of family members like Mr. Harrison and Dr. Kleinman.

They started with a word: caregiver. A search on the word "caregiver" in databases such as Medline or Google's n-gram, which track year-to-year trends in words, shows a remarkable result. This term that is now ubiquitous was once upon a time—but not so long ago—unknown. Prior to the mid-1970s, "caregiver" doesn't appear in scholarly writings. What was unspoken was unstudied. By 1980, however, the word "caregiver" appears and then becomes increasingly prevalent.

Why?

It was around this time that economists, sociologists, and feminist scholars were asking a simple but provocative and politically charged question. What's the value of work done in settings other than places like a factory, office, or farm? One of these settings was the home. What, for example, was the value of the labor of being a homemaker or, in other words, a housewife?

For much of human history, this time was not counted as labor. The work of providing care at home for a chronically ill family member was simply not among the harms of a disease or a cost to society. This "informal care" was simply just what families did, meaning what women did. "Formal care," such as paying the staff of a nursing home or asylum to provide care, was counted as a cost. Lewis Thomas, in making his plea that Alzheimer's is the disease of the century, cited the $10 billion cost of nursing home care. He didn't speak of the cost to caregivers because he couldn't. The word didn't exist. Yet.

What if the care taken on by families was also classified as work? Researchers began to categorize the tasks and the time required to complete this work. Their answers in turn begat other seemingly simple questions, such as how much could a person who performs this work earn?

To answer this, researchers tallied the hours a person devotes to caregiving and then multiplied the hours worked by an hourly wage. Simple math to be sure, but it led right up to a complex and politically charged question in the cross hairs of ideas about the family, economics, culture, and ethics or, in a phrase, "family values."

What should be the wages of caregiving? What price should we attach to the daily hours Dr. Kleinman and Mr. Harrison devoted to being present with their wives to ensure they were safe and engaged, to helping them get dressed and ready for the day?

Should it be the wage typical for a person hired to undertake such tasks? This job is called a home health aide, and in 2019, her (nearly *all* are women, many from minority or immigrant communities) hourly wage was about $12.18.[9] Economists call this a replacement cost. The term describes the cost of paying someone else to perform the work of caregiving: that is, what Dr. Kleinman would pay to replace his labor with the work of a home health aide.

Or should the caregiver's wage be what he'd earn for his usual work? For Kleinman, that would be his work as a physician and professor on faculty at Harvard. For Mr. Harrison, who was retired, the economists look to the typical wage earned by a man at his age.

Both calculations may seem odd. The work of assisting with instrumental and basic activities of daily living—picking out her clothes, preparing breakfast, and driving her to the doctor—is really quite different from the work of a psychiatrist and anthropologist. And yet, the hours Kleinman spent caring for his wife were hours he could have been working at Harvard. In some sense, he was giving up or otherwise losing the wages he could have earned. Economists call these foregone wages.

A study of the annual costs of Alzheimer's disease to the United States produced a staggering, headline-grabbing result.[10] The disease's total yearly cost in 2010 was as much as $215 billion. Even more arresting was the breakdown of the components of this total. Costs to Medicare—the tests and the limited number of prescription treatments doctors order—were a small fraction. The costs of informal care drove up a total to rival the costs of cancer and heart disease.

Notably, the total cost of informal care depended on the wage the economists assigned to the work of care. Informal care—the work of spouses and adult children—made up from one-third to one-half of the total (the former was the sum of foregone wages, and the latter was replacement costs).

These figures are an entrée into expansive reflections over the wages of caregiving.[11,12] It's a protracted commitment. Over these years, as caregivers gain skills to care, their skills to perform other kinds of work atrophy much like their relative's brain. Promotions and wages stagnate. The result? Savings don't accumulate as they might. The experiences of life are delayed or even foregone, experiences such as dinner out with friends, a vacation, and retirement. The staggering cost of a college education for children or grandchildren adds to the debt.

Depending on the economic methods, such as what is counted and over what time period, the "costs of caregiving" differ, but they consistently point in the same direction. The Alzheimer's crisis is a crisis of uncompensated labor and lost income. It is a crisis of the American family.

THE STIGMAS OF ALZHEIMER'S DISEASE

Time and task are the common experiences of caregivers of persons disabled by any chronic disease. It is a third feature of the caregiving experience that distinguishes an Alzheimer's caregiver from other caregivers: the caregiver controls the truth.

This control allows caregivers to shape the world around the patient. In the mild and moderate stages of dementia, they try to do this in collaboration with the person with dementia. Over time, though, authority shifts. The caregiver removes the person's name from his or her checkbook, chooses where they will eat out for dinner, where they will go for an outing, and what they will wear on that outing.

The design and practices of a memory center facilitate this control. The training we provide the caregiver, done either privately or to a group of caregivers, includes instructions on how to tell a patient the truth.

As Mrs. Harrison's disease worsened, she began to ask when her mother would visit. The old but for her novel news that she had died would precipitate hours of furious grief: "Why didn't you *tell* me!" We instructed Mr. Harrison to practice a "loving deception." Tell her that her mother was fine and would be visiting soon and then to move on to a different and pleasant topic.

I once cared for a couple who dined off large platters instead of the customary dinner plates. The husband, my patient, had become obsessed that he was eating too much. He refused to eat. His wife became distressed. He was losing weight. And then she discovered a solution. The same portion of food served on a large platter seemed like a smaller portion. And so he became calm and ate his seemingly modest supper.

This practice of "loving deceptions" is morally fraught. An essential feature of all moral relationships is trust. Deception subverts trust.

This moral anguish caused Larry Ruvo to construct a structure the world would remember, a building he hoped would change the course of Alzheimer's disease. After his father, Lou Ruvo, died of Alzheimer's disease, Larry—his only child, caregiver, and a multimillionaire wine and liquor wholesaler—commissioned the architect Frank Gehry to design the Lou Ruvo Center for

Brain Health, an $80 million memory center in his home city of Las Vegas, Nevada.

With his signature curvaceous design style, Gehry erected a structure that stands out even among Las Vegas's ostentatious buildings. The bright steel facade is a multiplicity of wavy, nonlinear, gravity-defying walls. The shiny steel seems to be melting under the desert sun. The design also reflects Larry Ruvo's desire to redeem himself before his father. Larry had lied to his father.

It happened as he and his father were waiting to see the doctor who diagnosed Lou Ruvo with Alzheimer's disease. "In the waiting room there were three patients: one in diapers, one in a wheelchair, and another with his head bent over, out of it. My dad was still cognizant, and he said, 'This is what's happening to me?'"

Larry answered no. Those patients, he explained, were seeing the doctor for other problems.

"You knew what was coming, that my father was going to die," Ruvo recalled. "But there was no dignity. So I told myself that very day that I wanted to build a facility where patients never saw other patients, where people's dignity was preserved."[13]

The center opened in 2009. There is no common room where patients and families wait. Ruvo ordered Gehry to design individual "tranquility rooms." Patients and their families enter and exit through private doors. A patient never sees another patient.

Lou Ruvo's question and his son's response, both in word and, years later, in a grand architectural deed, are vivid examples of how brains affected by Alzheimer's disease—patient and caregiver—are also affected by the stigmas of Alzheimer's disease. Larry Ruvo was enacting public stigma.

For patients and caregivers, public stigma causes isolation. Friends start to disappear. Walter Annenberg explained that he no longer saw his friend Ronald Reagan. "You have a living person who ostensibly is all right and he is just out of it, and I do not want to see him in this light anymore. I prefer to remember him as a vigorous fellow."[14] I expect that meant Reagan's former ambassador to the United Kingdom kept away from Nancy Reagan as well. Health care practitioners commit similar acts of avoidance and distancing. Families tell me physicians talk about the patient in the third person, as though she weren't present in the room.

Self-stigma describes a person having feelings of shame and disgust about herself and, in response, avoiding others or withholding information about oneself. "We deal with Alzheimer's by not dealing with it," a caregiver explained to me. "We just try to be as normal as we can." Family members tell my research assistants their relative with Alzheimer's disease can participate in studies as long as the research assistant does not say "the A word." Colleagues swap out "dementia" with expressions such as "progressive memory loss" or "memory problems."

Others talk of Alzheimer's as "an extreme form of dementia." This, I think, explains President Reagan's nuance in his handwritten public letter to the United States disclosing his diagnosis. The Great Communicator explained, "I have recently been told that I am one of the millions of Americans who will be afflicted with Alzheimer's disease." The "will be" stands out. It distanced him from his diagnosis.

For him, perhaps having Alzheimer's disease meant that more extreme form of dementia, even perhaps a loss of identity, and he couldn't identify with either condition. He explained to America: "At the moment I feel just fine." And yet, he offered a vision of his and his wife Nancy's future. "I only wish there was some way I could spare Nancy from this painful experience."

Lurid words fuel these stigmas. Larry Ruvo told the story of his promise to his father in the CNN documentary titled *Unthinkable: The Alzheimer's Epidemic*. Alzheimer's is "a natural disaster," "a plague," "a tsunami that will bankrupt the country." The disease is "a demon that attacks the brain." Perhaps the most potent image is that patients become "living dead." They are "zombies."[15]

I use my words to push back against these words and so against the stigmas. Many years ago, I ceased calling my patients demented. They were instead "persons living with dementia." This is my effort to denote humanity to people with a disease that some say "robs us of our humanity."

In 2010, as I turned Mrs. Harrison into a person living with dementia probably caused by Alzheimer's disease and her husband into a caregiver, I was practicing the standard of care at a memory center at an academic medical center. No dementia, no Alzheimer's disease.

I knew, however, that this tight linkage was rupturing. Researchers were discovering ways to diagnose Alzheimer's disease *before* a person had dementia. Storytellers like me writing detailed and vivid histories were going to be replaced by doctors proficient in ordering and interpreting tests that quantify what's happening inside their patients' brains and then transforming that information into a history of the future of yourself. Even more inspiring, these discoveries promised "disease-slowing treatments," drugs that slowed the patient's relentless decline from independence to dependence.

The beginnings of this revolution converge on a specific place and time. In the small midwestern city of Rochester, Minnesota, in 1984, an eminent senior researcher assembled a team of young researchers. He commanded them to run a study he would lead. It was a kind of census. They were to count how many people had Alzheimer's disease in Olmsted County, Minnesota.

They set to their task with no intention to revolutionize the diagnosis or treatment of Alzheimer's disease. Some of them didn't even want to do the study. But by the close of the century, they'd made an extraordinary finding, a result that would begin the irrevocable unbinding of Alzheimer's disease from dementia.

2

NO ONE SAYS NO
TO LEN KURLAND

A great deal of interest has been generated concerning the topic of a boundary or transitional state between normal aging and dementia, or more specifically, Alzheimer disease.
> —Ronald Petersen and colleagues, "Mild Cognitive Impairment: Clinical Characterization and Outcome," *Archives of Neurology*, 1999

RITA PHILIP AND her daughter were among my first participants in the revolution of how we diagnose Alzheimer's disease. I first met them in the spring of 2012. While Mrs. Philip underwent cognitive testing, her daughter and I took our catty-corner seats at the small desk in my examination room at the Memory Center. After I asked my opening questions—"What's the problem? How can I help you?"—she looked at me like she was about to cry, then looked at the floor and said, "I'd like to make sure my mom doesn't have something neurological."

Her mother, a retired homemaker, was aware of cognitive changes, though she minimized them. "Senior moments," she explained. "What do you expect? I'm seventy-eight."

And perhaps she was right. Whatever was going on was mild. Her daughter told me her mother needed more time to complete complex day-to-day activities, like preparing a family dinner. She was also making mistakes, such as forgetting to take medications, but she was catching them. Her cognitive testing showed scores that were low, but for a homemaker with two years of college (she left school to marry and raise a family), the scores were within the range of normal.

Her cognitive changes seemed to be more in degree than in kind. She wasn't doing as well as she once did, but she wasn't abnormal. She certainly did not have dementia.

Both wanted to know what caused her mild cognitive problems. Was it just aging or, as her daughter asked, "Is there something neurological?"

Much of their visit, just two years after the Harrisons', was quite similar to the Harrisons' but for two respects. Now there were brain scans that had not been available when I saw the Harrisons, and there was also a revolutionary new way of thinking about Alzheimer's disease. When I put these together, I was able to confirm her daughter's suspicion. Her mother did have something neurological. She had Alzheimer's disease, but unlike Mrs. Harrison, she *did not* have dementia.

The science that allowed me to diagnose her with Alzheimer's disease without dementia can be traced back to a spring afternoon in 1984 when the psychologist Bob Ivnik bumped into Len Kurland while crossing the intersection of Second Street and Fourth Avenue in Rochester, Minnesota.

YOUNG MEN AND SCIENCE

"It was bright, sunny, and clear, a nice day. I was walking to a meeting when Len Kurland pulled me aside at an intersection and said very quickly: 'I wanted to let you know I submitted a grant and put your name on it.' I was like, OK, whatever, and just kept walking," Bob Ivnik recalled.[1]

Ivnik, thirty-six years old, was just six years into his job as the Mayo Clinic's first neuropsychologist. A dedicated clinician with a calm but serious demeanor, his typical day was spent helping physicians care for patients with epilepsy. Caring for patients was his dream job. He had no desire to do research.

"I wasn't happy when I found out that Len had me on his grant. I thought that wasn't my interest. I felt like I was being pulled into something I didn't want to do, but you can't say no to Len Kurland at the Mayo."

Looking back in an interview thirty-four years later, he came to understand how singularly important that afternoon was not only for him but also for all aging people. He would become part of a team of researchers who, after fifteen years of work, published one of the most cited papers in the history of Alzheimer's. Its results upended how doctors talk about normal aging and Alzheimer's disease.

Dr. Leonard Kurland was an American success story. The youngest of ten children of Russian immigrant parents, he was born and raised in a crowded row house in Baltimore, Maryland. Forty-three years later, when he joined the Mayo Clinic faculty in 1964 to chair the Department of Medical Statistics and Epidemiology, he was internationally recognized and lauded as the creator of a new field of medical research that combined his doctoral training in neurology and epidemiology, or, in a word, neuroepidemiology.

Epidemiology is the study of the patterns of diseases. Epidemiologists use a sort of statistical detective work to explain how common diseases are (that is, their prevalence). They track the spread of an infectious disease in a country, such as the corona or influenza viruses, to determine the risk of infection to its population and whether the count of patients has achieved epidemic dimensions. Epidemiological studies also discover the causes of diseases. They showed, for example, that cigarette smoking causes lung cancer.

Kurland was particularly interested in discovering whether environmental exposures caused neurological diseases. His discovery, for example, that exposure to methyl mercury caused a neurological disease among the residents of Japan's Minamata Bay region led to government reforms to industrial pollution.

At Mayo, he set up the Rochester Epidemiology Project for epidemiologists to understand the patterns and predictors of diseases. His reputation was of a take-charge autocrat. Facing an impossible eleventh-hour deadline to submit a grant application on time to the National Institutes of Health via the US postal system, Kurland, a licensed pilot, flew the application from Rochester to Washington, DC.

The grant Kurland had mentioned in passing to Ivnik was an ambitious, first-of-its-kind application to the National Institute on Aging's recently formed Alzheimer's disease research program. Leveraging the resources of the Rochester Epidemiology Project, they would identify older adults with well-characterized cognitive abilities, divide them into two groups—those with and those without Alzheimer's disease—and then follow these hundreds of people for years. The data would allow answers to simple but foundational questions: How many people have Alzheimer's disease? What are the risk factors for getting it? How fast does it progress? It would also discover better instruments to diagnose patients.

Kurland was to lead the epidemiology part of the project. He chose Ivnik to lead the cognitive testing. To complete his team, he needed someone to recruit the hundreds of subjects and on each to perform detailed exams to decide whether the person was normal or had Alzheimer's disease. He needed Alzheimer's doctors.

In the fall of 1984, Ron Petersen received a telephone call at his office in the behavioral neurology section at Boston's Beth Israel Hospital (now Beth Israel Deaconess Medical Center). It was Len Kurland. "Ron, I'm putting in a grant application to the NIA [National Institute on Aging] to develop a registry for dementia. You're coming back in the summer. Would you like to participate in this grant?"

Reflecting on the call some thirty years later, Petersen recalled with his characteristic self-deprecatory wit: "I really didn't know what he was talking about. I kinda knew about grants but not really. I'd never written one. So, I said to Len: 'Sure. Love to!'"[2] That weekend, he set to work typing out the text Kurland assigned him to write about how the study would diagnose dementia.

Petersen was in the last year of his training as a physician, finishing up his Mayo Foundation Scholar–supported fellowship in cognitive neurology at Harvard. Kurland's out-of-nowhere invitation to the young neurologist was the latest in what was already a peripatetic academic career marked by similar sudden switches.

Petersen had started college studying mathematics, but came to find the work too theoretical. A summer job at Honeywell inspired him to switch to studying human factors psychology. Researchers in this branch of applied psychology seek to improve human function. They might, for example, study how people can best use multiple and sometimes contradictory bits of data, some from observation, some from a computer, to make decisions that minimize errors and maximize productivity.

The job at Honeywell was exciting work for the young man. "We'd do things like simulate an anti-warfare submarine environment where you used Bayesian theory to say, 'OK, you're in enemy waters, the probability there is a bad guy out there is thus and such,' and so you've got sonar information that may be semi-reliable and you've got to decide whether you fire your torpedoes or not, given you only have a few torpedoes."

The Vietnam War scuttled his plans to attend the University of Michigan's doctoral program in psychology. "I'd have been drafted the moment I set foot on that campus." He enrolled instead in the army's psychology training program and was assigned to a psychopharmacology lab at its Aberdeen Proving

Ground in Maryland. There, he tested how drugs affected soldiers' cognition. "It was so much fun that the guys I was working around said, 'If you really like doing this you should become a doctor.'"

By the cool fall afternoon in Boston when Len Kurland called Petersen, he was a young doctor with multiple, even competing interests: neurology, memory and the effects of pharmaceuticals on cognition, and also probability theory and the science of integrating information from multiple sources to make a tough-call decision. With such a multiplicity of interests, he risked a scattered career, but he was uniquely equipped to work for Kurland. His many interests would serve him well in a study that required doctors to make a life-altering decision: whether to label a person as a "normal older adult" or as a "patient with Alzheimer's disease." Remember, this was the era of "no dementia, no Alzheimer's disease." A person had to be diagnosed with dementia to then decide the cause: Alzheimer's or some other disease?

In September 1986, the Alzheimer's Disease Patient Registry was launched, and in the custom among medical researchers who transform their study's name into an abbreviation, like a kind of brand name, they called it the ADPR. In addition to Ivnik and Petersen, the ADPR investigator team included the geriatrician Eric Tangelos, the neurologist Emre Kokmen, and, a few years later, a second neuropsychologist, Glenn Smith, whom Ivnik had recruited from the University of Alabama. Smith recalls the day he and his family completed their road trip to Rochester, Minnesota. The date and the temperature matched. It was December 23, 1989, and 23 degrees.

The design of an epidemiology study can be creative, but its execution must be a dull set of routinized practices. Along the way, there is no room for creative invention. Data must be consistently gathered in a well-defined population of people. "Consistently" and "well-defined" are essential.

The subjects must all complete a common set of assessments whose results are systematically applied to classify persons as either a "case" or a "control." In the ADPR, a case meant a person with dementia, most commonly caused by Alzheimer's disease, and a control meant a person without dementia, or, in a word, a normal.

These data, together with meticulous measures of personal characteristics and health, such as gender, race, age, and medications, were collected. In time, as subjects returned for reassessments, the data set would record any changes in their health, such as normals (i.e., the control subjects) becoming patients with Alzheimer's disease. Kurland's skill was teasing out patterns from these data to discover the characteristics that predict whether a control will become a case.

The ADPR set up protocols to identify and recruit older adults and to perform a systematic exam. Then the investigator team met weekly at a consensus conference to decide as a group if the subject was normal or had Alzheimer's disease. The Mayo Clinic was the ideal site for such a study.

A MOST PECULIAR INSTITUTION

The city of Rochester is small. The 1980 census records fifty-seven thousand people. And in the largely rural Olmsted County, just thirty-four thousand more people reside. In 1989, when the ADPR started, the typical older adult was a descendant of settlers from Scandinavian countries. They worked in farming, manufacturing (IBM opened a plant in 1956), or with the county's largest employer, the Mayo Clinic. Their residents' trust and attachment to "the clinic" was profound.

The clinic is perhaps the most unusual medical center in the United States. It blends nationally recognized departments equipped with the latest medical technologies (for a time, Mayo had more MRI machines than the entire nation of Canada) and an organizational structure and record-keeping system that resembles Scandinavian socialized medicine.

How this came to be is the consequence of a disaster. In August 1883, tornadoes devastated Olmsted County. The accounts of the damage read like a scene from *The Wizard of Oz*. A house was lifted from its foundation and carried one hundred feet, leaving man and baby standing in the open air at the top of the steps of their now-unhoused basement. Property was scattered over a thirty-mile span. The experience of caring for the wounded, organized by the Sisters of St. Francis under the leadership of Mother Mary Alfred Moes, inspired a plan to create St. Mary's Hospital. Her collaborator in this effort was an English surgeon who'd settled in Rochester to examine Civil War draftees. His name was William Worrall Mayo.

The hospital built by Mother Mary, Dr. Mayo, and his sons William and Charles grew rapidly. By the early twentieth century, the "Mayo's clinic," as it was commonly called, had acquired a national reputation for the quality of its care and training. In 1914, it was renamed the Mayo Clinic.

Mayo faculty hesitate when asked to compare the clinic to other top-ranked academic medical centers. Midwestern modesty becomes them. In time, a common set of words slip out: "collegial," "collaborative," and "egalitarian."

The ethos is that of a top-down hierarchy, where everyone is equal and all get along, a true institution of e pluribus unum (out of many, we are one).

This unique ethos fosters research and clinical care and allows collective innovations unimaginable in the stereotypical academic medical center where a loose confederation of physician-scientists are constantly fighting over money and space. Among the most notable innovations—and one directly responsible for the creation and unquestionable success of the ADPR— was the Unit Medical Record.

The medical record, or patient chart, is where all clinical notes, labs and other tests, and correspondence are kept. In the twentieth century, this was a paper record, and it reflected the ironies and contradictions of American medicine. On the one hand, it was considered sacrosanct. Medical students were taught to respect it as an almost sacred document. No erasures or obliterations of text were allowed. Each record was a case and, gathered together, a set of records was an opportunity to discover diseases and even treatments.

In practice, however, the medical record reflected the chaos of the American health care and research systems. Patients often had multiple charts, one for each specialist. This precious property was kept locked away in each specialist's clinic. Separate charts for outpatient and inpatient care were common. Charts were routinely scattered about, even lost. A medical records department of a busy academic medical center was typically a dreadful basement room.

Research that used the medical record was fractured and siloed. The dermatologists' careful records allowed them to learn from and discover better ways to diagnose and treat their patients. So, too, the neurologists' records. A project that needed to gather information across specialties was a frustrating and resource-intensive exercise. It tested the limits of power and persuasion to negotiate with independent physician-scientists to surrender control over their charts and to obtain the consent of the patients to allow this.

The Mayo Clinic would have none of this. As the clinic grew in the early twentieth century, the medical record began to divide and break into separate charts. It was deviant behavior, at odds with the ethic of the group practice.

So, in 1907, a recent hire, a young polymath internist named Dr. Henry Plummer, was charged with bringing order to the medical records. Together with Mabel Root, who brought her expertise in filing, bookkeeping, and ledgers from E. A. Knowlton's dry goods store, they created the Unit Medical Record.[3]

On July 1, 1907, Unit Medical Record number one was assigned. Every

Mayo Clinic patient had one and only one medical record into which went every bit of medical information. The type of paper, the pen, and even the ink were all strictly prescribed. Its whereabouts were meticulously tracked. Years later, when vacuum tube technology came into use, the record was packed in a 7-by-10-inch folder, folded in half, and shot all about the clinic. It wasn't simply a filing system; it was an ethic of care and research embodied in a folder.

Patients came from all over the United States, Canada, and even the world seeking care, but for residents of Olmsted County, the clinic was special. If you were born in the county, raised in the county, and died there, your medical record was a complete cradle-to-grave document of your health. Which is why Len Kurland came to Mayo. He persuaded the other hospitals in the county to link their records with the Mayo Clinic's. It was an epidemiologist's gold mine: a stable population whose health was meticulously traced in a comprehensive medical records system administered by a trusted academic medical center whose practitioners prided themselves on collective, all-together action.

The ADPR was unfolding on perfect soil. This was an unmistakably unique opportunity to conduct a study of the aging brain, to count and compare the characteristics of persons without cognitive impairment and persons with dementia. As long as the team stuck to their methods and measures, the conclusions they would make about the epidemiology of aging, cognition, and Alzheimer's disease could speak to the nation. But first Bob Ivnik had to be inspired to make the best of what he felt was a bad situation.

For Ivnik, the ADPR was a distraction. He wanted to take care of patients. "I really enjoyed the testing and using objective measurements to make behavioral and cognitive predictions and to help with diagnosis." And yet, as he reflected on the clinical practice of psychology that he so enjoyed, he realized psychology was deeply flawed. The tests he used to measure older adults' memory really couldn't answer a patient's fundamental question: "Doctor, am I normal?"

"I realized that the normative basis for almost all of our cognitive tests above the age of seventy-four did not exist." The Wechsler tests, for example, "the absolute pinnacle of cognitive testing," lacked *any data* to say whether an older adult's score was normal.

Ivnik experienced a change of heart about the ADPR. It wasn't a distraction. It was instead an amazing opportunity.

The meticulous records made possible by Dr. Plummer and Mabel Root, Len Kurland's data factory, and a community of trusting patients willing to be subject to research allowed him to sort the normal from the not normal. Ivnik found his purpose. "I thought, 'I'll just collect all this normative data on standard tests and start publishing norms.'"

3

ACCURATE BUT NOT
PRESUMPTUOUS

No one with a modicum of medical and psychological knowledge fails to recognize the symptoms and signs of late-stage dementia; the symptoms and signs of early-stage dementia are, however, far from precise and predictive.

—Charles Wells, *Dementia*, 1971

THE TEAM SET to work. And Kurland left them alone. He'd mellowed, becoming grandfatherly to these young men, and he was also more interested in discovering the causes of a rare dementing illness seen in the residents of the Pacific island of Guam.

Their work required choreographing multiple people to follow well-established protocols. They convinced colleagues in the general medical practices to administer a short battery of cognitive testing to every patient fifty-five years and older, to refer to the study those whose scores were below a cutoff, and also to ask about cognitive complaints and refer those patients. Meanwhile, ADPR research nurses were hard at work. They scanned the meticulous Unit Medical Records for notes documenting cognitive problems, and for every case of Alzheimer's disease, they searched the Unit Medical Records to find a similar person in age, gender, occupation, and education who was healthy and therefore would serve as a control.

Being an ADPR subject required hard and time-intensive work. It included providing a detailed history; undergoing a careful neurological assessment, and Ivnik and Smith's "two plus two battery," two hours of well-known, but not-as-yet-normed cognitive tests; and two hours of experimental measures. In time, the work got even more intensive. The ADPR added genetic testing and MRI scans of the brain. Nearly everyone they recruited agreed to participate.

Hundreds of patients were studied. Each week, on a Friday around noon in the Mayo Clinic Baldwin Building, where the primary care practices were located, the team discussed that week's subjects, and, for each, they made the critical decision. Is this person normal or not? In the peculiar lexicon of the ADPR, a person was either a "000" or a "100," either a "normal" or a person with Alzheimer's disease.

They followed a cardinal rule. First the clinician diagnosed and then—and only then—could the clinician look at the results of Ivnik's cognitive testing. Further, they could not change the diagnosis based on those test results. Ivnik insisted on this. The expert clinicians decided an older adult is either normal or has dementia using their expertise with every bit of clinical information they could gather from the adult, their family, and whatever tests the clinician administered. Ivnik was using the neuropsychological test scores of the normal to define the range of normal cognition in older adults. If Petersen and his colleagues looked at those scores *before* they made their diagnostic judgment, they would most certainly incorporate the scores as one factor in their decision: 000 or 100. As a result, Ivnik wouldn't be able to use their independent assessments of who was a 000 or who was a 100 to determine which of the tests and the cutoffs best distinguished a 000 from a 100. His data would be corrupted. Their strict adherence to this cardinal rule would turn out to be critical to the discovery they made.

Never in the history of Alzheimer's disease had there been a more rigorous and thoroughly studied population of older adults living not in the hidden shelter of an asylum but in the community among family and friends, doing their best to live their aging lives.

"It was," Ivnik reflected in his characteristically understated manner, "a unique opportunity to look at who was normal."

And that's when things began to get complicated.

NEITHER NORMAL NOR DEMENTED

Years later, Ivnik recalled that something unexpected was happening.

"There were occasions when Ron and Eric would come together and say, 'Considering everything we know about this person, we consider him normal.'

And then they'd say, 'What do you think, Bob?' And I'd say, 'Well, let's make the diagnosis first.' And so they'd be listed as normal. Bang! Stamp on the chart. Normal. And then I'd say, 'Well, guess what, this guy has no delayed memory.' Back then we didn't know what that meant."

The "that" that didn't make sense was the following: the doctors had labeled an older adult as normal—a 000—but that same person had low scores on the psychologists' memory tests. Ivnik called it a focal cognitive impairment in one domain.

The confusion worked in the other and more mysterious direction. Petersen and Kokmen would report that the family had complained about the person's memory, that "they're not who they were." Something was going on. But Ivnik and Smith's testing was normal.

Glenn Smith remembered a growing frustration in Baldwin's fifth-floor conference room. "We were encountering this discrepancy between those who were weak but not clearly below the norm, and there was a concern by the patient or partner or the providers who'd say to us: 'There's *something* happening.'"[1]

A strange new group of people was taking shape. They were a kind of chimera of normal and abnormal. Normal on the doctors' clinical assessment but abnormal on the psychologists' memory testing, or they were normal on the memory tests but the people who saw them regularly—their spouses and adult children—were worried because something was different about their relative.

"We couldn't sort these people out," Smith recalled. "They didn't meet criteria for dementia. They certainly, based on our norms, didn't look normal. This happened time and time again until we couldn't ignore it."

They needed a name for these people. They called them the 002s.

What was happening? Were the 002s just bad test takers, the extreme of normal aging, people with a difficult family member who overreacted to the slightest memory lapse? Lifelong worriers and complainers now grown old?

In time, the data answered these questions.

"I have in my head a Kaplan-Meier curve," Smith recalled. The curve he was envisioning is a graph that depicts the chance of an event happening over time. In the case of an 002, it is the chance of becoming a 100, of being diagnosed with Alzheimer's disease.

All the 002s started without dementia. As time passed, some of the 002s began to change. After one year of follow-up, 12 percent were now labeled 100s, or people with Alzheimer's disease. After two years, the proportion who remained 002s dropped yet again, now closer to 75 percent. And so on. Relentlessly downward. Each year, 12 to 15 percent of the 002s changed from being an 002 to a 100, to a person with dementia probably caused by Alzheimer's disease.

This was the breakthrough. The 002s weren't just bad test takers, extreme worriers, getting old, or getting caught up in the tyranny of excessive scrutiny by their hypervigilant families. They were people at risk for Alzheimer's disease. If you followed them over time, many—not all, but enough to be concerned—developed dementia.

"We had been following them for years," Petersen recalled with boyish enthusiasm. "And I said, 'We should publish this stuff.'"

But what should they call them?

WHAT'S IN A NAME?

They looked to the literature, finding and rejecting a number of terms. "Age-Associated Memory Impairment" and "Late-Life Forgetfulness" suggested a condition caused by aging and so not of concern to a physician. "Benign senescent forgetfulness" was simply wrong—a 10 to 15 percent per year chance of developing Alzheimer's disease wasn't benign. "Alzheimer's disease" was inappropriate because the 002s didn't have dementia.

Petersen rejected qualifying the Alzheimer's label with words like "at risk" or "prodromal," a term to describe the earliest signs of a disease, such as a cough that precedes a pneumonia. "Once you say 'Alzheimer's disease,' that's all they'll hear. The prodromal stuff goes out the window," he insisted.

Befitting of midwestern modesty, Petersen wanted a term that was "accurate but not presumptuous." He found a term that had been circulating in the literature since the eighties. The 002s, he decided, would be called persons with mild cognitive impairment. The word "impairment" was essential, he explained. "It took away the rationalization that this was aging."

In March 1999, the *Archives of Neurology* published "Mild Cognitive Impairment: Clinical Characterization and Outcome."[2] The paper was not the first to report on the characteristics and outcomes of older adults with memory problems who did not have dementia—the paper cited several prior studies—but those studies all had notable limitations. Their subjects came from specialized memory clinics or had short follow-up or used memory test norms from younger adults. Each of these features limited their value. They were guideposts for further studies but not for clinical practice.

The Mayo paper didn't just change clinical practice. It was revolutionary. It changed how doctors thought about an older adult with a mild memory problem. This mild memory problem was like cigarette smoking. It was akin to a risk factor for a major medical illness: dementia caused by Alzheimer's disease.

The diagnosis took off.

Mild cognitive impairment became a brand. My colleagues and I called it not by its full name but by its abbreviation: MCI. In the years to follow the 1999 *Archives of Neurology* paper, a billing code, practice parameters for diagnosis, and continuing medical education talks on how to diagnose MCI all appeared quite rapidly. The concept expanded to include subtypes: a patient with only a memory problem had "MCI–memory only," and the finding of an additional cognitive problem was "MCI–memory plus other."

An exponential growth of research ensued. The paper became one of the most highly cited papers in the Alzheimer's field. MCI was added to the uniform data set gathered by the NIA-funded Alzheimer's Disease Research Centers. These studies of the characteristics and outcomes of persons with MCI recapitulated the Mayo results. MCI was a risk factor for Alzheimer's disease. Not all smokers get lung cancer, but smokers are at heightened risk of cancer.

Drug companies saw a large and promising market for a treatment that could prevent Alzheimer's. They began testing drugs in persons with MCI. Unfortunately, none of these studies discovered an effective drug.

Ivnik and Smith's work to create norms was also a great success. Their papers reporting on the ranges of normal performance on test scores from hundreds of older adults living in Olmsted County, Minnesota, filled the embarrassing void of data describing normal cognition in older adults. The Mayo Older Americans Normative Study, or MOANS, norms became the lingua franca for neuropsychologists.

Rita Philip—the woman whose daughter wanted to know if her mother had "something neurological"—had MCI. She met each of the five criteria. She had a memory complaint (really her daughter did about her). Although she needed more time to perform her complicated instrumental activities of daily living like managing her bills, she was still doing them without error. She performed well on most of the measures of her cognition (the pencil-and-paper tests and the questions I asked her), but on some measures she did not perform as well as I would have expected. Especially the measures of memory.

She wasn't normal. She didn't have dementia. She had MCI.

Memory centers such as where I practice rapidly adopted the MCI criteria into research and practice. MCI and MOANS freed us from a false dichotomy between "normal" and "dementia." There must be a space in between these. The challenge was agreeing on how to describe it and what to call the people in that space. MCI solved that.

It gave us a common language. And it was a large space, more prevalent than dementia. The Mayo team estimated that 10 percent of Olmsted County had dementia. Those with MCI were even more numerous: 15 percent.[3]

But then things got really complex and very controversial.

Diagnosing dementia was comparatively easy. My colleagues and I found diagnosing MCI a complex and time-intensive process that involved integrating multiple bits of information into a demanding human factors analysis. We had to figure out if a person was less efficient in performing their daily tasks. For every complex problem there is often a solution that is quick, simple, and wrong. Clinicians pushed for an easy-to-use, simple test, and they read the 1999 paper to find one: MCI patients' memory test scores were often at least one and one-half deviations below the average score.

What Petersen intended as just *one* of the features of a clinical diagnosis became, in the minds of many practitioners, *the* defining characteristic of the MCI diagnosis. Petersen's careful human factors analysis to arrive at the diagnosis was being reduced to just one simple test result: "MCI is performance on a cognitive test that is one point five deviations below the mean."

For patients, this shortcut had sometimes devastating consequences. The MOANS norms came from a population classified as "older Americans." In fact, they were just one and arguably a peculiar subpopulation of older Americans.

"Everyone used to say these are 'Norwegian norms,' that it was the 'Mayo Older American Norwegian Study,'" Ivnik explained. His colleagues at Mayo's Jacksonville, Florida, clinic showed the hazards of applying these norms into the quite different population of the elderly residents of Jacksonville.

They were discovering dissonance, especially in persons who were African American. The clinical assessment suggested the person was normal, but the norms said they had mild dementia. MCI was prevalent in Olmsted County, Minnesota, but it seemed to be missing in Jacksonville, Florida.

John Lucas, a neuropsychologist and one of the Mayo clinicians who discovered the problem, was also among the researchers who figured out what was happening.

Cognitive tests are like the tests we take in school. The more schooling a person has, the better they perform on the test. Good test takers score well; better test takers score better. The norms need to take this into account. And so, Ivnik's MOANS norms were anchored to the number of years of school a person reported. The problem in Jacksonville was that twelve years of schooling for one person was not equivalent to twelve years of schooling for another. It depended on the color of your skin.

Lucas summarized the disparities in the quality of education between those who were brown versus those who were not. "A Caucasian kid may have been in school for nine months, but African American schools only ran for seven months. Here in Jacksonville they had a system of education where the African American children only went to school half days. So you either came in the morning or the afternoon, whereas Caucasian kids got to go to school all day."[4]

The population in Jacksonville was quite different from Rochester's. A legacy of segregation and injustice reemerged decades later when these older adults sought a work-up for their memory problems.

The human factors analysis was thus unavoidable. The clinician who failed to exercise judgment and interpret a person's test score in light of a thoughtful assessment of the quality of their education took a terrible risk. They might misdiagnose a person who was normal as having MCI or, even more fraught, as having dementia.

Clinicians struggled to make the MCI diagnosis and to explain it to their patients and their families. Was it even a diagnosis or instead a risk factor for a future diagnosis of Alzheimer's disease? Patients and their families often experienced confusion and uncertainty: Am I normal or not? Do I have a disease? Is this bad news or just not-so-good news?

The husband of one of my patients complained to me. "It's like you told me she's wearing a pretty blue dress. I know she is, but what does it mean?" MCI was like the "tranquility units" in Larry Ruvo's center. By hiding the word "impairment" in an abbreviation and conveying no mention in the name of the risk for Alzheimer's disease, the term, for some, created a false sense of assurance.

Ronald Reagan was worked up at the Mayo Clinic by Dr. Petersen. His letter to America announcing his diagnosis of Alzheimer's disease did not in fact say he had Alzheimer's disease. He wrote, "I have recently been told that I am one of the millions of Americans who *will be* afflicted with Alzheimer's disease." Had he in fact been diagnosed with MCI? Or perhaps he held to the common view among some patients and families that the term "Alzheimer's disease" describes a more severe stage of dementia? That is, the mistaken concept of Alzheimer's disease as "full-blown dementia." Maybe he felt he had dementia or just memory problems that were not yet Alzheimer's disease.

Some clinicians exploited the ambiguity and confusion, using MCI rather than dementia as a term to deliver a softer blow to a patient who in fact had dementia in the mild stage. MCI eased a person into their Alzheimer's problem. It also kept a clinic visit short.

Other clinicians rejected the term. They argued MCI is "Alzheimer's disease" or "prodromal Alzheimer's disease" (terms Petersen cast aside as "presumptuous"). They cited papers such as "Mild Cognitive Impairment Represents Early-Stage Alzheimer's Disease," which showed results from MCI subjects evaluated at a university memory center.[5] These persons had a high likelihood of cognitive decline, and autopsy studies of their brains showed that most had Alzheimer's disease pathology.

The absence of a drug treatment only amplified clinicians' frustration with MCI, especially busy primary care clinicians. Why devote precious time to diagnose a condition that isn't causing obvious harm, might not get worse, and has no treatment? To them, MCI seemed a presumptuous medicalization of aging.

I told Mrs. Philip two diagnoses. She had MCI and its cause was Alzheimer's disease. And if she lived long enough, she would likely develop dementia. Was I being presumptuous? No. I was confident.

I didn't need to wait for her to die to tell her daughter that her mother's MCI was caused by "definite Alzheimer's disease." I possessed a test result that wasn't available when the Mayo team performed their research. I could see the disease in her living brain. This vision was replacing my profession's gothic horror mystery with a new story, an explosion of pure facts in an epic foretelling of her future:

"MCI caused by Alzheimer's disease."

Alzheimer's was becoming unbound from dementia. I was able to diagnose her with Alzheimer's disease because of the result of a test made possible by two singularly driven researchers' collaborative imagination and love of fly-fishing: a nephrologist who'd lost his job at Stanford and a very smart young neuropathologist eager to keep his field out of the morgue.

4

THE OLYMPICS OF PHARMACOKINETICS

Until this time, there has been no useful diagnostic test for Alzheimer's
Disease. A definitive diagnosis is possible only postmortem or during life
through a brain biopsy . . . Therefore, there exists a need for a definitive diagnostic test which can be performed on individuals suspected of having
or being at risk for Alzheimer's disease.

—From "Polypeptide Marker for Alzheimer's Disease
and Its Use for Diagnosis," US Patent 4,666,829,
by George G. Glenner and Caine W. Wong, 1987

THE STORIES TOLD BY THE DEAD

Edith Harrison lived for five more years after the January afternoon in 2010
when I diagnosed her with probable Alzheimer's disease. Her husband and
daughter cared for her at home. In the last months, hospice helped them.
They moved a bed to the first-floor living room, close to the bathroom. Aides
assisted them to bathe, dress, and groom her.

In the end, she lay in the bed, largely unable to move, her skull visible beneath her flesh, her knees like clubs, taking hours to eat. And then one day
she simply stopped eating. Late in the severe stage of dementia, some call it
advanced-stage dementia, problems with feeding are nearly universal. They
include taking in less and less food, trouble swallowing, and a cessation of
the drive to eat.

Mr. Harrison's call to our autopsy on-call team initiated an orchestrated
and methodical procedure. The autopsy coordinator called the funeral home
and ordered the body taken to the hospital's basement morgue.

Within twenty-four hours, a laboratory technologist "harvested" her brain. The skin at the back of the skull was sliced and then peeled away from back to front, so as to allow the skull to be neatly sawed open like some gigantic nutshell. The brain was then extracted, skull replaced, and skin folded back and sewn up. Her body, now brainless, appeared untouched and was returned to the funeral home for an open-casket viewing.

Her brain was set in preservative and remained in the lab. In the ensuing weeks, the autopsy was performed. The report read in part: "Sections reveal marked loss of neurons . . . Other major findings included large numbers of senile plaques and neurofibrillary tangles." History and pathology were finally united into one coherent story. "Senile plaques" described dense deposits of a protein called amyloid set between the neurons. "Neurofibrillary tangles" described twisted filaments inside neurons of a protein called tau. A "marked loss of neurons" described dead brain cells. According to the 1984 diagnostic criteria, she had "Alzheimer's disease, definite."

Her history and autopsy were a retelling of a typical case of Alzheimer's disease. The first was told in 1907 by the psychiatrist and neuropathologist Alois Alzheimer. He had cared for Auguste Deter—like Mrs. Harrison, a housewife brought in by her distressed husband. Dr. Alzheimer diagnosed her with dementia and after she died five years later, he examined her brain.

"Many neurons, especially the ones in the upper layer, have completely disappeared," he wrote. "Inside of a cell which appears to be quite normal, one or several fibrils can be distinguished by their unique thickness . . . Distributed all over the cortex, but especially numerous in the upper layers, there are minute miliary foci, which are caused by the deposition of a special substance in the cortex."[1]

In the decades to follow his case report, researchers discovered what made up "minute miliary foci"—Dr. Alzheimer's "special substance"—and the fibrils tangled up in the shell of a neuron, "only a tangle of fibrils indicates the place where a neuron was previously located." The "special substance" was the first to be figured out.

Around 1930, the Dutch psychiatrist and pathologist Paul Divry discovered it was a protein. He, like Alzheimer, had observed how difficult the substance was to stain, and so his insight was to try a dye that was recognized for its unique ability to attach to a protein called amyloid. Amyloid occurs naturally in the body and when it is overproduced in an organ, it slowly destroys the organ. It is notorious for its resistance to staining.

The dye was called Congo red, branded in the late nineteenth century by the German dye manufacturer AGFA to celebrate the German colonization of the African Congo. Congo red colored cotton fabrics a brilliant red. When applied to a thin slice of brain tissue, it lit up the "special substance" with the same characteristic appearance as when it was applied to amyloid. The special substance was therefore most likely amyloid.

Thirty years later, advances in microscopy made it possible to examine the plaques' ultrastructure, that is, to directly see the special substance's shape and confirm it was in fact amyloid. Using electron microscopy, the neuropathologist Robert Terry and colleagues described the plaques, and his results, together with the Congo red studies, added up to a definitive discovery. Senile plaques were most certainly amyloid.

But which kind of amyloid? Amyloid is like a term from geometry such as "triangle." It describes the unique shape of a protein. Just as there are several types of triangles—obtuse, equilateral, and right angled, for example— there are several types of amyloid proteins. They vary in their composition depending on the organ they are building up in and slowly destroying.

The discovery of the specific kind of amyloid in senile plaques was made by George Glenner and Caine Wong. In 1984, using the techniques of biochemistry—a meticulous set of steps to separate, concentrate, and purify the protein and then break it into its daisy chain of orderly amino acid constituents, sort of a dissection of a molecule—they reported the exact sequence of amino acids that string together to form the dense plaques. They called it amyloid beta, or A-beta or A-β. The full name for this pathology is "beta-amyloid neuritic plaques." Hereafter, the widely used nicknames "amyloid" and "amyloid plaques" will be used.

Glenner championed his discovery. This was the key to diagnosing Alzheimer's disease. In 1987, he filed a patent on a blood test he hoped to develop to detect the specific sequence of the amyloid beta protein he'd discovered. The preamble of his patent application summed up the frustrations experienced by clinicians, patients, and families. "Until this time, there has been no useful diagnostic test for Alzheimer's Disease. A definitive diagnosis is possible only postmortem or during life through a brain biopsy to reveal the presence of the characteristic plaques, tangles and cerebrovascular deposits which characterize the disorder." Misdiagnosis, he noted, was common. What followed was a visionary idea. "There exists a need for a definitive diagnostic test which can be performed on individuals suspected of having or being at risk for Alzheimer's Disease."[2]

Glenner would not live to achieve his idea. In 1995, he died of systemic amyloidosis, the accumulation of an amyloid protein throughout his blood vessels and heart, a protein different from the kind of amyloid that accumulates in the brains of persons with Alzheimer's disease.

Three-quarters of a century after Dr. Alzheimer's case report, the "special substance" riddling his patient's brain was named and its precise molecular structure written out like a sentence in a pathology report. Similar advances in stains, ultrastructural studies, and biochemistry would reveal the name and amino acid code of the tangles he observed. By 1986, they were discovered to be broken bits of a protein called tau that when not tangled up is part of a healthy neuron's structure.

By the end of the 1990s, researchers had achieved great progress in defining the pathologies of Alzheimer's disease. Its three-part pathologic signature was two so-called proteinopathies—amyloid plaques and tau tangles—and the absence of neurons, or what is called neurodegeneration. "Proteinopathy" describes a disease caused by a protein that has misfolded from its normal functional shape into a damaging molecule.

They also identified the enzymes that sliced and diced the body's normal protein into the toxic fragments of amyloid beta (the protein was aptly named "amyloid precursor protein"). Manipulating these secretase enzymes offered a potential target for treatments that might prevent the destruction of the precursor protein.

Clinical practice, however, wasn't keeping pace. None of these pathologies were detectable in a living person. A diagnostic work-up followed essentially the same standard of care as in Alois Alzheimer and his colleagues' early twentieth-century standard. We performed a careful history and exam and then tried to follow the patient until death, when our pathology colleagues then extracted the brain from the cadaver and sliced, stained, and examined it.

This standard of care was woefully antiquated compared to the diagnostic methods used in cardiology and oncology. The problem was an unsurmountable, unbreakable castle wall. The brain is behind the human skull. Brain biopsies are simply impracticable and highly dangerous. That wall is made further impenetrable by a kind of border patrol of elegant, thin tissues that create the "blood-brain barrier." It blocks many molecules from getting either into or out of the brain, thereby limiting the ability to measure pathology in blood or to inject a radioactive tracer that could illuminate the pathology in the brain.

How, then, to get into the living brain, examine it, and take away a diagnosis?

TWO MEN, ONE MOLECULE,
AND COUNTLESS FISHING TRIPS

Chet Mathis really didn't want to meet with Bill Klunk. Mathis was busy, very busy, running the Department of Radiology's PET facility at the University of Pittsburgh.

"I'm working with the chair of psychiatry and other big names in psychiatry, three of four other full professors with very large funding portfolios. They're the reason I came here,"[3] he recounted in an interview twenty-four years later.

PET stands for "positron-emission tomography." When a patient says "my scan lit up," she's describing the results of her PET scan. "Positron" refers to radioactive labels and "tomography" is a technique to detect these labels and print a picture showing where the labels have concentrated—that is, "lit up" in the body.

Chet Mathis was an expert in developing radiotracers, compounds that link a radioactive label with another molecule that works like a bloodhound, seeking out the tissue it is engineered to bind to. Mathis was developing radiotracers that visualized the whereabouts of serotonin in the brain of a person with depression.

He was well funded and busy. For a researcher in academic medicine, this is the state of well-being. Klunk was junior faculty, and "junior faculty" meant lots of extra work—even hand-holding—with the potential of little reward. Mathis didn't need more work, particularly work with a junior faculty member.

Klunk, bespectacled and preternaturally youthful, was thirty-eight and in his fifth year as an assistant professor in the Department of Psychiatry. Following his residency in psychiatry and a doctorate in medicinal chemistry from Washington University, he'd been hired on to faculty to work in a large lab studying brain metabolism in patients with Alzheimer's disease. His days were taken up with this work, but in his off time, he was pursuing other interests.

He was keen to discover molecules that bind to amyloid in the brain of a living person, and he'd become interested in whether he could engineer Congo red to do just that.

"I was getting ready to write up our papers on our Congo red derivatives we were playing around with and the senior vice chancellor says, 'You ought to talk with Chet Mathis in the PET facility.'" In the spring of 1994, he called Mathis, wondering: "Is he even going to *care* about this?"[4]

They met in the conference room of the PET center. Klunk got straight to his idea.

"I think I want to image Alzheimer's disease in a living person. You probably don't know about Congo red?"

Mathis cut him off. "Yeah, I know about Congo red. I radiolabeled it, and it doesn't get into the brain."

Klunk cut him off, saying the words that launched their decades-long relationship. "That's exactly right. It's charged. But I've got this *other compound* called Chrysamine G and it's an analog of Congo red and it gets into the brain."

"This was a distraction in a way, but it was a distraction I was interested in," Mathis recalled.

The idea Bill Klunk was on to was to make a radiolabeled compound that binds to amyloid plaques in the brain not of a dead but rather a living person. Eight years later, this distraction, an idea his mentors judged secondary, would produce a discovery that transformed not simply the tests doctors use to diagnose Alzheimer's disease but also the very definition of the disease and who is called a person living with Alzheimer's disease.

Klunk saw medicine as, in part, a chemistry problem. His doctoral research in chemistry at Washington University in Saint Louis made him proficient in manufacturing molecules. His dissertation was a study of compounds that, depending on how he manipulated their structure, would either treat a seizure or cause one.

He and his colleagues experimented with redesigning the molecules and then testing them in mice. They'd place bets on whether a molecule would cause a seizure or treat it. The prize was a can of Coke. Klunk quickly learned by smell. Coincidentally, seizure-inducing drugs smelled sweet and fruity, and drugs that treated a seizure smelled bitter and unpleasant.

"I won a lot of Cokes in those days."

Mathis's training was more unusual. He was proficient at using radionucleotide imaging to measure brain function. He'd been a member of the investigator team whose study was the first to report how PET measures of brain blood flow differentiate persons with Alzheimer's from age-matched persons without dementia.

He perfected these skills studying compounds that are more provocative than seizure medications. Every Friday afternoon, Chet would drive to the Shulgin Road Lab to work with Alexander T. Shulgin, or Sasha, the Godfather of Ecstasy.

Sasha, a designer drug chemist, had invested his fortune—earned from developing pesticides for Dow Chemical—into a private lab located on his family ranch at the end of Shulgin Road in Lafayette, California.

This was in the Bay Area, near Berkeley. The drug culture was everywhere, and Sasha was inspired by his experiments with methylenedioxymethamphetamine, or MDMA (later known as the club drug "ecstasy" or "Molly"). His research was devoted to designing hallucinogens and other psychoactive compounds. Mathis's job was to radiolabel these compounds in order to study their trip through the brain.

These drugs, Mathis argued, alone or in conjunction with psychotherapy could help people overcome long-standing depression or anxiety. With his skills in molecular synthesis and human experimentation—performed on himself and volunteers—he understood their behavioral effects. The experience of the "twinkle," a subtle change in alertness and perception, signaled the lower end of the dosage likely to produce a behavioral effect.

What he didn't understand was how they worked. What parts of the brain did they affect?

Mathis explained Sasha's science. "Sasha said he used hallucinogens to experience life from the inside out, but he wanted to look from the outside in. That's what we were about, looking from the outside in." Sasha wanted to get inside a brain on MDMA and figure out what the drug did, where it went, the receptors it bound to. In short, what caused the twinkle.

Sasha, like Klunk, would manipulate the MDMA molecule and test these compounds in rats and then in himself, looking for the twinkle. Mathis would radiolabel the compound, so they could measure where it was active in the brain.

Mathis had one other experience without which he likely would have turned Klunk away. It was a side experiment done in what would be his last years at Berkeley.

A colleague had suggested he radiolabel Congo red to PET image Alzheimer's disease pathology. "So, I read about Congo red. I got it. I radiolabeled it and cleaned it up and injected it in some rats to see if it got into the brain, and lo and behold, none of it did. It didn't enter the brain at all."

On reflection, he realized that if he'd simply thought over Congo red's structure, he could have predicted this negative result before he'd sacrificed a single rat. Congo red is charged, and the border patrol of the blood-brain barrier doesn't admit charged molecules. Mathis, like Klunk, thinks about molecular structures like a chef approaches ingredients she uses to construct a recipe.

Well funded, busy, far away from the Shulgin Road Lab, immersed in serotonin, he set aside research to image amyloid in the living.

But then he got the phone call from Bill Klunk.

Their meeting in the conference room of the PET center was the beginning of a true collaboration, a moment akin to the synthesis of a new molecule, a conception.

IMAGING THE GARBAGE CAN

The idea of a "test for Alzheimer's disease"—meaning a test to identify the pathology in a living person—had been circulating around the Alzheimer's field since at least the early 1980s. Glenner and Wong, for example, were explicit in their intentions with the protein sequence they discovered. The close of their paper summarized the next step. They were going to develop antibodies that bind to the protein in order to create a blood test for Alzheimer's disease. But they never achieved their invention.

There was a precedent for the approach of injecting Congo red into a patient to visualize amyloid. Among the tests that were once used to work up a case of suspected amyloidosis in organs such as the spleen, liver, and kidney was to inject the patient with Congo red, biopsy the tissue, and look at slices under the microscope. Mathis and Klunk both knew, however, that Congo red bound to a radiotracer couldn't get into the brain. The blood-brain barrier kept the molecule out of the brain.

What they were setting out to create was a compound—a radiotracer bound to a ligand—that did what Congo red did when applied to the tissue of a dead brain: stick to amyloid and only to amyloid. Their compound would, however, detect amyloid in the living. The plan was to inject it into the blood, have it cross the blood-brain barrier, circulate through the brain, attach to amyloid and only to amyloid just long enough to light up in the PET scanner, and then be cleared from the brain and body. All this would have to unfold without causing harm to the patient.

The chemistry was intimidating and so, too, was securing financial and moral support for the research. Pitt was among the leaders in a revolution in psychiatry. America was embracing a new zeitgeist, and not just in psychiatry. Mental illness was the result of disorders in how neurons communicated or, in a word, neurotransmission. Both men were working in well-funded labs led by prominent scientists dedicated to this line of investigation. These senior researchers commanded their time.

And it was exciting work. Discoveries of the role of serotonin in depression had led to breakthroughs in understanding the biology and treatment of depression. Drugs like fluoxetine—marketed by Lilly as Prozac—captured wide attention. The psychiatrist Peter Kramer's bestselling *Listening to Prozac* made the case that brain diseases were caused by imbalances in neurotransmitters. Suicide was, for example, conceptualized as a "serotonin problem."

PET imaging was a valuable tool for this research. Researchers used it to study how the brain functions in health and disease. Mathis's radiotracers allowed the comparison of neurotransmitter activity in the brains of persons with depression to persons without depression.

What Bill Klunk and Chet Mathis were thinking about was quite different than the zeitgeist. They didn't want to use PET to label brain activity but instead to label inert deposits of proteins, what their colleagues called debris or even garbage.

Mathis has a gruff side and a sharp wit. He grew tired of the criticisms. "I was told: 'You can't say that measuring how something bound to an inert protein was a receptor-ligand interaction.' And so on. It was like, 'Yeah, whatever . . .'"

"It was different," Klunk recalled. "The idea of imaging amyloid was like imaging the garbage can."

Their idea was considered a misuse of the technology and therefore judged a waste of their time and effort. Klunk, a junior faculty member in a well-funded lab, was kept and bound to receptor-ligand work, a situation, Mathis reflected, that "was like an abused wife."

This would have to be a side project done on their own time, but they were the ideal collaboration to take it on.

They started making Valentine cards.

MAKING VALENTINE CARDS

Klunk and Mathis had a conceptual model to explain the engineering task they faced. It came from watching their daughters make Valentine cards. The girls would draw a heart on a card using a glue stick, coat the paper with glitter, wait for the glue to dry, and then shake the paper. The glitter all fell away. Except for the glitter bound to the glue. The result was a glittering heart.

Their task was to get enough glitter (a radiolabeled molecule) onto the page (the brain), and let it bind to the glue (the amyloid) while the rest cleared so that what remained was the radiolabeled dye attached to amyloid.

Their work, however, wasn't child's play.

Klunk was passionate in his account of the work. "It was the Olympics of pharmacokinetics. You have to get in and get out of the brain. You have a short time to measure these things, and you can only give a patient so much radioactivity, but the PET scanner can only detect so much radioactivity. So, a big proportion of the dose you give a person has to get into the person quickly and it has to get out of them quickly so that you have a specific signal."

Guided by the laws of chemistry and physics and mindful of their colleagues' skepticism that this project would succeed, they composed a detailed, step-by-step set of experiments that a molecule had to pass in order to reach the final experiment: injection into humans with and without dementia caused by Alzheimer's disease. Success would be PET images of their brains that showed a signal in persons with Alzheimer's disease and no signal in persons without Alzheimer's disease.

They began with the "grind and bind experiments." Does the manufactured molecule bind to amyloid fibrils in a test tube solution, and if it does, does it bind to amyloid recovered from a ground-up human brain of a person with Alzheimer's disease?

Next came the experiments in the living. They started with mice. Inject the compound into the tail vein, wait, then sacrifice the animal, remove and dissect the brain, chop it up, and place the bits of brain under a gamma counter to measure if the compound was getting into the brain. Next came baboons—injecting and then scanning the living animal—to show whether the compound circulated through the entirety of the cortex, the brain region where amyloid accumulated in a human. The work was laborious, multi-stepped, and promising—but not promising enough to move on to humans.

Months passed. Years. Grant funds supported them but like a couple in a long-term relationship, habits sustained their relationship. They found one of those habits when they discovered the reason why each was unable to meet the other on Fridays: fly-fishing trips to catch salmon and trout. They started fishing together and soon lived by the rule: you can talk about fishing at work, but you can't talk about work while fishing.

They studied four hundred compounds. Still, there wasn't enough glitter on the page.

Klunk recalled the frustration. "We were almost there, but we couldn't seem to get over the goal line."

The opening came when a junior faculty member working with them needed a grant. The Congo red derivatives were bound up in licensing agreements with Aventis, the company that owned them. The fellow needed to submit a grant application quickly. There just wasn't time to secure all the reviews and signoffs Aventis required and still make the grant deadline. They assigned him to make derivatives of thioflavins, a compound that was like Congo red, but unlike Congo red, no company owned it.

The junior faculty member set to work. In time, he came back with compounds for Mathis and Klunk to radiolabel and run through their multistepped experiments.

The mouse brain lit up. The thioflavin compound circulated through the baboon brain and then cleared out in just enough time to scan. The page was bright with glitter.

Success!

After years of work, they'd engineered a molecule that got into the brain in quantities large enough to be measured by a PET scanner. But would it stick to the glue and only to the glue? That is, would the compound bind to amyloid and only to amyloid?

Mathis recalled the rising feeling that success was imminent. Things were lining up. The next experiment was the critical one. The "transgenic mice" experiment.

Alzheimer's disease is an unusual disease. Some aging nonhuman animals, such as dogs, develop cognitive impairment, but no animal other than humans develops cognitive impairment caused by Alzheimer's disease. Mice and rats—the preferred animals for experiments in living animals as they are cheap and relatively efficient to raise—have to be genetically engineered to develop the two proteinopathies, the amyloid plaques and tau tangles. These "transgenic" animal models are costly. At the time Mathis and Klunk were working, a single wild type mouse cost about $1. A single transgenic mouse cost several hundred dollars.

These engineered animals were the essential step before testing an Alzheimer's disease drug or radiolabeled compound in a human. They are the "go-no-go" doorway through which drugs pass from bench to bedside. Meaning, to support experiments in humans, mouse model results must show safety or signs of benefit. If the mice suffer harms or fail to show signals of benefit, then drug development stops. Back to the bench.

Klunk and Mathis were confident. The counts of glitter in wild type mice were intense. Thioflavin avidly bound to amyloid obtained from the ground-up brains of humans who died with Alzheimer's disease. The transgenics were loaded with amyloid—twenty-five times the amount found in the brain of a human with Alzheimer's disease.

Klunk remembered the wind-at-their-back feeling. The mouse experiments were going to be a sprint to the finish, a pro forma, necessary, and logical step before crossing the finish line: injecting the compound into a human with Alzheimer's disease.

"We got the mice. We bred 'em up and got them old enough to have lots of amyloid. The first thing we always did, just like we do with the brain tissue from a person with Alzheimer's disease, we do the grind and bind experiments with the mouse brain." Meaning, take the brain of a mature transgenic mouse, grind it up and mix it with the radiolabeled compound, wash the glitter from the page, and then count the glitter. If any glitter is there, then it was bound to the glue, to the mouse amyloid.

They were expecting to see glitter. Instead, they saw nothing.

"No signal," Klunk remembered. "Next to nothing. Maybe a little blip compared to the wild type mice. It was a great disappointment."

"A huge disappointment," Mathis concluded.

"Crap," Klunk thought. "We don't have a model."

According to the rules of science this negative result should have sent them back to the starting line. Other labs working on similar projects to discover an amyloid PET tracer also encountered this same disappointing result. They stopped their research. Klunk and Mathis, however, decided to keep on going. And with this decision, they entered uncharted scientific territory.

Up until this step in their laborious process, they'd been following the rules of science like accountants, requiring little need for judgment and taking no risks. Their machines were providing the results that decided whether to move along. Now, however, they faced a critical human factors decision.

Should they listen to the machine—that is, the mouse model whose signal was a resounding "no go"—or should they "go" into humans?

If they decided to go, they placed themselves—their careers—at tremendous risk. Obeying the mice results was following the rules of science. The experiment was a failure, but it was failure in the conventional sense. They'd have moved on as scientists with their reputations intact.

Going forward put them at risk of unconventional failure. If the brain of a human with Alzheimer's disease did not glitter, they would've failed as scientists. This presumptuousness, this hubris, would have harmed their reputations. It might even be judged unethical.

They engaged in a lot of thinking, deep thinking and back-and-forth exchanges drawing molecules at the whiteboard. They were confused. Why didn't the compound bind to the mouse amyloid? They were thinking, but they were also feeling.

Klunk, a psychiatrist, reflected on researchers doing similar work as theirs who'd encountered the same disappointing results in their transgenic mice experiments. Those researchers decided to stop. He could empathize with their decision and in doing so he came to recognize: he and Chet were different from other researchers.

"They're not the parents of these compounds. They don't believe in them like their parents do. They're like: 'We're not going to put our resources into this if it doesn't work in transgenic mice. We believe in the mouse we developed more than the compound.' Chet and I believed in the human tissue."

"We were committed," Mathis remembered. "And so we went ahead and we did it."

"It" meant injecting the compound into a human. "It" meant calling the Swedes.

A BALL HIT OUT OF THE PARK

A few years before the failed transgenic experiments, after presenting their research in progress at a radiopharmacology meeting in Uppsala, Sweden, Mathis was approached by a large man with a great beard. His trousers were held up by wide suspenders. "He kinda looked like a Viking," Mathis recalled.

"I'm Bengt Långström."

Långström was the director of the PET center in Uppsala. He explained his operation. Mathis was impressed. "It was a new tracer factory."

They had perfected a method to test PET radiotracers in humans they called micro-dosing. This approach cut out years from the time required to perform the human toxicology studies that were required by the FDA. Testing in Sweden promised results not in years but in months.

Bengt Långström liked what he saw. "Let me know when you're ready to inject into humans."

In December 2001, Mathis and Klunk sent the Swedes detailed instructions on how to make the thioflavin radiolabeled compound. The Swedes set to work. They synthesized the compound and began recruiting persons with Alzheimer's disease and persons without the disease to undergo an injection of this novel radiotracer.

Late in the evening of February 14, 2002, Bill Klunk received a call. It was Bengt Långström. "He said to me: 'Bill, I think we have something to celebrate.' I said, 'Really?' Because we were on pins and needles all day waiting for what happened, and so I'm immediately like: 'Yes!'"

The next day, via an email attachment, Klunk received his Valentine glitter card. It came from a fifty-seven-year-old nurse and a patient with Alzheimer's disease. "I like to think of her as my Auguste Deter," Klunk reflected.

The cortex of her brain was bright red, signaling avid uptake of the amyloid labeling compound. Radiolabeled thioflavin was lighting up just where amyloid should be in her brain.

Nearly two decades later, Klunk still recalls his excitement. "I get the image and I'm like: 'This is where it should be!' I'm like *immediately* saying, 'This works!'"

Mathis, however, was characteristically less enthusiastic. "We haven't seen a control yet. What if the person without Alzheimer's looks just like that?"

They postponed the celebration.

On Monday, the control brain images arrived. Cool blue. No glitter in the brain.

The two men gazed at the image. Mathis was convinced. A decade of work was done. "OK, I'll celebrate.'"

They celebrated not with Cokes as Klunk did in his fellowship years but with beer. "Monday we went out and I had my first Belgian beer. I had a Delirium Tremens." Klunk keeps the bottle in his office. The date of their celebration is penned on the label.

Five months later, on July 24, 2002, Henry Engler, one of the Swedish collaborators, stood before a packed auditorium at the annual international meeting of Alzheimer's disease researchers (which, by coincidence, was held in Stockholm, Sweden).[5] Bill Klunk and Chet Mathis were in the balcony. When Engler advanced to the slide showing the first image of amyloid in the brain of a living person with Alzheimer's disease, there was a collective gasp. The image was sublime.

"It was like when a batter hits the ball and you know, as soon as they do, that it's going to go out of the park."

Bill Klunk and Chet Mathis's child was sent off into the world. She was called Pittsburgh compound B. The name came from the Swedes' prosaic naming convention: first the city where the investigators worked, then a letter to indicate its place in the sequence of studies (Pittsburgh compound A had failed).

5

THE REPUBLIC OF ALZHEIMER'S DISEASE

We the people . . . in order to form a more perfect Union.
—Constitution of the United States, Preamble

THE ALZHEIMER'S FIELD was ecstatic and united in its unqualified praise for Pittsburgh compound B. Brad Hyman from Harvard University gave the first comment from the audience. "This is going to change the field." *Science* magazine quoted Mark Mintun, a PET imaging researcher at Washington University in Saint Louis, Missouri. "People are going to point to this particular presentation and say, 'This is when we started making progress on visualizing Alzheimer's disease.'"[1]

Like MCI, the amyloid imaging radiotracer Pittsburgh compound B became known by its abbreviation: PiB. "Positive PiB uptake" became a shorthand for the detection of amyloid in a living person's brain. Also like MCI (mild cognitive impairment), PiB was revolutionary.

PiB wasn't simply a radiotracer. It was an idea at the vanguard of a new way of thinking about Alzheimer's disease. A single word captured the collective scientific imagination: "biomarkers." The term describes biological measures of a disease in action. PiB was among a growing set of technologies that measured Alzheimer's biomarkers in the brains of living humans.

Biomarkers opened researchers' minds to new ways of thinking about what is Alzheimer's disease and therefore who is a patient and how to diagnose and treat her. The idea of PiB spread throughout memory centers across the world, instigating hundreds of novel studies.

The most exciting studies were in persons with MCI. Petersen and colleagues had shown how, each year, about 15 percent of persons with MCI declined from MCI to dementia. Could "positive PiB uptake" identify who was among this 15 percent?

Even more revolutionary were the studies in persons without cognitive impairment. Could PiB identify persons who, while normal, were on the trajectory of decline from normal to MCI and, in time, dementia?

Other biomarkers included images from magnetic resonance imaging (MRI) that showed the brain's structure, shape, and size. Advances in computational technologies allowed a researcher to measure the annual rate of brain atrophy, that is, the loss of brain tissue. The radiologist's interpretation of an image—"it looks a little atrophied"—gave way to a machine's precise measurement of just how atrophied the brain was. At the same meeting where PiB was premiered, Nick Fox from London's National Hospital for Neurology and Neurosurgery demonstrated just how precisely MRI can quantify brain atrophy: 4 percent per year in a person with Alzheimer's disease compared to 1 percent in a person without Alzheimer's disease.

Another biomarker was FDG-PET, shorthand for fluorodeoxyglucose, a PET radiotracer that displayed the blood flow throughout the brain. A brain region with low blood flow suggested there were fewer living brain cells there compared to regions with a brighter FDG signal. Researchers used this, like MRI, to quantify just how much atrophy was present. Studies of spinal fluid were able to detect amyloid and tau proteins, and studies measuring amyloid in the blood were showing provocative results: the protein might be detected with a simple blood test.

Each biomarker was quite different, but their outputs shared a common feature: numbers, counts, and measurements. Alzheimer's disease was becoming digitized and quantified, measurable not simply in persons with dementia but also in persons with MCI and even, perhaps, persons with no cognitive impairments.

THE WATER AROUND THE FISH

Researchers in both universities and pharmaceutical companies began to converge on a vision. Biomarkers—rather than the clinical history—could diagnose Alzheimer's disease. This vision also offered a new paradigm for treatment. A biomarker test would determine who should get a drug treatment and show whether the drug was effectively treating the patient. Numbers—a slowing in the annual rate of brain atrophy measured using MRI or the decrease of FDG-PET–measured blood flow or a reduction in the uptake of PiB—would show both the disease and its successful treatment.

My colleagues and I entertained visions of cardiology dancing in our heads—a "cholesterol test of the brain" to simultaneously guide an Alzheimer's diagnosis and treatment and to measure the outcomes of that treatment. The term of art was "disease slowing."

One of these early researchers was Dr. Mike Weiner. He recalled the state of excited confusion. The year was 1999. The occasion was an advisory board meeting convened by the pharmaceutical giant Pfizer in the suburbs of Washington, DC. "There was a whole bunch of academic people all talking about their biomarkers. Someone was talking about plasma amyloid, and someone was talking about MRI, and so on."[2]

The problem Weiner identified wasn't difficult to perceive.

"There were all these different talks about different technologies," Weiner recalled. "But you couldn't make any sense of it. There were different technologies and different centers. The same technologies being used in different ways. You just couldn't figure it out."

Somehow, all these great ideas needed to be harmonized. The problem started with the lack of standardization. The results of spinal fluid studies that measured amyloid and tau proteins varied widely from center to center. There was no uniformity of cutoffs, error rates, or predictive values. The collective data delivered lots of signals but also a lot of noise.

This loose confederation frustrated Pfizer's scientists and executives. They and their colleagues at other pharmaceutical companies were eager to pursue the billion-dollar market for a "biomarker-based" diagnosis and treatment for Alzheimer's disease, but they were all stuck on the same question: among the multiplicity of biomarker measures, which one tells doctors and patients that the drug treats Alzheimer's disease? Put another way, how could they connect the dots between biomarkers, cognitive test scores, the stories of what's a typical day, and an effective treatment?

Leaving the meeting, in the car ride to Dulles International Airport, inspiration struck. Weiner took out his laptop. Order was needed. The technologies needed to talk to each other, and everyone needed to use them in the same way in a common group of patients so that, in time, the data would show what biomarkers accurately measured the disease.

Six hours later, he landed in San Francisco with a proposal. He would write a grant application to the NIA to fund a yearslong study of hundreds of persons with dementia, MCI, and normal cognition. Everyone would undergo the same set of biomarker measures according to a meticulous set of instructions. Like the ADPR, there would be no room for creativity. Over time, as people changed—as some persons with normal cognition became persons with MCI and some persons with MCI became persons with dementia—the study would show how best to measure the biomarkers that explained those persons who changed.

Weiner's multiyear, multimillion-dollar idea was a tremendous undertaking not so much in science as in scientific politics. He wasn't simply creating an infrastructure. He was changing the culture of how scientists designed and used that infrastructure. He had to persuade researchers committed to their favorite biomarkers, multiple pharmaceutical companies beholden to their boards of directors and shareholders, and the taxpayer-funded NIA to come together and pool their resources to support a common effort to gather biomarker data in the same way and to make it publicly available.

He was perhaps uniquely qualified for the task. He'd come to Alzheimer's out of a personal and professional crisis, a kind of scientific refugee determined to succeed in his adopted country. Trained as a kidney specialist, he was well along the path of a successful academic career at Stanford University studying kidney metabolism when in 1979, disaster struck. Stanford denied him tenure.

He was out of a job.

In an interview forty years later, Weiner recounted the details with an incredible vividness. He descended into a crushing, near suicidal depression. "It was hugely humbling. It made me much more aware of how people are reacting to me and what people are thinking and to look at people's motives and what people are doing. It changed my whole way of dealing with the professional world. As my mother used to say, 'It's not what you know. It's who you know.' I wasn't a good politician then."

Colleagues in nephrology at the Veterans Administration found him a position running a dialysis unit at the San Francisco veterans hospital. At least he had a job. Alone at this work, he longed to return to research. Inspiration came at a lecture on a novel technology called, at the time, nuclear magnetic resonance imaging, or NMR, developed by physicists to measure the properties of atoms (it would be renamed "magnetic resonance imaging," or MRI, to cut short the misunderstanding that the machine used not magnetism but radiation). Weiner was among the cadre of early researchers who saw that MRI technology could image not just atoms but whole organs such as kidneys.

Weiner was inspired.

He obtained grant funding so as to divide his time between the dialysis unit and the MRI lab. He let the nascent technology lead him like a muse into all kinds of possible studies. He imaged his arm before and after exercise. He imaged his fifteen-year-old son and then himself. The work had an almost playful, "let's image this" aspect.

After several years, he realized a new career problem was taking shape. He decided he needed to get serious with his MRI studies because if he didn't, he risked a repeat of the debacle at Stanford. He was a doctor, and doctors researched diseases.

He needed to study a disease. But what disease?

He made a resolution. Every morning, from Monday to Friday, he went to the UCSF library until he knew what disease to study. After four hours of browsing, he'd leave to take care of patients at the hemodialysis unit. He carried on like this for six weeks. And then the light bulb went off.

"I was sitting in the library and I thought, 'Of course, it's Alzheimer's disease.'" He'd been reading that you couldn't diagnose the disease until death. He'd also learned how radiologists weren't interested in it. In fact, in 1988 few investigators were interested in the disease.

He was going to use the MRI to study how to diagnose Alzheimer's disease.

Nearly a decade after being fired from Stanford, he'd become one of the first MRI researchers focused on Alzheimer's disease. Ten years later came his inspiration on the flight home from DC. He was by then a better politician, keenly aware that people are motivated by distinct blends of public interests and self-interests. He was also adept at getting the right people in the room at the right time and at following the money. Personal qualities helped, too. He possessed a singular drive and an indefatigable and persistent work ethic (email replies come rapidly and at all hours). That he was six feet, three inches tall and wore his dark hair pulled back into a ponytail lent him additional gravitas, a kind of George Washington standing head and shoulders above others, a leader determined to create a republic out of the confederation of Alzheimer's scientists.

He started shopping the idea to colleagues. Key leaders of the scientific community came around. This could be the infrastructure to prove that a drug slowed the disease. The discovery of PiB imaging three years later added high-octane fuel to launch the idea.

In 2004, Weiner's inspiration was born. The NIA funded him to lead the $67 million Alzheimer's Disease Neuroimaging Initiative (ADNI). Thirteen pharmaceutical companies contributed $20 million, and the NIA and two foundations paid the rest. It was a rare alignment of private-public-academic interests on a project whose budget, at that time, was staggering.

For the academics, it was an opportunity to discover the natural history of Alzheimer's disease. Patients like Mrs. Harrison and Mrs. Philip would undergo both careful histories and clinical exams and a battery of biomarker tests. The promise was an early and accurate diagnosis.

For the pharmaceutical companies, it was an opportunity to discover the best design for a drug study targeting an Alzheimer's biomarker, and it set up a multisite infrastructure of research centers trained and ready to perform their drug studies.

Fifty-seven memory centers began studying eight hundred persons ages fifty-five to ninety balanced among the cognitively unimpaired, MCI, and probable Alzheimer's disease dementia. Each year, the participants underwent cognitive testing, MRI, FDG-PET, PiB, blood, and spinal fluid measures. When they died, their brains were autopsied.

The rules were uniformity of measurement and immediate public access to the data. All sites followed strict protocols on data collection (each MRI machine must be calibrated and tuned alike using a plastic head, or "phantom image"; the tubes for spinal fluid must be polypropylene, not polystyrene, and so on), and the data were entered into a common online, open-access database. Independent centers were now organized into a common enterprise following a meticulously proscribed protocol to gather Alzheimer's biomarkers across a continuum of older adults.

Weiner even persuaded the researchers to adopt a novel name for the study. Like AD, MCI, and PiB, researchers called the Alzheimer's Disease Neuroimaging Initiative by its abbreviation, ADNI, but Weiner insisted they pronounce it not *ad-nigh* but *ad-knee*. The name stuck, and not just in the United States. Like democracy in the nineteenth century, ADNI became a model of scientific organization and governance that spread across the world. By 2011, there were ADNI projects in Australia, Europe, Japan, South Korea, and China.

Weiner described this "worldwide ADNI" network as the "water around the fish." And the fish—the researchers—prospered. Ten years after US ADNI launched, the project had generated some six hundred papers. Researchers discovered methods to standardize Alzheimer's biomarker measures and then used these measures to show how the biomarkers changed over time and to map these changes on the subject's cognitive and functional abilities. MRI, spinal fluid, and PET results were understood using numbers, as volumes of brain regions or the concentrations of tau and amyloid. These mathematical methods led to algorithms to predict which persons with MCI or dementia were likely to decline and, most provocatively, which persons without cognitive impairment were likely, over time, to develop MCI or dementia.

In 2009, ten years after Ron Petersen and colleagues' landmark MCI paper in *Archives of Neurology*, they revisited their concept. "Mild Cognitive Impairment: Ten Years Later" opened: "During the past decade, a major transition in the clinical characterization of cognitive disorders has taken place . . . We may be able to identify the earliest clinical features of these illnesses before functional impairment is evident."[3] They were being characteristically modest. The field was beginning to converge on a redefinition of Alzheimer's disease. Alzheimer's would be defined and diagnosed by biomarkers.

Alzheimer's disease had leaped into the twenty-first century.

SEPARATE AND UNEQUAL

Alzheimer's biomarker science was truly exciting. Memory centers were transforming into modern digitized and quantified operations. This great leap forward was, however, qualified.

The centers' clinical side was stuck in the slow, early twentieth-century practice of storytelling and waiting until death for a definitive diagnosis. None of the biomarker measures—amyloid PET scans, spinal fluid studies, or volumetric MRI readings—were routinely used in clinical practice. The reasons were multiple and interconnected.

ADNI was the water around the fish, but the water was unusual. The subjects weren't assembled using the rigorous recruitment of a population-based study like the Mayo team's ADPR (Alzheimer's Disease Patient Registry). Instead, ADNI enrolled a sample of very unique patients with MCI or dementia, people who'd been diagnosed at academic memory centers. The subjects who were cognitively unimpaired were typically the spouse and caregiver of those peculiar patients.

These subjects were generally healthy (aside from Alzheimer's disease), college educated, and married. Ninety-one percent were Caucasian and not Hispanic or Latino. Clinicians were understandably reluctant to conclude that results from these subjects accurately described how Alzheimer's disease biomarkers behaved in the millions of far more diverse older adults.

There were also interrelated practical challenges.

The amyloid imaging tracer PiB was complicated and costly to manufacture and deliver to a patient. The radiotracer rapidly decayed and so PiB could only be used at centers equipped with an expensive cyclotron capable of manufacturing the radiotracer and quickly injecting it into the patient. GE, its owner, therefore chose not to pursue the elaborate steps needed to assemble evidence to make a case to the FDA to approve marketing the tracer to doctors.

Spinal fluid is obtained from a spinal tap, a procedure that requires special expertise to insert a needle into a person's lower back and, drop by drop, extract the fluid. While generally safe and far less expensive than a PiB scan, a "spinal tap" is not as convenient and risk free as lying on a scanner. These risks and costs are treated quite differently across countries as, for example, in Scandinavian countries, spinal taps are routine.

In the United States, the culture of research was comfortable with keeping Alzheimer's disease biomarkers out of the clinic. Keen to preserve a sharp distinction between research and clinical care, research centers routinely declined to return to subjects their Alzheimer's biomarker results. There were two reasons for this.

First, in research, data are gathered to understand phenomena not to diagnose and treat a patient. Research results belong to the scientist, not to the subject who gave them to the scientist. Centers kept their biomarker data segregated from the clinical records. We might—and sometimes did—sneak results to selected research subjects, especially those with dementia. They were bothered by symptoms that demanded an explanation. In general, though, we kept them secret.

This provided a scientific advantage. If patients didn't know their biomarker results, the data were unblemished by their knowledge of biomarker results. Emotions and ethics were also at work. Clinicians felt a perhaps understandable disquiet about telling a person her biomarker results. A lot was known, but even more was unknown. Of particular concern was disclosing biomarkers to a person with MCI. We lacked precise numbers to explain her risk of developing dementia. We were even more uncertain over what to tell persons who were cognitively unimpaired. Remember, the ADNI data weren't designed to answer questions about populations.

The limitations in the data were only part of the problem. We also lacked a vocabulary and practice in how to tell a person with MCI that her PiB scan looked like the scan of a person with Alzheimer's disease dementia. We were largely ignorant in how to explain this information to persons who were cognitively unimpaired. The peculiarities of the ADNI subjects—their cultural and social distinctiveness—only added to our discomfort.

Second, and beyond all these reasons, however, there was one overarching one: money.

The market to sell an Alzheimer's biomarker test had millions of potential customers, but the business case to expend time and money to move a biomarker from the research lab to a motivated sales force wasn't obvious. Insurers, especially Medicare, would have to be persuaded that the test results were worth their cost because most of the market were over sixty-five years of age.

Something was missing to make that financial case.

The "cholesterol test of the brain" analogy only worked so well. A doctor's prescription for a cholesterol test foreshadowed another prescription: a treatment, a drug to lower cholesterol and thereby reduce the risk of a person suffering a heart attack. At the time, no such drug for Alzheimer's disease was available.

Alzheimer's disease biomarker tests were caught up in a maelstrom of evidentiary, cultural, ethical, and economic uncertainties. Biomarkers seemed stuck on the research side of the memory centers.

But then a young neuropathologist decided to take a big risk to bring amyloid imaging to clinical practice.

6

A YOUNG MAN IN A HURRY

I don't like going down into the morgue and cutting up brains. Of course it's important for research, and I understand that, but I never felt like I was helping the patients. It's helping their doctors and maybe their families, but it's too late for the patients. If we're good at diagnosing patients, we shouldn't need autopsies for diagnosis.

—Dan Skovronsky, MD, PhD

What is truth?

—Pontius Pilate, John 18:38

DAN SKOVRONSKY WAS a young man in a hurry. And he was also intensely smart, hardworking, and willing to take big risks. Less than a decade after high school, lean and fit, he was a rising star in academic medicine. He'd graduated from Yale University in three years with not one but two degrees (biophysics and biochemistry). Two months later he moved south, from New Haven, Connecticut, to Philadelphia, to the University of Pennsylvania to earn two doctorates: one in medicine and the other in neuroscience, followed by training in neuropathology. His impeccable academic pedigree set him on the fast track to becoming a tenured Ivy League professor of medicine.

But then he walked away from it all.

In July 2005, he left his office on Spruce Street on Penn's campus and walked three blocks north to a new office on Market Street off Penn's campus. Skovronsky was thirty-two years old, married, and the father of a newborn daughter. He'd quit academics. He'd quit medicine.

Skovronsky was determined to solve the problem that kept amyloid imaging from clinical practice. He was now the founder, president, CEO, and lead investor of a small (there were just a handful employees) company. He named it Avid Radiopharmaceuticals.

Friends and colleagues questioned his judgment. He recalled in an interview thirteen years later how disappointed his mentors were.

PiB wasn't practical. The problem was the cost and complexity of its manufacture. Chet and Bill had created it using carbon-11, or C_{11}, a form of radioactive carbon that decayed quickly. This decay means no more than an hour can elapse between manufacture in the cyclotron, the machine that manufactures radiolabeled compounds, and injection into the patient. The solution would be to have an on-site cyclotron, kept close to the scanner. The money and personnel needed to purchase and maintain a cyclotron, however, were and remain simply prohibitive to most hospitals.

Surveying the situation at that time, Skovronsky was surprised at the impact of PiB. "Maybe it's a testament to how important amyloid imaging is that PiB had such a big impact because I saw C_{11} as so impractical and so difficult to use that I thought it would never have an impact on patients, but the impact on research has been good."[1]

His vision was to discover a more practical, hence marketable, PET amyloid imaging agent. Unlike Bill Klunk and Chet Mathis, who'd faced indifference about their idea and therefore carried out their research as a side project, Skovronsky's vision was caught up in the complexities of a large lab. The pace of academics was frustrating but developing an amyloid radiotracer using a business instead of grant-funded academics presented its own challenges. He had to line up investors, hire employees, and build a lab.

Avid's focus was developing a molecule attached not to C_{11} but to radiolabeled fluorine, called F_{18}. Unlike carbon-labeled compounds, these compounds last longer after manufacture in the cyclotron. If C_{11} is a frail and evanescent mayfly, F_{18}, the compound Skovronsky worked with, is a vibrant firefly.

Avid worked through multiple compounds. They landed on one that seemed to work. It was the forty-fifth compound and so they named it AV-45, or florbetapir. Like PiB, AV-45 passed the steps in human brain tissue and wild type mouse models (and courtesy of Mathis and Klunk they knew to skip the transgenic mice step).

By 2006, in collaboration with researchers in Australia, they were testing it in humans with and without dementia caused by Alzheimer's disease. Just like PiB, the glitter was sticking to the page. Unlike PiB, Skovronsky had one more step to go, one great leap before he could sell AV-45 to physicians like me to prescribe in our diagnostic work-up of patients like Mrs. Philip and Mrs. Harrison.

He needed permission from the FDA.

THE YOUNG UPSTARTS

PiB has never been subjected to the rigors of FDA approval. Consequently, its use was solely in research to measure amyloid in living humans. Without FDA approval, a company could not sell it to diagnose patients. The hundreds of patients in ADNI who'd undergone PiB scans did not routinely learn their results. The hundreds of thousands, perhaps millions, of patients who would undergo florbetapir imaging would do so in order to learn their results.

Avid faced competition. GE and Bayer were also developing compounds. All these companies were competing in uncharted commercial territory. In FDA parlance, the agency had never approved a "label" for a radiotracer to measure brain amyloid or any Alzheimer's biomarker.

The term "label" describes the multifolded document inserted into the package that contains the drug. FDA staff joke that they know no one reads the label—the tiny font is discouraging—but the text of a drug's label is of immense medical and commercial importance. It's a kind of rule book for a drug. It explains what the drug does, the kinds of patients who should receive it, its risks and benefits, and its appropriate uses. Insurers, including Medicare, look to the label for guidance on whether to pay for the drug.

The label for an amyloid imaging radiotracer would be an entirely new language. It would set a standard for how doctors, patients, and insurers such as Medicare talk about and use the biomarker. The agency presented the three companies with an essential question whose answer would determine whether they could obtain an FDA label: how will you prove what your drug does, that it works, that it images amyloid?

This question was a monumental conundrum for the three companies.

From PiB's inception, in the very first publication reporting the results of scans done at Bengt Långström's radiotracer factory, there were "outliers," science talk for data that don't make sense. Three patients with dementia thought to be caused by Alzheimer's disease were PiB negative and one "normal" had PiB uptake typical of a patient with Alzheimer's disease (the authors described him as an "asymptomatic amyloid positive case").[2]

Results from ADNI and other studies like it showed these outliers were in fact quite common. By 2008, it was well understood that about one-third of patients with either dementia or MCI that clinicians said was caused by Alzheimer's disease didn't have positive amyloid scans. They couldn't therefore have Alzheimer's disease.

Expert clinicians at the research centers found this result disturbing. They prided themselves on the accuracy of their ability to use their patients' history and exam to diagnose dementia or MCI and determine that it was caused by Alzheimer's disease. Chet Mathis recalled how these findings wounded their pride. "They were full of themselves and their clinical abilities to make these calls and be right almost all the time, but here was a test showing maybe they weren't so right all the time. Especially with MCI."

Even more challenging were the results of amyloid scans done in cognitively healthy persons. Some people an expert clinician said were cognitively unimpaired, commonly called normal, in fact had amyloid uptake that looked like a scan from a patient with dementia.

"Back then," Skovronsky recalled, "these results were controversial. People say AV-45 is not very sensitive because twenty percent of your patients with Alzheimer's dementia are negative and it's not very specific because twenty percent of your normals are positive. And so we had to somehow prove that it works."

For the FDA, "works" meant a very simple thing: prove that an image that showed amyloid in fact was measuring amyloid. The agency wanted proof the glitter was sticking to amyloid. They wanted a standard of truth.

On October 23, 2008, Avid, GE, and Bayer all came before the FDA to present their standard of truth. The occasion was the meeting of the FDA's Peripheral and Central Nervous System Drugs Advisory Committee in the Hilton Hotel in Silver Spring, Maryland. They came bearing three very different ideas about what is truth.

Bayer said truth was the consensus of expert clinicians at memory centers. Not one but a group of clinicians would determine that a person had dementia that was caused by Alzheimer's disease, and this consensus diagnosis would set the standard of truth against which the amyloid scan would be compared. In the Alzheimer's field, the concept of a consensus diagnosis was and remains a well-accepted standard of truth. And yet, autopsy results showed that at even the best of the centers using consensus diagnosis, the human factors analysis that led to a diagnosis of Alzheimer's disease was wrong about 20 percent of the time. For the question of validating an amyloid scan, Bayer's proposal seemed to wrap the problem right into the solution.

GE said truth was PiB. The results of a PiB scan would determine whether a patient did or did not have amyloid in her brain. A "true" amyloid scan, such as AV-45, was a scan whose result matched the results of a PiB scan done in that same patient. This undermined the FDA's authority. It meant a non-FDA-approved tracer was the standard for FDA approval of other tracers. Even more unpalatable, it made GE, a private company, the central banker of amyloid. The gold standard was available, provided GE manufactured PiB and made it widely available.

Avid said truth was pathology. The moment of truth is in the morgue—when a dead person's brain and history up until death come together. They proposed to compare the results of an AV-45 brain scan to the results of that person's brain autopsy. Truth would be the correlation between what is seen on the scan and what is seen under the microscope. Where the scan showed amyloid, did the neuropathologist see amyloid and, vice versa, where the scan did not show amyloid, did the neuropathologist not see amyloid?

The idea was conceptually elegant, but it seemed practically bizarre. To answer this question, the time interval between the amyloid scan and the brain autopsy needed to be short, just a few months at most. This short time interval would ensure that the brain of the living person at the time of her scan was similar to the brain of her cadaver. To answer this question, they needed to study dying people.

Avid's proposal shook up the room.

Dr. David Brooks, the head of neurology in clinical development at GE Healthcare, said the study was unethical. "I don't know how it works in the US because I am based in Europe, but we would have big problems taking end-stage Alzheimer patients, who really are not sure what is happening around them, and putting them in the scanner and imaging them in this way."[3]

Even those supportive of the idea found putting it into practice challenging, perhaps unworkable. Avid proposed to recruit people who were terminally ill not from end-stage Alzheimer's but instead from cancer and other diseases—people enrolled in hospice programs.

The logistics were daunting. The terminally ill patients would have to undergo an exam and cognitive testing and travel from the comfort of their homes to a hospital to undergo an AV-45 scan. Then, immediately after death, their grieving families would have to contact a pathologist on twenty-four-hour call who would travel across the country, harvest the brain, prepare it, and then deliver it to a central facility for an autopsy.

This autopsy would not be to make a diagnosis of Alzheimer's disease. Instead, the neuropathologist would count the location and the amount of amyloid in the brain tissue and compare those meticulous counts with the amount of amyloid measured using the PET scan. The more the two counts agreed, the more certain was the truth that an amyloid PET scan measures amyloid. This correlation of what was seen on the scan with what the pathologist saw in the autopsied tissue was called "histopathological correlation."

The committee members questioned all three proposals for the standard of truth to prove an image in fact measures "truth." At day's end, they came to a decision. The dry language of the minutes read: "In regards to the indication of detecting amyloid in the brain, the committee overwhelmingly agreed that histopathological correlation should be the 'standard of truth' in phase 3 clinical studies. There was discussion about the feasibility of obtaining 'enough' pathological studies or the ability to follow study patients to autopsy."

Avid won the day, though FDA's message to them was a sort of : "OK, give it a try. Good luck." Avid was so confident in their idea that they'd decided not to wait for the FDA's decision. They'd already started the autopsy correlation study.

"We were the young upstart," Skovronsky explained.

7

HOW DO YOU CAST
A BROKEN BRAIN?

Obviously, Alzheimer's disease is more complex than a femur fracture.
—Qi Feng, MD, PhD, Food and Drug Administration,
October 23, 2008

ON APRIL 6, 2012, four years after the 2008 FDA "standard of truth" meeting in Silver Spring, Maryland, seven years after Skovronsky walked away from a career in academic medicine, he and his colleagues achieved success. The FDA approved florbetapir for the detection of brain amyloid. Their standard of truth study of terminally ill patients found that the more amyloid the pathologist observed in a slice of brain, the brighter were the florbetapir images of that same brain.[1]

Skovronsky had reached his goal, and he'd achieved it quicker than the years needed to obtain tenure at Penn. Generous rewards followed. In 2010, the multibillion-dollar pharmaceutical company Lilly purchased Avid for $300 million. Pending the success of florbetapir, another $500 million would follow. FDA approval was the dawn of that success. With it, Lilly could advertise and sell florbetapir to physicians. Ten years after Chet Mathis and Bill Klunk's Valentine card from Sweden showed the first images of brain amyloid, amyloid imaging was coming to the clinic.

They named her Amyvid. Lilly's press release described Amyvid as "the first and only radioactive diagnostic agent approved for PET imaging of beta-amyloid neuritic plaques in the living brain."[2] With the resource of Lilly to support Amyvid's marketing and distribution, the millions of older adults with memory complaints, people like Mrs. Harrison and Mrs. Philip, would finally have a test for Alzheimer's disease. The hours of storytelling at a memory center, the surrender of privacy to an informant, the uncertainty of the diagnosis, the ghoulish trip to the basement morgue to obtain a final answer—it seemed the gothic horror story was ending.

Not quite.

A HOT DAY IN WINTER

Wintertime in Baltimore is typically cold. The city has experienced snowstorms severe enough to shut it down for days. But Wednesday, January 30, 2013, was a most unusual winter day. Temperatures rose into the seventies. Runners dressed as if it were summer. People walked around in short sleeves enjoying the warmth.

At the headquarters of Medicare, temperatures were rising indoors, too. The instigator was an argument unfolding in a meeting called PET Beta Amyloid Imaging in the Context of Dementia.

Skovronsky and his colleagues weren't done. FDA approval was not the last but rather the next-to-last step before they could sell their practical radiotracer to physicians caring for patients with cognitive impairment. The last step was to convince America to pay for the scan. They had to go before the Medicare Evidence Development and Coverage Advisory Committee, or MEDCAC (commonly pronounced *med-kack*) and convince it that there was adequate evidence to determine that PET imaging of brain beta-amyloid changes health outcomes.

MEDCAC is Medicare's independent adviser. Its expert panels review and evaluate evidence of a service's benefits, harms, and appropriateness. MEDCAC's charge is to ensure Medicare's coverage decisions are evidence based. When Medicare faces a decision about whether to provide a service fraught with controversies over its value, it turns to MEDCAC, and the decision whether Medicare should pay for an Amyvid scan was laden with controversy.

MEDCAC was picking up where the FDA had left off in 2008. At that standard of truth hearing, the FDA had asked the three companies to address not one but two questions. The second question was left unanswered: "To what extent, if any, would the detection of cerebral amyloid provide useful clinical information?" The FDA wanted to know the value of an amyloid scan. It was a simple question, but it didn't have a simple answer. Dr. Qi Feng of the FDA's Division of Medical Imaging and Hematology Products opened the 2008 meeting comparing an amyloid image to a much more common image. The X-ray image of a broken bone.

"For a femur fracture we use X-ray. You see it right away," Dr. Feng remarked.[3] His point was, the image of a broken bone speaks for itself. A man falls, he cannot get up, and he is complaining of excruciating pain in his thigh. An X-ray shows his femur bone is broken. The bone needs to be set in a cast. The value of the X-ray is self-evident.

But what was the value of an image of amyloid in the brain of a person with dementia or MCI? Feng reflected, "Obviously, Alzheimer's disease is more complex than a femur fracture."

The standard of truth study showed that an Amyvid scan measures amyloid. The truth was made evident. What was not self-evident was the value of that truth. How does a physician use the image to help a patient? How do doctors like me at a memory center cast a broken brain?

Amyloid images were without precedent. My colleagues and I had never used the results of a radiotracer scan of brain pathology to care for our patients. The more valuable the image, the more America would want to pay for it.

The stakes were enormous.

By 2013, the Alzheimer's Association reported in its annual *Facts and Figures Report* that they estimated 5.2 million people in the United States had dementia caused by Alzheimer's disease and as many as 8 million, MCI.[4] A 2011 Centers for Disease Control and Prevention study estimated 16 million Americans had cognitive impairment.[5] All totaled, 30 million people might be eligible for an Amyvid scan at a per scan price of about $3,000.

If just a fraction of these people sought a prescription for a scan, the dollars spent would add up to hundreds of millions—even billions. Because most of these people were sixty-five years and older, Medicare would pay that bill. No wonder the Centers for Medicare and Medicaid Services, known commonly as CMS, the administrator of the Medicare program, turned to MEDCAC for advice.

In the histories of Alzheimer's disease, January 30, 2013, is not typically included. It is a date most would like to forget. That preternaturally warm winter day was the first time the value of a diagnosis of Alzheimer's disease was subjected to public scrutiny. And it did not go well. Until this MEDCAC hearing, Alzheimer's doctors practicing at academic medical centers had been living a kind of prolonged life of a graduate student. Discoveries of MCI,

PiB, and Amyvid and the common language created by ADNI gave them an exciting new way of thinking about Alzheimer's disease. With biomarkers, they could diagnose it not after death but in life, and using the MCI criteria, they could diagnose it before a person was disabled. In time, with more research, a diagnosis might be possible before a person had MCI, akin to the work of our colleagues in cardiology and gastroenterology with their blood tests for cholesterol and colonoscopies for cancer.

The field was inspired by an iconic image created by a series of curves arranged along a horizontal line. Imagine a series of left-to-right swooping curves that start out flat, rise, and then flatten once more, one curve following the other in a harmonious sequence like waves racing to the shore. This image was the work of Cliff Jack, a neuroradiologist at the Mayo Clinic who'd been puzzling over the myriad of Alzheimer's biomarker data. In an interview, he explained his inspiration was "a staggering in time, a sequence of events staggered in time."[6]

He was uniquely talented to experience this inspiration. Since boyhood, he'd played jazz guitar, and he continues to at Rochester's Redwood Room. "You have to have a lot of stuff swirling about and then you execute a line. You use the unexpected to create something beautiful out of dissonance."

The "dissonance" in Alzheimer's biomarkers was that some people had elevated amyloid and were cognitively unimpaired and other people had the same amount of amyloid but were suffering from dementia.

Cliff put all the data together. What fell out was this series of curves, an ordered sequence in time, unfolding some one to two decades before a person was suffering like Mrs. Philip or Mrs. Harrison. The first note is tau, and then amyloid comes in, at first slowly, but then amyloid accumulation rapidly picks up, its accumulation answered by tau starting to rapidly accumulate. Then comes the third note, the wail of dying neurons as seen by atrophy on the MRI. Finally, the fourth and most resonant of sounds, the voices of people like Mr. and Mrs. Harrison and Mrs. Philip and her daughter.

The curves seemed to settle this dissonance: people with the same amount of amyloid but vastly different cognitive abilities were on very different points on their tau curve.

These elegant curves were called the Jack curves. They were a fascinating and inspiring intellectual exercise. They were the opening image of research seminars and conferences, but they hadn't been put into practice. This MEDCAC hearing was the chance to make the case to do just that.

�֍

Mrs. Philip was among the first of my patients to whom I relayed an Amyvid scan result. She was in a research study that used the scan, and I was willing to tell the result to those subjects who asked for it. I was using a set of new diagnostic guidelines prepared by a collaboration between the National Institute on Aging and the Alzheimer's Association. The 2011 criteria, as they came to be known by their date of publication, were intended to replace the 1984 criteria that I used to diagnose Mrs. Harrison. Remember, hers was a "clinical diagnosis" that relied solely on her history and exam.

The 2011 criteria debuted biomarker tests. Biomarker results, paired with a clinical diagnosis of either MCI or dementia, allowed me to tell the patient and her family whether their cognitive problems were caused by Alzheimer's disease.

Mrs. Philip's amyloid scan was positive. There was vivid uptake of Amyvid in her cortex. The computer's analyses of her MRI produced a precise measure of the size of her hippocampi. They were shrunken from years of cell death.

I did not have a measure of tau in her brain (such scans were being developed but in 2013 were not yet available). The available data showed, however, a compelling story of a clinical biomarker–defined case of Alzheimer's disease. My answer to her daughter's question was that her mother did have something neurological. She had MCI caused by Alzheimer's disease or, more simply, she had Alzheimer's disease.

With this diagnosis, I prescribed donepezil, a medicine shown to treat the symptoms in a fraction of patients with dementia caused by Alzheimer's disease (the drug's origins are described in part 2). I explained that studies hadn't shown it helped persons with MCI, but they were willing to give it a try.

The family was mobilized. They met with our social work team. They began to make plans for where she would live. They set up a system to monitor her finances and medications. They agreed to keep an eye on her driving and although she did not know how to use a cellular phone, she would carry one in her purse. It allowed her daughter to track her mother's location.

I closed the diagnostic follow-up visit with words I routinely deliver: "You're the same person today as you were the day before I first met you. All I've done is put a name to the cause of your memory problems. I expect to see you back next year and the years after that just as you are now, talking with me and telling me about your grandchildren."

They thanked me, and then they went home. I'd delivered a biomarker-based diagnosis of MCI caused by Alzheimer's disease, the emerging standard of care my colleagues would argue for on that unusually warm Wednesday in January in Baltimore.

It did not go well for either my colleagues or me.

"THERE'S BEEN SOME CONFUSION HERE TODAY"

The fifteen-member MEDCAC blended experts. Five worked in Alzheimer's disease (psychiatry, psychology, and neurology), and ten worked in assessing the value of a medical service. This group included Mark Fendrick, an internist and researcher at the University of Michigan. His concept of "value-based insurance design" examines how the ways doctors are paid and patients are engaged impact patients' access to care, its quality, and its costs. Other members included a cardiac surgeon and director of a patient-centered comparative effectiveness program, a professor of behavioral health, and a health-outcomes researcher from Bayer HealthCare. Rita Redberg, the chair of the committee and a professor of cardiology at the University of California–San Francisco, was an expert in biomarkers and biomarker-based therapeutics for heart disease.

Their charge was to answer a question. "How confident are you that there is adequate evidence to determine whether or not PET imaging of brain beta-amyloid changes health outcomes (improved, equivalent, or worsened) in patients who display early symptoms or signs of cognitive dysfunction?" If they were sufficiently confident, they would go on to answer other questions, such as their confidence in the characteristics that predict which patients experience improved health outcomes after receiving the test.

Most of this group weren't Alzheimer's experts, but they were experts in assessing value and the delivery of health care. They needed to be educated and persuaded. In the time allotted and strictly enforced with flashing red lights, they listened to stories from the Alzheimer's community intended to show the value of an Alzheimer's disease biomarker test for patients with early symptoms and signs, patients like Mrs. Philip with MCI.

Among the presenters were doctors, clinicians whose years of practice at memory centers made them well versed in the time-intensive history taking from both a patient and an informant to arrive at a diagnosis of dementia and the nuance and judgment needed to tease out MCI from aging or dementia. They were keenly aware of the limited kinds of medications available to treat Alzheimer's disease dementia and the lack of medications to help patients with MCI.

Dr. Paul Aisen started the presentations. Aisen, a geriatrician, led a large NIA-funded cooperative study based at the University of California–San Diego dedicated to discovering treatments for Alzheimer's disease. He was immersed in the worlds of clinical trials and the promise of Alzheimer's biomarkers as a target for drug therapy, and he was bullish about the promise of amyloid imaging. He described it as "an enormously important advance, perhaps the most important advance in therapeutic research in AD. In the clinic, it means that we no longer have to talk about probable Alzheimer's disease dementia. We can establish the presence of amyloid and make a definite diagnosis of Alzheimer's dementia and eliminate the substantial error rate in Alzheimer's dementia diagnosis."[7]

He showed the Jack curves and explained the paradigm shift they represent, the sequence of biomarker events beginning years before symptoms arise.

Notably, he focused on the care of patients with MCI, hailing the scan's "extreme prognostic value" because persons with MCI and a positive scan, persons like Mrs. Philip, were at increased risk of progressing to dementia. These patients with a positive scan, he explained, were best categorized not as having MCI but rather having "prodromal Alzheimer's disease."

He even gestured to the scan's future use to screen and treat persons in their fifties who did not exhibit cognitive impairment. Once anti-amyloid drugs were discovered, a positive scan would lead to a prescription for a drug to prevent developing MCI or dementia.

The momentum picked up.

Experts told stories of patients whose lives were transformed by their amyloid scan result, especially patients with MCI whose scan was negative. The ability to deprescribe the marginally effective and "off-label" use of the medications for Alzheimer's disease was noted, but even more impressive was how the result impacted their very selves. There was an executive whose negative scan meant "he didn't have to resign from life" and a seventy-two-year-old primary care physician whose negative scan dramatically reassured him and so he "returned happily to his practice."

The stories of persons with positive scans were darker. The presenters told of mobilizing families to begin monitoring and arranging affairs and referring patients to clinical trials to test drugs for Alzheimer's disease.

Michael Devous, a radiologist at the University of Texas Southwestern Medical Center in Dallas, summed up the stories he had gathered from his talks to patient and caregiver groups. "I hear heartbreaking stories about the consequences of incorrect and uncertain diagnoses and heartwarming stories of the incredible relief and value that an amyloid scan has provided by yielding greater diagnostic certainty."

Steve Salloway, a neurologist at Brown University, summed up his colleagues' sentiments. "Should I tell my patients that we have a test available to help clarify their diagnosis, but we can't use it because Medicare doesn't cover it? Instead we have to wait a few years to see how symptoms develop. That's the approach from the last century when these tools were not available."

The presentations finished, Dr. Redberg opened the floor for the committee to question the presenters.

The back-and-forth exchanges displayed struggles over understanding what Alzheimer's disease is, how it is diagnosed—especially at the "prodromal" or MCI stage—and the value of the available interventions. Concerns of stigma permeated the exchanges. A presenter cited the *New York Times* profile of Awilda Jimenez, a person with MCI who described her positive amyloid scan as "devastating news." She and her husband worried about their future and regretted she'd taken the test.[8] Curtis Mock, a committee member, family medicine physician, and MBA, worried about how the information might impact not just his patients' but their families' economic well-being. "I didn't hear anybody say here that they're a lawyer, but I'm wondering about my patient and family members that are going to get scanned that are going to have implications on the future of their coverage decisions for insurance and life and jobs. Is this a cart before the horse for beneficiary protections?"

The back-and-forth became angry. Howard Fillit, a geriatrician who specialized in Alzheimer's disease, implored the committee: "What do you think I've been doing for thirty-five years?" Then he answered his question: "I've been taking care of patients."

Redberg cut him off. "Dr. Fillit, I think that we all agree that Alzheimer's is a terrible disease and we would all like to do everything we can to improve the care of our patients with Alzheimer's. I'm sure that you have been doing that and that's what many doctors have been doing. The question before the committee is what evidence do we have that the beta-amyloid imaging test is going to help us improve the care of patients."

One exchange stood out in the efforts to answer this question. It was between Redberg and Salloway. Redberg was a cardiologist whose career was devoted to the rational use of the multiplicity of cardiovascular diagnostics and therapeutics. She was clearly troubled over whether the scan would improve health outcomes.

"What's not clear to me is what is the impact on patients of telling someone that they have a seventy percent change or whatever it is, because we don't know, of getting a disease we are all terrified of getting . . . because clearly there is going to be at least, I would say, thirty percent who are never going to have that terrible thing happen, but they will have to go through the trauma, the labeling, and everything else associated with it."

Salloway stepped up to the microphone. "I'm so glad you bought that up," he began. "Because I think there's been some confusion here today."

He set out to settle the confusion. He explained how appropriate-use criteria for amyloid imaging only allow the scan to be prescribed for patients who have cognitive impairment where the diagnosis is uncertain.

Redberg then asked him, the Alzheimer's doctor, "the question." It was the question of a patient with MCI, a person like Mrs. Philip, whose doctor has offered her the opportunity to have a brain amyloid test.

"And what would I do differently then?"

Salloway explained that a positive scan would allow him to explain that her MCI is likely due to Alzheimer's disease. He would mobilize the family and start preparing that person immediately. And if the scan was negative, he wouldn't mobilize all those resources or counsel them in the same way.

Redberg pushed back. "Based on their scan but not on their clinical presentation?"

"No," Salloway replied. "Based on the whole clinical evaluation including the scan." He proceeded to develop this important nuance. "The other point of your question is extremely important, something that I deal with every day. You really order tests for one patient at a time. You always want to assess what the impact of that test might be for the patient and how finding out that they have an amyloid-positive scan and a higher risk of Alzheimer's would have on them. And that we wouldn't routinely order that."

This exchange plainly illustrated how appropriate use of the scan required nuance and sophistication, time and effort. It was not in fact a one-and-done "test for Alzheimer's disease." It was just one important bit of information in a complex human factors analysis of the multiple bits of information needed to arrive at a diagnosis of MCI caused by Alzheimer's disease. Following that, the clinician needed to devote time and effort to explain the result to the patient and family. Care was needed to make sure they understood the probability of MCI progressing to dementia.

In the face of this sophistication, the committee was clearly worried. What clinicians possessed the skills and resources to do this? The appropriate-use criteria Salloway referenced recommended the scan only be prescribed by an Alzheimer's expert, but the definition did not include board certifications or other Alzheimer's-specific credentials because formal credentialing didn't exist. The criteria defined an expert as a geriatrician, psychiatrist, or neurologist who devoted at least one-quarter of her practice to the care of persons with Alzheimer's disease.

A doctor like Salloway, who devoted his practice to patients with Alzheimer's disease, was going to properly use the scan. The problem was there were very few doctors like him in America.

A worry ran through the discussion like a minor chord in a dark musical score. Repeatedly throughout the meeting, committee members expressed concern that the scan would be used in a widespread and indiscriminate manner. There would be massive overuse. Steven Pearson, a cost-effectiveness researcher at the Institute for Clinical and Economic Review and the Massachusetts General Hospital's Institute for Technology Assessment, emphasized that based on his perspective as a primary care physician, "I anticipate nearly every single patient over the age of fifty would expect to get this test, like a colonoscopy." These patients, he worried, "will include many patients with the earliest, if any, signs of MCI."

THUNDER IN WINTER

It was time to vote on the question. "How confident are you that there is adequate evidence to determine whether or not PET imaging of brain beta-amyloid changes health outcomes (improved, equivalent, or worsened) in patients who display early symptoms or signs of cognitive dysfunction?" This vote was critical. A mean score of 2.5 or more out of 5 would signify at least intermediate confidence and therefore move the committee on to vote on other questions, such as their confidence in the evidence about patient characteristics that predict improved health outcomes from the amyloid test.

The mean score was 2.167. Amyvid failed to make the cut.

After the voting, each committee member explained his or her vote. Ed Faught, a neurologist at Emory University, summarized the day. During the period of questions and answers, he worried over the nuance and judgment needed to make a diagnosis of MCI. He expressed concern, for example, about how cognitive impairment is defined in clinical practice. The failure to take the time and effort to perform testing and interview a patient and their informant and the nuance needed to interpret cognitive test results all risked mistakenly labeling a person as impaired. Frustrated clinicians might simply forgo these efforts and accept the patient's complaint of memory problems as proof enough of cognitive impairment and so order the scan.

His vote of a 3 was enough to move the committee forward but only two cheers for amyloid imaging. He explained his rationale.

"As a neurologist, I think this would change the way we manage patients, and I would like to have it available from that point of view. On the other hand, I see a big potential for overuse and misuse if everyone has this like a colonoscopy, so I found it a little vague."

It was that "other hand" that gripped him. He worried about how to enforce the criteria for the appropriate use of the test, especially the requirement that the test only be ordered by an Alzheimer's expert. His sentiment was one I shared. In the hands of clinicians like him or Dr. Salloway or me, this test would be used appropriately, but we were unusual. American medicine had—and still has—a habit of consuming a test like teenagers consume a keg of beer.

Several of the committee members explained that their lack of enthusiasm was because something was missing. They couldn't "connect the dots." The limited benefits of treatments for Alzheimer's disease dementia and the lack of treatments for MCI, the stigma, the lack of experts who would properly prescribe the tracer, the nuance needed to tease out MCI from normal aging—the evidence wasn't convincing that adding a costly amyloid scan would improve the quality of care for the millions of patients who might receive it.

The day ended with Amyvid just short of success. Dan Skovronsky and his fellow neuropathologists would still be called to visit the basement morgue. As the attendees gathered their belongings to depart, they received a warning. The unusually warm January day was ending with an even more unusual meteorological event: thunderstorms.

Five months later, the Centers for Medicare and Medicaid Services issued its decision. "The evidence is insufficient to conclude that the use of PET amyloid-beta ($A\beta$) imaging improves health outcomes for Medicare beneficiaries with dementia or neurodegenerative disease."[9] The FDA approved it, but Medicare wouldn't pay for it. America wasn't ready for an Alzheimer's biomarker.

Mrs. Philip and her daughter weren't either.

Three months after her new patient visit, they returned to the memory center for a routine follow-up visit. Something was terribly wrong.

Mrs. Philip was nervous and anxious. "I felt better before I came here. Now, if I do something that's not one hundred percent, I worry."

She explained she was scared about dementia (she struggled to even say the word). She described counting and recounting the change at the gift shop where she volunteered, double-checking to be sure she hadn't made a mistake. Seated at the edge of her chair, ready to leave, she announced this would be her last visit with me.

Her daughter in her private time with me told me how she worried about her mother, how she saw some of her friends with their parents walking about like zombies.

That ghastly word. I was devastated.

Implicit in the question that opened our relationship—"How can I help you?"—was that I and my team at the Memory Center could do just that. My biomarker-based diagnosis and our efforts to mobilize the family, however, had helped neither Mrs. Philip nor her daughter. My center offered them no room for tranquility.

The stigma of Alzheimer's disease dementia was spilling into their lives. Mrs. Philip was preoccupied by negative beliefs about herself and her abilities to perform activities she once enjoyed. Her daughter was beginning to see her mother as less of a person than she was before the diagnosis. Fears of the future were corrupting their relationship.

"I had to drag her in here to see you," her daughter lamented.

I did my best to repair the mess I'd made. I listened. I walked back from the word "Alzheimer's" and never used the "dementia" word. I reassured her that she had "*mild* cognitive impairment," and I noted that her MRI showed some vascular disease. "Maybe *that* and not Alzheimer's is causing some of this, and you can do something about that." I repeated those lines I used at the close of her diagnostic follow-up visit ("You're the same person today as you were before I first met you . . .") and then I prescribed an antidepressant.

In the weeks and months that followed their visit, I returned again and again to that upsetting Friday afternoon. I thought I was skilled at explaining MCI and disclosing biomarker results, but Mrs. Philip and her daughter were a kind of fire bell in the night, warning me that I had a lot to master. I worried about the magnitude of harms that might be committed when Alzheimer's biomarker tests were prescribed by busy clinicians who lacked the time and resources available at a memory center.

I came to see that America was in a peculiar situation. Since the influential cancer researcher and essayist Lewis Thomas's 1981 proclamation that Alzheimer's disease was the "disease of the century," research had produced remarkable discoveries. MCI, together with amyloid imaging and other biomarker tests, was transforming Alzheimer's into a biological diagnosis. Progress had occurred, and yet, progress hadn't occurred.

In 2015, a survey of thousands of Medicare beneficiaries—people like Mrs. Harrison and Mrs. Philip—showed how bad the care was. The norm among physicians was not to tell the patient or their family a diagnosis of Alzheimer's disease.[10] I wasn't surprised. The typical new patient visit at the Penn Memory Center began with a family's frustrating story of months, even years, of searching for answers and struggling to get care.

There were several explanations for this. They included the stigma of this frightening disease and the scarcity of physicians skilled in making and disclosing a diagnosis and discussing a treatment plan with the patient and caregiver. Sadly, physicians with these skills lacked the resources to practice them. Memory centers were uncommon. Most were based at academic medical centers and staffed by clinicians juggling passionate but competing devotions to research and patient care. To function, they depended on generous philanthropy and research funds. Physicians didn't have effective pharmacologic treatments for the disease. They just had better ways to diagnose and talk about it. Alzheimer's disease really was a crisis.

Why? Why did even rich and powerful nations like the United States face the Alzheimer's crisis?

Part 2 explores the answers to this question. They form a maddening tale that involves world wars, economic recessions, dark and violent nationalism, and competing ideas about the family, self, autonomy, and what causes a brain disease. It is also about choices we've made—and failed to make—to live well and together as one nation with the loss of independence and productivity as we age.

PART 2

· · · · · · · · · · · · ·

THE BIRTH OF
ALZHEIMER'S DISEASE

In some ways disease does not exist until we have agreed that it does, by
perceiving and responding to it.
  —Charles Rosenberg, *Framing Disease: Studies in Cultural History*, 1992

8

THE OLD WOMAN
IN THE TOWER

Somewhere beyond the curtain
Of distorting days
Lives that lonely thing
W. B. Yeats, "Quarrel in Old Age"

I'LL NEVER FORGET her. I keep returning to that unusually sunny autumn afternoon in Chicago some thirty years ago, revisiting and reinterpreting what we did and said and, more importantly, what we neither did nor said.

I was a medical student, and she was a patient on the VIP floor of Northwestern Memorial Hospital. This was in the era of the ironically named "semiprivate hospital room." The cluttered space was divided in half by a curtain, on either side of which was a symmetric arrangement of two chairs, a nightstand, and a wheeled tray table placed around a hospital bed.

Her room, though, was truly private. It was a large, well-furnished space (upholstered wing chairs and polished side tables with Queen Anne legs). She had her own bathroom. Situated at the very top of the tower, its view of the Chicago cityscape and the vast, flat, blue calm of Lake Michigan was spectacular.

I was one of four students gathered at the foot of her bed under the tutelage of our attending physician. We were on teaching rounds, and this elderly woman was our teaching case. One of my fellow students, I'll call him Ron, had selected her as his bedside case presentation.

These presentations followed a ritual. First, the student presented the patient's history of illness that brought her to the hospital (accomplished students recited this from memory). That done, the physician asked questions, both to clarify the history and to provoke us to think over what might be the cause of the patient's illness and what physical exam findings we'd expect.

Next, the student presented that exam, and then the physician posed the question. "What's your differential diagnosis?"

We answered with a list of the possible diseases that explained the patient's history of present illness. Because we were astoundingly book smart, clinically ignorant, and young, we often called out unusual, even nonsensical causes. To avoid this, we tried to order our lists from the most to the least likely causes. We followed maxims such as "when you hear hoofbeats think of horses, not zebras. Unless you live in Africa."

The presentation ended with a discussion of the laboratory tests we would order and the results we expected. The results presented, the ritual concluded with the final question.

"So then, what's the diagnosis and how do you want to treat it?"

We sought out "good cases." A good case meant a well-told story of a common disease. The horses, so to speak. A good case, for example, was the story of a previously healthy man with two days of a cough productive of rusty-colored sputum, shortness of breath, and fever and chills. He ought to have crackles on his lung exam, a well-demarcated patchy haze on his chest X-ray, elevated white blood cell count, and a stain of his sputum should display lancet-shape diplococci. This was the story of a pneumonia most likely caused by pneumococcal bacteria and the treatment was a penicillin-based antibiotic, oxygen, and intravenous fluid.

As medical students, we started with these classics—acute illnesses like pneumonia and appendicitis or acute flares of chronic illnesses such as heart failure and gout—and then we moved on to the great cases. The stories of zebras.

There was the woman with fever, rash, renal failure, and lung nodules caused by a rare autoimmune disease. Steroids were her treatment. There was the man with an unusual bacterium infecting his blood, a bacterium normally found in the mouth. The source was a rotting cancer in his esophagus that allowed this bacterium that resides peacefully in our mouths to gain entry into his blood and therefore live violently. Antibiotics and consults to surgery and oncology.

"Great case."

That was the praise we desired.

Ron's case was of a very old white woman who'd been disruptive at home. After three days of shouting and pacing about, she was brought to the emergency room. Ron told us that his patient didn't know why she was in the emergency room. She spoke little, but she did say she was fine. She was without complaints of fevers, chills, pain, nausea, or vomiting. She had a past medical history of arthritis and a distant history of breast cancer treated with a radical mastectomy. Her exam was essentially normal save for the expected missing breast. Her labs were also normal. And today, on bedside teaching rounds, there she lay beneath a soft pink quilt.

Beside the bed, in one of the wing chairs, was a woman. She was much younger, Black, and she, too, was silent. She was dressed in the kind of uniform a maid wore. She, too, smiled at us. Ron explained that the younger woman lived with the patient.

Ron's presentation was unusually short because the physician didn't ask questions. He stood with his arms folded looking like a frustrated coach. When Ron reached the customary break points, the physician would nod and say, "Go on."

We all stood around the old woman's bedside entranced by her head. She kept it awkwardly flexed forward so that it hovered above her pillow. The sight was so uncomfortable that in time Ron patted her on the shoulder, called her sweetie, and urged her to lie back on the pillow. The woman just smiled. She didn't relax her head. Ron asked her how she was feeling. More smiles and silence. Her well-kept hair was chalk white like her skin and her lips bright red with lipstick.

Presentation done, the physician struggled. He said some words about how the absence of any signs of infection in the blood or ischemia on the cardiogram suggested the agitation didn't have an organic cause. We never discussed why she'd become agitated at home, why she didn't speak to us and needed the woman who was neither maid nor nurse beside her bed. Aside from Ron, no one spoke to the woman. No one touched her. No one spoke to the woman in the wing chair.

No diagnosis. No treatment. Not even a social call.

We stood about. Strangers in a strange place. We didn't know what to talk about. The view was spectacular. And then we left the room.

When I was a medical student at the close of the twentieth century, we cared for lots of older adults like the old woman in the tower, many of whom were quite forgetful and confused, and if the forgetful weren't confused at hospital admission, they became so. "*Watashi wa Amerika no heishi desu!*" ("I am an American soldier!") Veterans of the Second World War repeated the few bits of Japanese or German they'd been taught to recite to their captors. Women screamed, "Neighbor!" Others became lethargic and dull.

Some of these forgetful patients had a diagnosis of senility (the majority had no diagnosis). Few of them, however, had a diagnosis of Alzheimer's disease. I remember caring for one and only one patient with Alzheimer's disease—a very thin, dark-haired woman who was being seen at the geriatric medicine clinic.

Unlike the old woman in the tower, the physician who was caring for her (one of only four geriatricians on staff) talked to her. She told him vague bits about family members bothering her. He was attentive. He asked her for details. She looked at him and then to me and then she looked away. Names eluded her. Her lips pursed, she was done talking. We stepped into the hall.

The physician asked me: "What's her diagnosis?"

My answer was a psychoanalytic ramble about how a reaction formation had developed in her aging brain unable to resolve long-standing, sublimated family conflicts. Hardening of the cerebral arteries was no doubt contributing. A stroke was possible, though her speech betrayed no evident aphasia, and her gait, though slow, was steady.

He cut me off, shaking his head to signal: *Enough.*

"Wrong," he announced. "She has Alzheimer's. Alzheimer's disease." He tilted his head as if to signal: *Don't you get it?*

Our exchange was indicative of a revolution that was beginning to unfold in medicine—especially in the disciplines of geriatrics, neurology, and psychiatry—and was just beginning to spread into the rest of medicine and society. An enormous change was occurring in how we explained and labeled older adults with cognitive and behavioral problems. My answer—a mash-up of biology and psychodynamics—was the old order. I hadn't considered Alzheimer's because I'd been taught that it was an uncommon disease, one of the causes of the rare "presenile dementias," meaning dementia whose onset was before sixty-five years of age. It was caused, maybe, by two distinct but little understood pathologies, plaques and tangles.

"Senile dementia," or more simply "senility," on the other hand described a dementia caused not by a disease but by an extreme state of aging. Alzheimer's disease was not considered one of the causes. Senility was a convergence of physical, social, and psychological causes, some combination

of aging neurons, social isolation, vascular disease, and unresolved psychological conflicts. It was a kind of degenerative adolescence leading to a second childhood of infantile dependence. We were without any understanding
of the biology of what was happening to an aging neuron. Aging was dark
magic.

Older adults with senility were out of both our sight and our minds. They
were either cared for at home by wives and daughters or—like the old woman
in the tower—a hired helper, a maid who wasn't really a maid, or they lived in
nursing homes and the few remaining asylums. We only saw them if they got
sick from some other problem or, like the old woman, became too agitated
for family to care for them. Our interest in caring for them was minimal because, we were taught, a problem caused by aging and a matrix of social and
psychological factors was, unlike a disease, essentially untreatable. It certainly was not a medical problem.

We did care for older adults with brain diseases. There was the stroke unit
with the fascinating aphasias: patients who could speak but made no sense
or those who couldn't speak but could understand language. I remember the
thrill of seeing patients at the neurology clinic. A leonine-faced elderly man
shuffled along the linoleum hall to the exam room.

"What's the diagnosis!" the neurologist commanded.

"Parkinson's disease," I replied proudly.

We prescribed dopamine pills and, like a miracle, the symptoms abated,
at least for a while.

For the senile, we had little to offer save for chemical and physical restraints to palliate the extreme symptoms. The woman I saw in the geriatrics
practice was on the antipsychotic drug haloperidol. The old woman in the
tower was tied to her bed with a Posey vest (the name comes from the vest's
manufacturer, the J. T. Posey Company). We could do nothing to treat the
underlying cause of their rambling suspiciousness and agitation.

And then things began to change. Slowly and then all at once, senility
disappeared. In its place was Alzheimer's disease, and it seemed to be everywhere.

The commonly accepted explanation for why this happened is demography. For much of human history, there weren't a lot of old people, and
so there weren't many older adults with disabling cognitive and behavioral
problems.

The statistics that describe the twentieth-century transformation of the
US population are repeated throughout the industrialized world. In 1900,

4.1 percent of the United States' 76 million population—or about 3.1 million people—were sixty-five years old or older. By 1940, this proportion was 6.8 percent, and by 1990, it had doubled to 12.6 percent of the 281.4 million people. So, between 1900 and 1990, the number of Americans who were sixty-five years or older had increased from 3.1 million to 35 million.

Demography describes why senile dementia or senility, a problem that is closely associated with chronological age, became so common. It is estimated that about 15 percent of persons sixty-five and older have dementia. Assume that over the twentieth century this proportion was consistent. The numbers of persons with dementia has increased from about 155,000 in 1900, to 5 million in 1990.

Demography cannot answer a profound question about our responses to those numbers: why would the increase in the number of older adults with senility cause us to change how we label them from persons with senility—a biopsychosocial problem at an unfortunate stage of aging that medicine has little to offer as a solution—to patients with a disease caused by distinct brain pathologies in need of a medical cure? Why would a private family problem become a national crisis in need of a medical cure?

The answers to these questions are found in the transformation of a social, political, ethical, and scientific order. "Quarrel in Old Age," the poem that opened this chapter, recounts the sufferings of an enraged elderly woman who lives "distorting days." It was written in 1931. Since the beginnings of America, there were people living with dementia.[1] We just didn't think of them as people with a disease and so didn't respond to them as patients in need of medical attention. The problem we now call Alzheimer's disease was hidden from medicine and society.

And then, as the twentieth century drew to a close, within a span of just one decade, beginning in the United States and then spreading rapidly throughout the world—particularly in industrialized nations—this order collapsed. Older adults who were disabled from cognitive and behavioral problems transformed from the senile elderly into patients whose disease became inflamed by the rhetoric of a crisis that is bound to bankrupt nations' economies.

Before we look closely at those ten years that changed the world, we need to look even further back. In the closing decades of the twentieth century, medical students like me were learning about tremendous advances in the diagnosis and treatment of common diseases of older adults such as cancer and heart disease. But when we talked about Alzheimer's disease, if we talked about it at all, we traveled back in time, stuck at Dr. Alois Alzheimer's presentation on November 3, 1906, at the Saturday afternoon session of the Thirty-Seventh Assembly of Southwest German Psychiatrists, in Tübingen.

9

ALOIS ALZHEIMER:
AN UNWITTING REVOLUTIONARY

The question therefore arises as to whether the cases of disease which I consider peculiar are sufficiently different clinically or histologically to be distinguished from senile dementia or whether they should be considered under that rubric.

—Alois Alzheimer,
"On Certain Peculiar Diseases of Old Age," 1911

ALOIS ALZHEIMER WAS an unwitting revolutionary. One of six children of a German Catholic family, his father supported them comfortably with work as a royal notary for the Lower Franconian city of Marktbreit. Unlike his brothers, who chose careers in the clergy, teaching, or pharmacy, Alois was interested in the natural sciences such as botany, and so he chose to study medicine.

In 1883, at the age of nineteen, he enrolled in Germany's most prestigious medical school, the Royal Friedrich Wilhelm University in Berlin.[1] He liked his beer, but he didn't enjoy life in the cosmopolitan metropolis, preferring instead to live closer to his hometown. So after just one year, he transferred to the medical school in the more provincial city of Würzburg. He was a stocky, broad-chested six-foot-tall man—*ein Prügel-mannsbild* or "big brute"—who, for a time, enjoyed fraternity life more than his medical studies. A fencing injury scarred the left side of his face.

In time, however, he focused on his studies. Scientists can be divided into two types: foxes and hedgehogs. Foxes follow ideas and so wander across fields of study and methods. Hedgehogs never leave the field where they were born. They patiently focus on a topic and a method.

Alois Alzheimer was a hedgehog. Among the courses that most interested him was histology, the study of tissues, made possible by microscopy and recent and dramatic advances in techniques to stain tissues. His medical school thesis was a microscopic study of earwax (the substance was believed to be an excretion of the brain and therefore a clue to brain diseases). The thesis displays his notable talents as a microscopist. The work was meticulous, even tedious, requiring careful tissue extraction, preparation, slicing and staining, and then recording the wealth of results both narratively and with carefully executed drawings.

Over the course of his career, he would perfect these methods. His neuropathology results of a 1911 case study of a single patient's brain tissue take up seven pages of narrative derived from multiple stains and present ten meticulously drawn figures. His work is as elegant as Meissen porcelains.

He began practicing as a psychiatrist at the Asylum for the Insane and Epileptic in Frankfurt. He was twenty-four and one of only two physicians on the asylum's staff and so quite busy with patient care, but this was balanced with the opportunity to pursue his other interest: microscopy. Moreover, the other physician and the asylum's director, Emil Sioli, shared his passion to improve patient care. Instead of restraining and confining agitated patients, they adopted the techniques of restraint-free, calming interventions. These included hours-long temperate baths, mud wraps, talking to the patients, gardens where patients could wander or garden, and workshops for activities such as bookbinding, woodcutting, and straw weaving. They aspired to create a place to support, shelter, and even nurture the mentally ill—that is, a true asylum.

Their asylum was also a research center. There was an on-site autopsy room with an adjacent laboratory for microscopic study of deceased patients' brains. The arrangement allowed a thorough study of patients' illnesses from admission to death. Alzheimer and Sioli recorded the patients' clinical histories and then, after death, examined the brain tissue.

Alzheimer and Sioli were a participant in an emerging revolution in psychiatry and the definition of psychiatric diseases. Their inspiration was the work of the eminent nineteenth-century German physician Rudolf Virchow, who advocated careful dissection and microscopic study of tissues as the method to discover the causes of disease such as cancer. The psychiatrists wanted to apply these same approaches to diseases of the brain.

They were different from the psychiatrists of other European nations, Great Britain, and the United States. Unlike these colleagues—who often

practiced in out-of-the-way asylums and called themselves alienists to capture their role in treating the socially isolated, or alienated, asylum patient—
these German physicians preferred the novel title of "psychiatrist."

Together, psychiatry and pathology allowed them to practice "clinical-
pathological correlation." By combining the results of their careful clinical histories—some unfolding over years and made possible by residence
in their comfortable asylum—with their detailed microscopic studies to
discover pathology in the brain, Alzheimer was among a small cadre of
clinician-scientists who sought to classify and understand mental illnesses
as the consequence of organic diseases in the brain.

It was a revolution facilitated not only by recent advances in the technology of microscopes and stains but also by nation and culture. Alois Alzheimer was part of an emerging group of German physicians that included Max
Bielschowsky, Oskar Fischer, Emil Kraepelin, Franz Nissl, and Gaetano Perusini, who all wrote and published in German-language journals and textbooks. They were well acquainted with one another not only from scientific
conferences but socially as well. Nissl was best man at Alois Alzheimer's
wedding. He also discovered the stain that visualized distinct nerve cells in
the brain, a discovery of particular significance for Alzheimer's research, a
discovery akin to PiB.

Nation and culture meant this revolution was quite dependent on the sta-
bility, well-being, and support of their asylums, a circumstance that faced
substantial challenges after the spectacular destruction of World War I and
the economic and social upheavals that followed imperial Germany's defeat.

By the dawn of the twentieth century, German psychiatry had arrived
at an auspicious moment. Technologies such as Nissl's stain, asylums with
built-in laboratories and university linkages, and a German-speaking scientific intelligentsia would soon converge to make the discovery of Alzheimer's
disease possible.

Alzheimer performed numerous clinical-pathological studies of the asylum's
resident patients. In 1906, at the Thirty-Seventh Assembly of the Southwest
German Psychiatrists, he presented the results of one of these studies. "On a
Peculiar Disease of the Cerebral Cortex" recounted the case of Auguste Deter,
a patient he'd admitted five years earlier.[2] Her husband, Carl, a railway clerk,
was overwhelmed by her disruptive behaviors. He could no longer have her
at home. Her once-meticulous house was in disorder, and she was accusing
him of infidelity.

She was "unusual" because her history of illness didn't match any of the stories of the typical early twentieth-century patient with dementia. At that time, dementia was used to describe the extreme stage of disabling mental deterioration, and there were just a handful of recognized causes of dementia. The most common, constituting from one-quarter to one-half of an asylum's residents, were patients with dementia paralytica, also called general paresis of the insane. They were diagnosed using an extensive literature that described the common behavioral and distinct physical signs and symptoms such as unusual pupillary reflexes, weakness and unsteady balance (hence the "paralytica"), and characteristic findings on neuropathology. By the end of the nineteenth century, the cause was suspected to be a late stage of syphilis infection, and this was confirmed in 1913.

Other common causes were chronic mental illnesses (dementia praecox, later understood as schizophrenia), epilepsy and other developmental brain disorders, strokes, alcoholism, and finally senile dementia (dementia senilis or *Altersblödsinn*, "aged insanity"), the diagnosis of persons like the old woman in the tower. No doubt many patients' histories and exams blended these causes, leading to diagnostic uncertainty.

Auguste Deter's story fit into none of the common categories. She lacked the characteristic neurological findings seen in dementia paralytica, such as unusual eye reflexes and movements. She had grown up normally, been raised a healthy child, and ran an ordered house. She had no evidence of alcohol abuse, stroke, or vascular disease.

This previously mentally healthy woman was clearly disabled from progressive cognitive and behavioral problems that resembled aspects of dementia senilis: "Her memory is seriously impaired . . . When reading a text, she skips from line to line . . . In speaking, she uses gap-fills and a few paraphrased expressions ('milk-pourer' instead of 'cup') . . . She does not remember the use of some objects."

But she wasn't elderly. When Dr. Alzheimer began caring for her she was just fifty-one years of age.

Her autopsy four and a half years later confirmed she was unusual. There was no evidence of dementia paralytica or the other common causes of dementia that Alzheimer was quite familiar with from the wealth of his pathologic studies of his Frankfurt asylum patients. There was something present, however, something made visible courtesy of the recent advances in stains developed by Nissl. Alzheimer saw fibrils inside and outside her neurons and "minute miliary foci which are caused by a deposition of a special substance in the cortex."

He concluded his presentation with the directive: "Considering every-thing, it seems we are dealing with a special illness . . . This fact should per-suade us not to be satisfied with classifying clinically undetermined cases by forcing them into the categories of recognized illnesses."

In other words, he was telling his colleagues, this patient was not elderly, so she can't have senile dementia. To say she did would force a square peg into a round hole. Do not, however, diagnose her with an uncommon presenta-tion of a common disease well described in the textbooks: dementia paralyt-ica. Alzheimer's message was: let us call her "unusual" and see what we learn from her and other similar cases.

Alois Alzheimer was on to something, and he wasn't alone in his pursuit. By 1907, research by him and his German-speaking colleagues on "unusual dis-eases of the cerebral cortex" was taking off. Among the most accomplished investigations were those done by Oskar Fischer, a psychiatrist on faculty at the German University in Prague, then part of the Austro-Hungarian Em-pire.

Over the course of five years, from 1907 to 1912, Fischer published three studies that compared, collectively, hundreds of patients, some with and others without dementia. He also compared the brains of young patients like Auguste Deter to the brains of older patients with what was then called se-nile dementia. He produced detailed microscopic studies of the miliary sub-stance Alzheimer observed, even developing a six-stage classification system for these plaques. His work led him to conclude that the plaques, which soon came to be called Fischer's plaques, were the cause of the dementia and that what was seen in the unusual "presenile" cases was strikingly similar to the more common "senile" cases of dementia.

Dr. Alzheimer followed Fischer's research and in 1911 he made use of it when he revisited the conclusion of his report on Auguste Deter. The opportu-nity was a second case report, of Johann F., a previously healthy man with dementia.[3] Now, though, Alzheimer had studied the work of Fischer and other psychiatrists and "stainers" with which to compare his findings. Like Auguste Deter, Johann F. had a dementia with notable problems with memory, language, and performing tasks. Like her, his pathology showed abundant plaques (Alzheimer used the term Fischer's plaques). And like her, he was middle-aged: fifty-four years old.

Reading his century-old case report, I feel I'm reading the work of a physician and researcher who was clearly recognizing the need to rethink the distinction between presenile and senile dementia. The histories of presenile and senile cases of dementia often differed, particularly in the severity of their symptoms. The presenile often declined faster and with more notable problems with language than did the senile. And yet, these differences seemed more of degree than of kind. Moreover, the finding wasn't consistent. Some senile cases had notable problems with language and declined quickly.

Alzheimer's conclusion to his report of Johann F. is strikingly modern. He foreshadowed a common conclusion in twenty-first-century Alzheimer's research. He wrote: "These observations . . . demonstrate to us in an impressive way how difficult it is to define diseases solely with respect to their clinical features." Even more provocative were his and his colleagues' studies that compared the brains of the presenile and senile cases. He'd used his friend Nissl's stain to show that the plaques he saw in Auguste Deter were *also* found in his patients with senile dementia. He concluded: "It cannot be doubted that the plaques in these specific cases do in all relevant aspects correspond to those which we find in dementia senilis."

This statement, that senile and presenile dementias may in fact be the same disease, was utterly revolutionary.

Alzheimer wasn't ready, though, to assert this because the evidence didn't consistently point to this conclusion (Johann F. lacked the tangles he saw in Auguste Deter, for example). He was willing to pose a revolutionary question: "The question therefore arises as to whether the cases of disease which I consider peculiar are sufficiently different clinically or histologically to be distinguished from senile dementia or whether they should be considered under that rubric." In other words, presenile and senile are not distinct but the same.

Every Alzheimer's doctor reads the Auguste Deter case (I read it as a fellow). Few read the case of Johann F. I recall the first time I read the above sentence. "My God," I thought, "Alzheimer was entertaining a question that was strikingly aligned with the views of the physician who corrected my misdiagnosis of the paranoid woman at the geriatrics practice." Alzheimer was an unwitting revolutionary.

He called for more research, a kind of "ADMI"—or Alzheimer's Disease Microscopy Initiative. "It will therefore have to be the task of future research to collect a large number of such cases." He likely planned to perform this research, but other events intruded.

THE DARK AGES DESCEND

With the outbreak of World War I in 1914, as physicians enlisted in the kaiser's army, the clinics and asylums were depleted of doctors. Alzheimer, fifty years old, remained in civilian practice and took on increased clinical duties. His health began to fail. His research slowed. A stay at the Wiesbaden spa provided comfort but no cure. In 1915, he died of kidney failure.

There were of course others who could have taken up his call for more research. Since 1903, he'd been head of the histopathology laboratory at the prestigious university-based Royal Psychiatric Clinic at Munich. There, he trained numerous physicians. Clinicians were using the diagnosis of Alzheimer's disease in both senile and presenile cases of dementia.[4] He also had a champion: the Royal Psychiatric Clinic's leader was his mentor, the internationally prominent German psychiatrist Emil Kraepelin.

Kraepelin's system to classify psychiatric diseases dominated early twentieth-century psychiatry worldwide. It was disseminated in multiple editions of his canonical text *Compendium of Psychiatry: For the Use of Students and Physicians.* The eighth edition included Alzheimer's 1907 case report, naming it "Alzheimer's disease."

Poor eyesight prevented Kraepelin from performing microscopic studies. His tools were boxes of annotated index cards that charted the natural history of each patient's illness. He sorted and re-sorted these cards according to their features and outcomes until a clear category emerged. Among his discoveries was the category of mental illness now called schizophrenia.

The work of colleagues like Alzheimer added the strength of biology to his clinical categories. Psychiatric illness, Kraepelin asserted, could and should be grounded with the same approach as diseases of the body; that is, a careful description of the essential clinical features tightly correlated with clinical outcomes and, ideally, the findings from pathology.

The influential Kraepelin was therefore a champion of Alzheimer and his research. Kraepelin was effusive in his support of Alzheimer's application for a faculty position at Munich's Ludwig Maximilian University. He wrote: "His attempt to place diverse anatomic images beside the finer clinical differences of individual disease processes distinguished by him, practically for the first time, makes it possible for psychiatry to be equal to other forms of medicine in its modes of research and results."[5]

Munich was not the only center of psychiatric research capable of carrying out the large-scale studies Alzheimer called for. Oskar Fischer, whose research skills were arguably more sophisticated and productive than Alzheimer's, was a faculty member in a prominent Department of Psychiatry at Prague's German University, led by the eminent Arnold Pick. Fischer lived until the 1940s. He and his colleagues could have taken on the task of research to collect a large number of cases.

At the start of the twentieth century, researchers who questioned the distinction between the presenile and senile dementias were beginning to change clinical practice. Kraepelin, for example, included Alzheimer's case report in his text's section on *senile* dementias (*Altersblödsinn* or *Das senile Irresein*) not the *presenile* dementias (*Das präsenile Irresein*), implying it was a disease predominantly found in the elderly. Clinical records of patients seen at the Munich clinic show the psychiatrists used the diagnostic label of Alzheimer's disease (*Alzheimersche Krankheit*) in both middle aged *and* elderly patients.

And then this all stopped.

Why it stopped is a story of events—some scientific, most not—that crippled progress in the diagnosis and care of frail older adults suffering from progressive and disabling cognitive and behavioral problems. Some of these gruesome events are set in time past. Others, however, still linger like ghosts. They're the causes of why Alzheimer's disease became a crisis and a disease to be feared.

We are still paying the price for these events. If psychiatry had persisted in gathering clinical histories and microscopic studies of presenile and senile dementias, it is entirely possible that the 1984 criteria I used to diagnose Mrs. Harrison would have been written forty or fifty years earlier. My colleague Ron's bedside case presentation would have been about his patient with dementia, and our differential diagnosis would have included Alzheimer's disease. In answer to the physician who asked me the cause of the elderly woman's delusions and hesitant speech, I would've explained how her brain was being destroyed by Fischer's plaques.

But none of that happened.

As the twentieth century unfolded, Dr. Alzheimer's 1907 and 1911 case reports and Fischer's work were all forgotten, of interest only to the few neurologists who specialized in cognitive disorders.

Senile dementia—the most common cause of dementia—fared poorly, too. The dominant theory was that senility was the end stage not of a disease but instead of a hodgepodge of causes—a breakdown in a psychodynamic balance among various pathologies, including vascular disease, personality, and, most importantly, relentlessly aging neurons. Senility was a difficult, unavoidable natural event. Like the winter, there wasn't much to do except bundle up and tough it out.

For millions of older adults and their families, this state of affairs presented tremendous and vexing consequences. By the close of the twentieth century, when my colleagues and I graduated from medical school, the few who pursued psychiatry or neurology had scant interest in Alzheimer's disease. The disease had disappeared into oblivion.

10

OBLIVION, OR WAR
AND MADNESS

These are men whose minds the Dead have
  ravished.
Memory fingers in their hair of murders,
Multitudinous murders they once witnessed.
        —Wilfred Owen, "Mental Cases"

ON FEBRUARY 4, 1917, Wilfred Owen, second lieutenant in Britain's Manchester Regiment, stationed in Abbeville, France, wrote to his mother, Susan, of the "ugliness" of the battlefield:

> Hideous landscapes, vile noises, foul language and nothing but foul, even from one's own mouth (for all are devil ridden), everything unnatural, broken, blasted; the distortion of the dead, whose unburiable bodies sit outside the dug-outs all day, all night, the most execrable sights on earth. In poetry we call them the most glorious. But to sit with them all day, all night . . . And a week later to come back and find them still sitting there, in motionless groups, THAT is what saps "soldierly spirit."[1]

Owen was witness to and a participant in mechanized, industrial warfare that exacted carnage on a scale never before seen in the history of war. To this day, the numbers of military and civilian dead are astonishing: by war's end, 20 million had perished. Owen was among them; the soldier and poet

was killed in action just days before the November 11, 1918, armistice that
ended the brutal war.

War's end found Germany defeated and plunged into social, political, and
economic turmoil. The 2.7 million disabled German soldiers, 600,000 wid-
ows, and 1,192,000 orphans created immediate, immense, and persistent
demands on pension and welfare systems. The national debt doubled, the interest rates on loans reached double digits, and inflation escalated into hy-
perinflation. As the value of the deutsche mark plummeted, the Weimar
government printed more and more money.[2]

Tram fare rose weekly. Food disappeared from store shelves. A day's pay
for work became valueless. Outside Berlin's central Reichsbank, crowds gathered demanding to withdraw their savings. They needed baskets and wheel-
barrows to carry home their increasingly worthless deutsche marks. Political
unrest spread. In Saxony and Thuringia, communist demonstrations turned
violent, and in Bavaria, an angry young veteran named Adolf Hitler gathered
more and more dedicated followers.

Under these conditions, German psychiatry suffered. Alzheimer, a civilian, was taken up with added clinical work while his younger colleagues such
as Franz Nissl and Oskar Fischer ran military hospitals. Alzheimer's friend
and close collaborator in Munich, Gaetano Perusini, was killed attempting to
help a wounded soldier. Perusini arguably would have carried on Alzheimer's
research. After the war, the persistent problem of limited research resources—
time, money, and researchers—only worsened.

The meticulous and time-intensive clinical pathological studies especially
suffered. The raw materials for such work required patients with a carefully
charted clinical story of their years of care from the day of diagnosis to the
day of death. In resource-depleted Germany, asylums were unstable and un-
reliable institutions to support research.

The financial resources needed to perform research were also scarce.
Before—and ever more so after the war—physician researchers were so
poorly supported that they often relied on their own wealth to fund the work.
Alzheimer, independently wealthy from his marriage to the widow of a dia-
mond merchant, twice intervened with financial support to thwart Auguste
Deter's husband from moving her to a cheaper state asylum. For several years
as head of the microscopy laboratory in Munich, he worked without pay. He
even used his personal wealth to pay staff salaries and purchase equipment.

Perusini, independently wealthy from an inheritance, similarly worked without a wage.

Psychiatric clinical-pathological research required resources: physicians with time to undertake research instead of patient care, subjects with well-documented case histories and brain tissue, and a lab with microscopes and other equipment. The lack of sustained and steady access to these resources was one reason why Alzheimer's disease remained stuck as the unusual disease of the cerebral cortex that he presented after lunch at the 1906 meeting in Tübingen. Other factors were at work as well. One of them was present the very afternoon after Alzheimer stepped away from the lectern: Sigmund Freud's psychodynamic theory of mental illness.

A VAST, DARK, IRRATIONAL NIGHTMARE

After Dr. Alzheimer ended his presentation, no one asked a question. The silence of an assembly of ninety ambitious academic physicians was notably peculiar. The November 5, 1906, issue of the *Tübinger Chronik* reported in its From City to Country section that the case that generated discussion was the one that followed Dr. Alzheimer's presentation: "On the Analysis of Psychotraumatic Symptoms."

That case instigated a vigorous debate over the cause of mental illness. No doubt this engaged a prominent audience member, Carl Jung, who was at the time Sigmund Freud's anointed intellectual protégé (though within six years their relationship would cease with an irrevocable separation).

Jung and Freud advanced a very different theory of disease than the organic theory being advanced by Kraepelin, Alzheimer, and their colleagues. This theory posited that mental illness was a disease of the mind caused by suppressed traumas. Freud identified suppressed childhood sexual traumas as a main culprit. This focus arguably kept the theory the preoccupation of academic debates such as the gathering in Tübingen. But then came the vast and unprecedented madness of the First World War.

Two months after Wilfred Owen wrote to his mother about the dead whose unburiable bodies sit outside the dugouts all day, a shell exploded a few yards from his head as he slept one evening, blowing him in the air. He lay in a hole near a dead fellow soldier, disemboweled, covered in dirt. In the weeks to follow, he became shaky and tremulous, his behavior "peculiar,"

and his memory confused. Now a soldier whose mind the dead had ravished, he was removed from battle and began treatment at Craiglockhart
War Hospital.

Hundreds of thousands of cases of neurasthenia, or "shell shock," became
case studies on the effects of trauma on otherwise healthy brains. Despite
any physical wound, young men were blind, tremulous, mute, or paralyzed.
The Battle of the Somme left some thirty thousand cases. They were living, brain-damaged proof that trauma to the psyche—to the mind—causes
mental illness. Freudianism—or more generally a psychodynamic theory of
mental illness and its treatment—not only gained legitimacy, but it also dominated other theories of psychiatric illness. Alzheimer's revolutionary idea
that presenile and senile dementia might be caused by a distinct, biological
disease was supplanted by a more urgent and overwhelming crisis.

Even Oskar Fischer became swept up in psychodynamic theories. After
his wartime experiences, he returned to Prague and made a study of a man
who claimed clairvoyant and telepathic powers. The historian Andrew Scull
argues that "it was that awful war, more than anything else, that helped to
advance the psychoanalytic cause."[3] It was an understandably attractive frame-
work, promising both an explanation and treatment for many of the previously healthy but now desperately wounded young men. Biological psychiatry
in contrast only offered an explanation—not treatment—and that came after
death.

Larger social forces were also at work. After the First World War, Germany
became increasingly consumed in a vast, dark, irrational nightmare.

In 1919, just two years after his promotion to associate professor at the German University in Prague, Oskar Fischer was denied tenure. The reason was
not his academic skills but rather his religion. He was Jewish.

Forced to leave the university, he worked in private practice, retaining only
an appointment as a lecturer. Without the resources of a university laboratory, his elegant clinical-pathologic studies of his eponymous plaques ended.
In 1923, as he was campaigning for the German Democratic Liberal Party,
anti-Semites assaulted him. Sixteen years later, the Nazis occupied Prague,
and SS member Kurt Albrecht took over as chair of the German University's
Department of Psychiatry, revoking Fischer's lectureship. In 1941, Fischer
was imprisoned by the gestapo at the notorious Theresienstadt prison. One
year later, at the age of sixty-five, he was tortured to death.

In the aftermath of World War I, German psychiatry and neurology began to collapse under the weight of anti-Semitism and Nazi eugenics. Kraepelin—devastated by imperial Germany's defeat and the social and economic disorder that ensued—became disillusioned with democracy. He embraced dark ideologies.

In his 1919 essay "Psychiatric Observations on Contemporary Issues," he wrote, "a great misfortune has befallen us."[4] He assigned blame to people whose unchecked "primal dispositions" caused mass hysteria: "dreamers and poets," "busybodies," and the "infirm and decrepit" (his term for criminals). He singled out the Jews.

"The frequency of psychopathic predisposition in Jews could have played a role, although it is their harping criticism, their rhetorical and theatrical abilities, and their doggedness and determination which are most important." He bemoaned how "the war had carried out a terrible selection among our most able and self-sacrificing men; it was above all the unfit and selfish individuals who remained unscathed." He regretted the "humanitarian efforts" that had helped "the suffering, sickly and the decrepit" and explained how "they load the shoulders of the able-bodied (on whom our hopes for the future rest) with ever greater burden under which the latter's energies must ultimately expire."

His solution was medical. The "physical, mental and moral regeneration of our people" would require the work of doctors. "Attention must be focused above all on the fight against all those influences threatening to destroy future generations, in particular hereditary degeneration and genetic defects resulting from alcohol and syphilis."

Writings such as these eugenic and anti-Semitic tracts would sink Kraepelin's reputation and consequently the influence of his textbook that championed Alzheimer's disease.

Kraepelin died in 1926. His successor and mentee at the Munich clinic, and Alzheimer's colleague and peer, was Ernst Rüdin. He picked up where Kraepelin left off.

A proponent of hereditary degeneration, he argued that genetic defects explained much of mental illness. Treatment was purging society of those genes. Residents of the underfunded and overcrowded asylums were no longer patients to be cared for and studied. Rüdin and colleagues, such as the psychiatrist Alfred Hoche, who coauthored the 1920 book *Allowing the Destruction of Life Unworthy of Life*, regarded them as so-called *unnütze Esser*, or "useless eaters" who needed to be purged from the human race.

After the Nazis seized the German government in 1933, Rüdin became the *Reichskommissar*, meaning "governor" or "leader," of the Deutsche Gesellschaft für Rassenhygiene (the German Society for Racial Hygiene). He insisted on the fusion of psychiatry and neurology in order to advance a "fundamentally new attitude of the German state to the art of healing."[5] Serious neurological and psychiatric illnesses were, he argued, hereditary and so prevention was better than cure. Nicknamed the "Reichsführer for Sterilization," Rüdin organized and participated in Nazi programs to either sterilize or euthanize the chronically mentally and neurologically ill, including persons with dementia.

By war's end, Kraepelin and his textbook were cast aside. The Royal Psychiatric Clinic of Munich where Alzheimer and Perusini had worked and trained psychiatrists in the clinical-pathologic model of psychiatric disease was a reputational cesspool and an academic wasteland. Alzheimer's disease was a casualty of war and madness.

DR. WILL'S PSYCHODYNAMIC REVOLUTION

The story moves overseas from Europe, exhausted by three decades of economic instability bookended by two world wars and a descent into fascist brutality, to a victorious postwar America. There, a set of medical, social, and cultural forces collectively kept the problem of dementia in older adults hidden from both medical and public concern.

After the Second World War, when America was the undisputed world power, if American psychiatry had taken up the biological concept of mental illness advanced by the likes of Alzheimer, Nissl, Fischer, and Kraepelin, arguably their vision of studies of hundreds of cases of senile and presenile dementia from diagnosis to death would have been fulfilled. Rather, Freud and psychodynamic theories about stress as a cause of pervasive mental illnesses and the focus on "neuroses" (that is, anxiety and depression) enthralled not only the profession of psychiatry but all of American culture.

Psychodynamic psychiatry crowded out the work of Alzheimer and his colleagues. The diagnosis and treatment of chronic and severe mental illnesses such as dementia, let alone understanding the biological basis of these diseases, were of little interest.

In 1948, a psychiatrist achieved American celebrity. Dr. William Menninger, the "rangy, friendly, 49-year-old Kansan," made the cover of the October 25 issue of *Time* magazine. As chief of the Menninger Foundation in Topeka, Kansas, he led a family-run medical institution, a kind of Mayo Clinic for the mind, dedicated to the diagnosis and treatment of persons with mental illness. This self-described "psychodynamic psychiatrist" was now president of the American Psychiatric Association. As president and chairman of the Group for the Advancement of Psychiatry, *Time* gushed that "Dr. Will" was traveling across America to boost the profession and the psychodynamic approach to treat the millions of Americans he said were suffering from neuroses.

A companion *Time* story, "The Lingo," set out the "correct definitions" for psychiatry's "technical jargon" such as Oedipus complex ("a male's feeling started in babyhood of rivalry with his father, and excessive attachment to his mother") and inferiority complex ("conscious suffering from an unconscious feeling of unworthiness or guilt").

After the war, as psychiatrists described themselves as Freudians (none chose the moniker "Kraepelinian"), America was swept up in variations on Freudianism. Freud himself would have been devastated. He hated America. Psychodynamic theories of disease and the application of the talking cure to treat them gained wide acceptance in America. By 1976, membership in the American Psychiatric Association had grown from 4,400 in 1948 to 27,000, and the chairs of most departments of psychiatry were proponents of a psychoanalytic definition of mental illness and its treatment.

The model of psychiatric practice was an outpatient office to care for persons who were conversational and sufficiently well off to pay for years of treatment. The essential technology was a dark leather couch or chair to comfortably situate the patient as she narrated her story with a few specific questionings or prompts from the doctor. Patients with dementia, especially those with psychoses, were typically unable to participate in this "free association" designed to unearth from the unconscious the hidden conflicts, suppressed desires, or wishes that cause mental illness.

This practice of psychiatry had little reason to care about persons with senility. Interest in it was confined to the small cadre of psychiatrists who still practiced in the underfunded and overcrowded state asylums. A leader of this work was David Rothschild.

Working out of state asylums in Massachusetts, he argued that senile dementia was a distinct disease caused by a psychodynamic interplay among the aging brain, pathologies, and personality. The crux of his argument was the finding that continues to vex the field: the imperfect correlation between the presence of pathology and the severity of dementia; that is, brain autopsies of some cognitively normal older adults showed pathology, particularly the plaques Alzheimer and Fischer observed, that therefore ought to have caused symptoms.

This model led to treatments that mixed biological interventions—including electroconvulsive therapy and sedative medications—and social and psychological interventions to reduce stress. It dominated psychiatry's understanding of dementia in older adults and sustained the distinction between senile and presenile dementia.

Neurology had little interest in dementia, particularly senile dementia. The essential term of their science and practice was the "lesion," meaning a brain disease was the consequence of damage by pathology—such as a tumor, inflammation, stroke, or head injury—to a specific region of the brain. The mantra to both define and diagnose a neurological disease was "find the lesion."

Parkinson's disease, for example, is a lesion to the substantia nigra, a distinct black-pigmented streak in the brain stem. Broca's aphasia correlates with stroke in the anterior portion of the brain's temporal lobe. The patient's speech is effortful, slow, and drops essential words. And so on.

Neurology was grounded in the practice of the "neurological exam." Their signature technology was the neurologist's black bag, a purse-size bag containing a collection of tools such as rubber-tipped hammers to tap reflexes, pins and brushes to test sensation, tiny lights to assess pupillary reflexes. The neurologist's expertise was using the results of this detailed exam to identify the location of the lesion in the nervous system and then reflecting on the cause.

Senile dementia did not fit into this lesion-based model of brain disease. It had a variable pattern of signs and symptoms caused by lesions throughout the brain rather than in one place, and the causes were uncertain: aging, psychological traumas, plaques, and vascular disease. Notably, the stereotypical description of senile dementia was a patient with a "normal" neurological exam, meaning normal motor, sensory, and reflexes. It was the cognitive and emotional exam that was abnormal, an exam that was more the practice of psychiatry than neurology.

Therapeutically, unlike psychiatry with its talking cures, neurology was a comparatively bleak field. For much of the twentieth century, few brain diseases, save for infections such as syphilis, were treatable. The discoveries of dopamine for Parkinson's and antiepileptic drugs were among the few breakthroughs that allowed a neurologist to treat the symptoms of these disabling and untreatable diseases.

Therapeutic nihilism was the norm. A quip in the field was "diagnosis and adiosis," meaning that after figuring out the cause of the patient's weakness, vision problems, tingling toes, et cetera, there was little more to offer and so adios, or goodbye.

Bobbie Glaze, an Alzheimer's activist who organized family support groups out of her Bloomington, Minnesota, home in the 1970s and was among the founders of the Alzheimer's Association, learned her husband's Alzheimer's diagnosis in the neurologist's waiting room. The doctor said it was progressive and untreatable, and then he asked her if she had any questions.

Throughout the world for much of the twentieth century, the diagnosis and treatment of dementia in an older adult essentially fell between the two professions who cared about the brain: neurology and psychiatry. It was neglected.

Other health and social service professions were also uninterested. Katie Maslow, a social worker in the mid-1970s at the Bethesda Health Center nursing home in Maryland, decided she needed training in how to assess and care for older adults, so she took a class at the Washington Psychoanalytic Institute: Therapy for the Older Adult. "Older" was defined as up to forty-five years of age. "That was considered old. Treating anyone who was old, really old, wasn't a topic. Dementia wasn't a topic."[6]

For the public, senile older adults were understood using ideas and attitudes not about disease but aging. Senility was unfortunate, but it was considered "natural." The senile were hidden away, either in asylums or in private homes in the care of homemakers, meaning women. When they died, the cause was often attributed to "natural causes," "old age," or common complications of advanced dementia such as pneumonia.

And then this world order began to change. Settled habits and customs of living and the social structures that sustained them began to fall apart.

As the twentieth century drew to a close, progressive, self-made, forward-looking America—where "go-ahead" isn't just a direction of travel but also a command for how to live—began to think differently about living with senility, whether as patient or family. It became a big medical problem.

Curing the problem of senility would become the means for all Americans—young and old—to continue to go ahead. But first senility needed to be rebranded from an extreme state of aging into a disease to be diagnosed, treated, and, ideally, cured.

11

THE ESSAY HEARD ROUND
THE WORLD

Senile as well as pre-senile forms of Alzheimer are a single disease, a disease whose etiology must be determined, whose course must be aborted, and ultimately a disease to be prevented.

—Robert Katzman, "The Prevalence and Malignancy of
Alzheimer Disease: A Major Killer," *Archives of Neurology*, 1976

IN APRIL 1976, with the publication of an essay, Alois Alzheimer's unusual disease of the cerebral cortex, one of the rare causes of the uncommon "presenile dementias," became a prevalent and malignant killer of older adults. With that, America needed to get to work and discover how to diagnose, treat, and care for the millions of ill and disabled older adults.

In the years to follow, efforts to achieve this would experience leaps of progress followed by stalls into dispiriting stagnation. Forty-five years would pass before January 4, 2011, when President Obama signed the National Alzheimer's Project Act and so launched a national effort to create a plan to address the disease. Eight years later, a National Institutes of Health call for studies to answer "high-priority research topics" in Alzheimer's summarized the state of care: "The current state of care for persons with dementia leaves room for improvement—there is little continuity of care, and health care and long-term services and supports are expensive but likely variable and ineffective."[1] Nonetheless, 1976—the bicentennial of America's birth and the declaration that all men are created equal—is rightly dated as the end of the oblivion. How this happened begins with the leadership and persistence of a socially conscious, polymath neurologist who'd been struggling to find a scholarly focus. His name was Robert Katzman.

In 1911, Alzheimer posed the question of "whether the cases of disease which I consider peculiar are sufficiently different clinically or histologically to be distinguished from senile dementia or whether they should be considered under that rubric." Sixty-five years later, Robert Katzman answered it in his essay in the *Archives of Neurology*, "The Prevalence and Malignancy of Alzheimer Disease: A Major Killer."[2] In just one thousand words, Katzman, chair of neurology at Albert Einstein College of Medicine in the Bronx, New York, argued that the distinction between presenile dementia caused by Alzheimer's disease and senile dementia was arbitrary. We should adopt a single designation for both: Alzheimer's disease.

The editorial was not a response to a breakthrough study published in that issue of the journal. He made his case by synthesizing selected research results from a short letter to the editor reporting on the outcomes of eighteen persons with presenile Alzheimer's disease and other case series. He cited the work of a small cadre of US psychiatrists and British "old-age psychiatrists" (a term used in the United Kingdom) working at asylums and with no interest in the dominant Freudian theories. They reported that clinical histories of older adults with senile dementia studied from diagnosis to death were similar to patients with Alzheimer's disease and that the extent of pathology and the severity of dementia were correlated.

In a sense, Katzman was picking up where Alois Alzheimer and Oskar Fischer left off in the early 1900s. They were entertaining a theory: senile dementia might not be the result of aging but instead a disease caused by the Fischer plaques. Katzman, with great confidence, perhaps even hubris, accepted this as true. He didn't address unresolved questions, such as the role of vascular disease or the finding that a notable proportion of older adults were cognitively normal when they died but still exhibited the obvious pathologic changes associated with Fischer's plaques.

To bolster his claim, he cited the results of more contemporary scientific methods, in particular electron microscopy studies that showed how the senile and the presenile brains appeared the same (Fischer had suggested the same in his studies). Katzman's point was that the data were good enough to support a revolutionary claim. Older adults' dementia was not caused by senility—an extreme stage of aging—but rather by a disease.

Dipping into epidemiology, he estimated there could be as many as 1.2

million patients with the newly redefined Alzheimer's disease and that it was the fifth leading cause of death. His numbers suggested a burden of disease on par with cancer and heart disease.

He closed with a call to action. "Senile as well as pre-senile forms of Alzheimer are a single disease, a disease whose etiology must be determined, whose course must be aborted, and ultimately a disease to be prevented."

Katzman was fifty-one when he published his essay. At his death thirty-one years later, memorials would describe the essay as "the shot heard round the world" and him not as a scientist but as a pioneer and an activist whose career reshaped medicine and the lives of older adults and their families.

His editorial caught the attention of leaders at the NIH, particularly Robert Butler, the inaugural director of the recently created National Institute on Aging, or NIA. Butler, a psychiatrist, was politically smart and a master communicator. His 1976 Pulitzer Prize–winning book *Why Survive: Being Old in America* was a fact-packed plea for American medicine and society to attend to the plight of the nation's elderly. Alzheimer's disease was an ideal vehicle to advance this mission.[3]

Within a year, Butler collaborated with Katzman to organize a meeting of researchers that launched the nation's scientific commitment to achieve his call to action. The NIA adopted Alzheimer's as its focus.

This was a clever strategy. Alzheimer's research was freed from the historical baggage of both psychiatry and neurology, each of which could have laid claim to the disease, psychiatry via the National Institute of Mental Health and neurology via the National Institute of Neurological and Communicative Disorders and Stroke. Alzheimer's disease soon took up as much as half the NIA budget, causing some gerontologists to complain it was the "National Institute on Alzheimer's."

Wherever Alzheimer's disease was being talked about, Katzman was there (often in the company of Robert Terry, his colleague who performed the electron microscopy studies he cited in his essay). He became an advocate for the recognition of Alzheimer's disease as a major medical problem and research as the solution to this problem. He chaired NIA grant-review committees and served on the institute's nascent National Advisory Council. He took on government roles. After the presidential election of 1980 installed a new Republican administration, he chaired the newly appointed Department of Health and Human Services secretary Margaret Heckler's Advisory Council on Alzheimer's Disease. Among the council's recommendations was that the NIH's annual spending on Alzheimer's disease research should be half a billion dollars a year.

Congress's Alzheimer's Disease and Related Disorders Treatment Act of 1984 authorized the now-decade-old NIA to establish a national network of Alzheimer's centers. These were essential infrastructure for the discoveries of MCI, PiB, and other biomarker measures, and the ADNI network. Katzman was a director of one of the first centers. He was a coauthor of the 1984 diagnostic criteria that the physician used to diagnose the woman I saw at his clinic and that I used twenty years later to diagnose Mrs. Harrison. His letters to NIH officials—as well as phone calls, meetings, and lunches with patients' wealthy and well-connected family members—instigated the creation of the national advocacy organization that would come to be the highly influential Alzheimer's Association.

Katzman didn't start his medical career with any of these ideas or ambitions. He started out as a physician who thought little about Alzheimer's disease. But then a series of personal and professional events collided to turn him into an Alzheimer's activist.

In medical school at Harvard, Katzman was torn between pursuing psychiatry or neurology, ultimately choosing the latter after his disappointing experience using psychoanalysis to treat a patient with major depression. He moved to New York to enroll in Columbia University's neurology residency program, hoping to study diseases with identifiable biological mechanisms amenable to diagnosis and, ideally, treatment. His talents as an academic and clinical leader were evident. In 1964, at just thirty-nine years of age, he was named chair of the Department of Neurology at Einstein Medical College, pursuing his interest in the chemistry and circulation of the fluid that surrounds the brain.

By 1970, he dropped this interest. Alzheimer's was his vocation. How this happened is not only the story of a person able to see the world differently by perceiving the importance of things that other people ignored or took for granted but also a story of taking advantage of enormous professional setbacks.

As chair of a department, Katzman was undoubtedly attentive to the department's balance sheet, and so when a colleague presented an opportunity to build a new and potentially lucrative treatment program, he listened. The many older adults with senile dementia, the colleague argued, have a treatable disease: "adult onset hydrocephalus."

Hydrocephalus, or "water on the brain," is a disease of newborns in which the inability to properly drain the fluid that bathes the brain causes damaging swelling of the spaces where fluid gathers in the brain, called ventricles. A shunt effectively drains the swollen ventricles and relieves the pressure. A 1965 paper from researchers at Massachusetts General Hospital in the prestigious *New England Journal of Medicine* claimed spectacular results in older adults with dementia and swollen ventricles.[4] The authors' nine-page report, "Symptomatic Occult Hydrocephalus with 'Normal' Cerebrospinal-Fluid Pressure: A Treatable Syndrome," concluded with a clear and inspirational message to neurologists and neurosurgeons. "Recognition and treatment of these cases is of great importance since it will result in what amounts to a 'cure' of a clinical condition that closely resembles presenile or senile dementia. It is in the large group of patients with late-life dementia that further cases must be sought."

Katzman's colleague agreed. The brains of senile older adults, with their enlarged ventricles and thin brain tissue, suggested the opportunity for a lucrative treatment. In 1969, they launched the "shunting program" for elderly adults with senility.

The initial promising results of the first few shunts did not play out in most patients (cases of hydrocephalus can occur rarely in older adults, but what was seen as swelling was in fact more commonly the artifact of fluid filling in the space left from brain tissue dying). The program closed.

Katzman's interest in dementia might have ended there but for three other events. The first introduces Robert Terry, a neuropathologist at Einstein. Since childhood, he was fascinated with photography. As a medical scientist, he channeled this interest to the nascent method of electron microscopy. His data were photographs of an object's molecular structure. He could have applied these skills to any number of diseases, but the departure of the head of neuropathology left a job vacancy.

For Terry and his wife, Pat, a scholar of French poetry, the job allowed the two Francophiles to enjoy a bottle of Château Talbot and rack of lamb at the Upper East Side's Le Veau d'Or restaurant. For Terry the researcher, though, the job presented a problem. He needed brain tissue, but a brain biopsy to obtain tissue is risky. Enter the failed shunting program. Each time the neurosurgeon inserted a shunt, a sliver of brain tissue was removed, frozen, and stored away. Terry examined these biopsies with his electron microscope. They showed a consistent result. Most of the patients with senile dementia had the pathology seen in Alzheimer's disease. From the hyperfocused vantage of the molecular ultrastructure of the amyloid plaque, senility looked a lot like Alzheimer's disease.

The other two events were personal. Throughout Katzman's entire medical training, he cared for few if any patients with Alzheimer's disease or senility. But then Katzman started to care deeply about one patient, a person he was quite close to, his mother-in-law, Elsie Bernstein.

He recalled in an interview in 2000 that "something happened at her grandson's wedding that led the family to realize that something was very wrong."[5] It wasn't an isolated incident. She couldn't name family members and roasts were found not in the oven but in the cupboard. A colleague diagnosed her with senile dementia. Terry's studies of the shunting program biopsies gave Katzman the idea what the cause really was: Alzheimer's disease. She died seven years after her diagnosis.

Her husband, Katzman's father-in-law, exhausted their savings caring for her. The impact of her illness on the family was unforgettable and enduring.

At the same time that his family was suffering, Katzman's career was suffering as well. While on sabbatical at Lund University in Sweden in 1969, he'd witnessed a miraculous result: the regeneration of injured neurons. Brain cells could regrow. He was determined to apply this to the discovery of a cure for Parkinson's disease. Witnessing the Nobel Prize in Medicine ceremony kindled a dream that he, one day, might receive that award.

Back in the United States, his dream became a nightmare. Every grant application he submitted was rejected. At first he was taken aback and depressed, but in time he applied his scientist's skills at contemplation and reflection. If senile dementia was Alzheimer's disease, then the number of patients, people like his mother-in-law, exacted a significant burden on society. He started to think about the importance of these numbers. The disease wasn't rare. It was common—a leading cause of death. And he knew personally that it was a cause of substantial suffering for patients and their families.

One summer afternoon in 1971 in his study at his home in Mamaroneck, New York, he said to his son Dan: "Alzheimer's is one of the biggest diseases around."[6] He dropped the promise of neuroregeneration and instead took up the problem of neurodegeneration.

Katzman saw Alzheimer's not just as a medical problem but also as a social problem. His politics were those of a progressive liberal Democrat with a deep commitment to civil rights and social justice (a regular donor to the

ACLU and Southern Poverty Law Center, he'd turned down a job in 1950s Little Rock, Arkansas, because the city was segregated). He believed that collective action, reason, and logic could solve a social problem.

Although reserved, even shy, he was committed, and so he began to speak up at conferences. A talk at a 1973 meeting in Houston, Texas, was covered by the *National Enquirer* under the headline: DOCTORS FIND NEW MAJOR CAUSE OF DEATH. Readers from all over the country sent him letters about their relatives with senility asking him: "Might they have this disease as well? What should I do?"

He knew he was on to something.

At meetings of neurologists and psychiatrists, he started to buttonhole colleagues to test out an idea. Senile dementia isn't an extreme end stage of aging. It's a disease like Parkinson's disease. They listened and encouraged him. By 1976, he decided he was ready to become an Alzheimer's disease activist.

The timing of his editorial's publication was auspicious. Psychodynamic Freudian theories of brain disease were collapsing and being replaced with "biological psychiatry" and its promise that hard sciences of molecular biology, neurochemistry, and genetics could lead to treatments for psychiatric and neurological illnesses with the same precision as treatments for cancer and heart disease.

The system of care was changing, too. Asylums were closing and nursing homes were under both state and federal pressures to discharge residents to the "least restrictive" (and, coincidentally, least costly to taxpayers) place of care, namely their families' homes or the street. Their social workers, largely untrained in how to assess cognition or dementia, scrambled to cobble together discharge plans. Senile older adults were discharged with no attention to their cognitive or behavioral problems. They started to show up in hospitals, brought in by distressed family members, financially strapped and at their wits' end over how to care for them.

Larger social and cultural forces were also at work. Between 1901—when Dr. Alzheimer began caring for Auguste Deter—and 1976, families were changing. America and other developed countries were living through a revolution in the values and structure that defined family, gender, work, and selfhood. In 1973, the same year Katzman first presented his idea that senility was Alzheimer's disease, the US Supreme Court ruled that newspapers' classified ads could not separately list "jobs for women" and "jobs for men." Courts were also tossing out as unconstitutional rules that kept women from certain kinds of jobs or from being employed and pregnant or a mother. In 1976, the same year as Katzman's editorial, the United States Military Academy at West Point admitted its first woman and the Equal Rights Amendment, or ERA, was moving swiftly toward ratification (just three states were needed to ratify it). The ERA would enshrine in the Constitution that a person's sex could not be used to deny them rights.

In the year following, 1977, President Carter, continuing the work of the Ford administration's International Women's Year commission, sent a US delegation to the National Women's Conference. For four days in Houston, every major media outlet covered this culmination of International Women's Year. In attendance were delegations from every state, White House and congressional Republican and Democratic delegates, First Lady Rosalynn Carter, and former first ladies Ford and Johnson. In addition to bipartisan support for the ratification of ERA, the detailed National Plan of Action included demands for home health and social services and geriatric training for all medical personnel. Coretta Scott King stirred the assembly of thousands to tears and applause when she proclaimed, "Let this message go forth from Houston and spread all over this land. There is a new force, a new understanding, a new sisterhood against all injustice that has been born here. We will not be divided and defeated again."[7]

Women were no longer the automatic caregivers for their elderly family members. Family sizes were shrinking, and their members were dispersed. Not only were there more and more older adults, but there were also fewer younger adults to care for them.

A new ethic was emerging that was changing societal expectations of being an adult. Characteristics such as race, gender, sexuality, and even age were becoming less and less acceptable as the organizing principle for what a person could or could not choose to do, such as where they ate lunch, lived, went to school, or the job they worked at. For older adults, this meant upending beliefs that the elderly are passive, quiet, dull, and unproductive.

Treating an older adult based on these beliefs should be replaced with respecting each person's exercise of her self-determination, her autonomy to create a life as she desired. Society had a duty to respect each person's autonomy and remove barriers to her self-determination. This ethical revolution made unpalatable the idea that with aging, loss of the abilities to make decisions and live independently was just a natural—and so normal—part of life.

The disabilities in older adults with senile dementia should be diagnosed and treated as disease. Alzheimer's disease was becoming a disease of the American way of living. As the historian Jesse Ballenger observes, "Senility haunts the landscape of the self-made man."[8]

12

A SELF-HELP GROUP FOR
THE SELF-MADE MAN

In the United States, as soon as several inhabitants have taken an opinion or an idea they wish to promote in society, they seek each other out and unite together once they have made contact. From that moment, they are no longer isolated but have become a power seen from afar whose activities serve as an example and whose words are heeded.

—Alexis de Tocqueville, *Democracy in America*, 1840

I haunted the major medical centers for help for my wife, my family and myself.

—Jerome H. Stone, "The Self-Help Movement: Forming a National Organization," Alzheimer's Disease and Related Disorders Association, 1982

LONNIE WOLLIN'S LANDLORD was furious. He called Lonnie, accusing him of lying. "I leased you space for a law office, not a mail-order business!"

Twice a day, the postman was delivering bags and bags of mail to Wollin's small office in New York City's financial district. The letters were piling up. The space was overflowing with mail, and unopened bags were left in the halls, stuffed into closets. Lonnie was in a bind. He was about to lose his lease, but he was far away from the office on a ski vacation, so he called the one man he knew could help: Jerry Stone in Chicago.

Stone reassured the tax attorney. "I'll take care of it." And he did. He was good at fixing things, taking care of problems, settling the fights, and keeping the peace. And writing the checks. Nothing seemed to bother Stone.

For Stone, the threat of Lonnie's eviction from his 32 Broadway office was among the best news of the last twelve months. It was a kind of anniversary present, as it came almost a year to the date since he'd gotten into this new business. He wished he could tell Evelyn, his wife, the good news, but as a result of her Alzheimer's disease she was too forgetful and confused to follow even a simple conversation. He'd come to accept that. This new business was all for Evelyn. The good news was the Dear Abby letter was a smashing success.

In October 1980, the nationally syndicated advice columnist Abigail Van Buren had received a letter from "DESPERATE IN NY."

Dear Abby,
About two years ago, I began to notice a change in my husband. He became increasingly forgetful and easily confused, even though he was only 50 . . . We saw several doctors before one finally seemed familiar with my husband's condition. He told us he had Alzheimer's disease, for which there is no known cure. Alzheimer's disease occurs in people as young as 40 and 50 as well as in some older people.[1]

Desperate went on to explain that her husband, although in excellent health, had memory problems so bad he could not drive, had to quit work, and needed to be watched every minute. Sometimes he seemed normal, but then he was once again dependent and forgetful. "I feel so helpless. How do others cope with this disease?"

Abby began her reply: "You are not alone."

In a few years, these four words would be the opener of caregiver support groups across the nation. She explained that "there are now groups of concerned friends and relatives who have banded together to provide support, develop and disseminate helpful information and encourage much needed research in Alzheimer's disease." She gave Desperate a simple instruction. Send a stamped, self-addressed envelope to Alzheimer's Disease and Related Disorders Association. The address was 32 Broadway, New York, New York.

Lonnie Wollin's office was the official address for the association because Lonnie used this address in the articles of incorporation and office for the Alzheimer Disease Society, the not-for-profit Lonnie established in 1978. The office had a desk and one staff person.

But Wollin was a reluctant organizer of his society. Alzheimer's was in his family, first his father's brother, Uncle Arthur, then his father. The exhausting experience of caring for his father left him emotionally drained. He just wanted to avoid the disease. It was not until Uncle Lou died of the disease that he decided to act on the advice of his father's doctor. Create an organization that would raise awareness and funds for Alzheimer's disease research.

This doctor was polite but persistent. He explained how "grassroots" patient advocacy organizations made great progress to raise awareness, change laws, and increase congressional funding for research. It worked for cancer and even less common diseases like epilepsy.

The doctor was Robert Katzman. It was Dr. Katzman who introduced Jerry Stone to Lonnie Wollin, a single meeting that ignited a cascade of meetings, a national network of relationships, and finally, the national self-help group for Alzheimer's disease. Stone's calls and visits to Dr. Katzman at Einstein were yet another stop in his quest for help for Evelyn. Like Desperate's husband, her symptoms began at age fifty.

Stone was a great American industrialist and a self-made man.

At fifteen, he began working for $12 a week at his father's small family business that made cardboard packaging. Within forty years, he was the CEO of the Chicago-based Stone Container Corporation, a Fortune 500 company that employed some ten thousand people in the manufacture and sales of shipping and packaging containers. Stone knew how to build a business, run it, and motivate people to work toward a common mission.

Stone knew a lot and he also knew what he didn't know and so he sought out the best advice and did research. When the doctors at the University of Chicago recommended a shunt for Evelyn, he sought out Dr. Raymond Adams at Massachusetts General Hospital, a neurologist and the lead author of the *New England Journal of Medicine* paper reporting on treatment by shunting. After a one-hour call with Adams, he decided against the treatment. He read neurology textbooks. Of the ten he checked out from the University of Chicago library, only three even mentioned the disease. This limited attention, the lack of treatments, and the indifference of most physicians added up to an enormous disappointment.

He persisted. He took Evelyn to the neurologists at London's renowned National Hospital for Neurology and Neurosurgery (at the time it was called the National Hospital for Nervous Diseases). He made calls. Who was doing research on Alzheimer's disease? "Terry at Einstein," was the answer. He traveled east to visit Robert Terry.

In an interview twenty-five years later about these early years, he recounted, "Bob [Terry] was glad to hear from me because he wanted money for his research projects. I said, 'Sure, I would be glad to give you money. All I want to know is what is the latest on research and who else is interested in Alzheimer's?'"[2] Which is how he ended up having lunch at New York City's Ritz Hotel with Lonnie Wollin and Terry's colleague and collaborator, Robert Katzman.

Networking and hard work came easily to Stone. So, too, did the capacity to gain a researcher's time and attention with a generous donation.

Katzman and Wollin decided that Jerry Stone was the solution to their problem. Their Alzheimer Disease Society faced competition. There were six other locally founded lay groups dedicated to the problem of dementia. Some featured Alzheimer's in their name. Others, dementia. Each of the seven organizations offered a model for a national organization. Two stood out.

With funding from the state of California, the San Francisco–based Family Survival Project, led by Anne Bashkiroff and Suzanne Harris, gathered data on the needs of brain-damaged older adults and began to develop support programs for caregivers. The organization took its name from the two women's yearslong struggles to find care for their husbands, Bashkiroff's from Alzheimer's disease and Harris's from a brain hemorrhage. "What we had been told by the doctors was 'take him home and love him,'" Harris recounted.[3] This and other frustrating experiences transformed and united them into fierce advocates for caregivers of adults with brain diseases or damage.

The Minneapolis-based Association for Alzheimer's and Related Diseases, led by Hilda Pridgeon and Bobbie Glaze, both caring for husbands with Alzheimer's disease, was also far along. Hilda used a one-year paid leave of absence from her employer, Control Data Corporation, to start the organization out of her home in Bloomington, Minnesota.

They started public meetings, support groups, public service announcements aired on local networks, and a newsletter. Their public meetings were, like the Family Survival Project's, packed. In those early years, Ryan, the youngest of Hilda and Al's three children, would answer the phone for the fledgling association. Among the calls the teenager took was from a man in New York eager to speak with Ryan's mother: Jerome Stone.

In an interview forty years later, Ryan recalled his mother's tireless work ethic, visionary leadership, and selfless dedication.[4] She took calls at all hours from families suffering as hers was, families at a breaking point over how to find answers and help for a loved one ill with dementia, senility, or some otherwise undiagnosed "brain disorder." As he recalled her boundless patience and empathy, Ryan wept.

When Jerry Stone called Hilda Pridgeon, she and Bobbie Glaze were already organizing a national association. Following a September 1979 meeting with NIA director Robert Butler, they produced a detailed vision, goals, and even a name for this national association: the Alzheimer's and Related Diseases Association. Pridgeon and Glaze were hardworking and very tactical. Leading with "Alzheimer's," they explained, would position the organization first in nationwide white pages telephone listings and so expedite their positioning in lists of local organizations.

Katzman was worried. Compared to the work of Bashkiroff and Harris and Pridgeon and Glaze, his Alzheimer Disease Society's accomplishments were modest. All he could claim was some calls and letters from neurologists replying to advertisements the society placed in neurology journals. A few donations had come in. Each organization had turf to defend and a vision for what a national organization ought to be called, what it should do, and where it should be located.

Jerry Stone was Katzman's solution. Stone was his own man, unattached to any of the seven organizations, he cared about Alzheimer's disease, he was a leader, he was well connected, and he was very rich. Jerry Stone just might be the man to bring the seven organizations together, a kind of founding father who could turn the seven colonies into one nation. Katzman just needed to get Jerry interested.

Jerry Stone's recruitment into the Alzheimer's disease self-help movement began over lunch at the Ritz Hotel and concluded over dinner at Germaine's. In late-1970s Washington, DC, this self-described "Asian-fusion" restaurant in Georgetown was a destination to enjoy inventive food in the company of powerful Washingtonians. An invitation to dine at Germaine's told you that your host was part of the Washington scene.

On October 28, 1979, representatives of all seven organizations gathered for the dinner. Wollin and Katzman made sure Stone received an invitation. To add further luster to the invitation, it came from the very well-known Georgetown resident Florence Mahoney, one-half of the Lasker-Mahoney team who were fiercely committed to expanding the NIH and the federal commitment to medical research. Mahoney was an early champion of the creation of the NIA, and the invited guests that evening included a friend she'd supported as the first director of the NIA, Robert Butler.

Butler, Mahoney, Katzman, and Dr. Donald Tower, the director of the National Institute of Neurological and Communicative Disorders and Stroke, had a plan. The representatives of the organizations would get to know one another over dinner and the next day attend a one-day meeting at the NIH campus to map out the idea for a national Alzheimer's disease organization.

Stone almost declined the invitation. It conflicted with a business trip to China, but he decided to meet them halfway. He'd attend the dinner and skip the meeting in Bethesda.

As the dinner wore on, he kept taking up his coat and attaché case as though to leave only to sit down again. Several times he announced, "I don't know if I can stay the night." But something was happening.

He stayed and he listened. Listening was among his skills. That and a great sense of humor would serve him and the association well when emotions flared and the whole thing seemed ready to fall apart.

Stories flew about of how families were struggling but no one seemed to care. These people, though, they cared. And they were angry. They shared vivid stories of the health care system's ignorance and indifference to their desperate efforts to find answers and help for their relatives and themselves. They were just like him.

They were intense and united in their passion to change the system, but they had differences. Where should the national organization be based? Should its focus be improving care, research, or both? Should it focus on Alzheimer's disease or all causes of dementia? What should it be called?

He changed his mind. "I bought a toothbrush and stayed at that terrible motel where everybody else was staying."

The meeting the next morning at a conference room at the NIH started with advice from Robert Butler. "You either sink or swim together," he said.[5] They nearly drowned each other.

It was after lunch, during the agenda's four-and-a-half-hour discussion of "Toward a National Alzheimer's Organization," when emotions flared. They argued over just about everything: their name, location, mission, and purpose.

In Stone's memoir, *The Self-Help Movement: Forming a National Organization*, he recalled: "During that day, with much good will dissipating into acrimonious debate, I could appreciate with full force the torment that our founding fathers must have gone through trying to satisfy 13 colonies who did not want to give up local autonomous rights for the national good."[6]

The discussion of the organization's mission created sharp and angry divisions. Each side offered passionate and compelling arguments. Ann Bashkiroff, of the Family Survival Project, wanted an organization dedicated to the needs of brain-damaged adults regardless of the cause of their impairments. This organization would advocate for all the families of these disabled patients. A focus on any one disease, she insisted, would exclude the caregivers and patients who don't have that disease.

Wollin and others argued for an organization dedicated to Alzheimer's disease. This would ensure the organization captured the attentions of researchers and Congress and, eventually, discoveries of treatments. Support and education could still be given to caregivers of all kinds of patients. The organization's name and its messaging, though, must be about what they argued was the most common cause of dementia.

In between were Pridgeon and Glaze, who strategically featured Alzheimer's disease but titled their organization and its services to capture all causes of dementia.

Emotions grew raw. Some twenty years later, in an interview with Katzman, Lonnie Wollin described Anne Bashkiroff and her colleagues as "idiots." Bashkiroff became so angry she snapped at Jerry Stone: "I'll trade my little house in Sausalito anytime for your paper box company."[7]

Stone said nothing. Nothing seemed to bother him.

Each of these people was caught up in a tense and deeply personal struggle. How to reconcile as many as four different perspectives on the self that this self-help group should help: the person with dementia, the family trying to care for that person, themselves one day as a person with dementia, or their child one day as a person with dementia?

Ann was among those who deeply identified with the raw and painful sufferings of the patient and family. They needed help and they needed it now no matter what the disease that caused the dementia. Wollin was moving beyond that experience. He'd already lost three family members, and his concern was his own risk of developing the disease. He wanted an organization dedicated to discovering the cure for the disease that threatened him.

Katzman championed the focus on Alzheimer's disease. He argued: "If we go before Congress and we want something—whether it's a change in the law or funds—and they see in our mission statement that we assist families that deal with trauma, then when we ask for money, Congress will say, 'Oh we had the trauma people in here last month and we gave them eight million dollars.' When we go to Congress, we're there for Alzheimer's."

The acrimonious debate ended with what might be called the Bethesda compromise. Each of the seven groups would send one representative to a national board meeting and within one year that board would develop bylaws and guidelines for a national voluntary self-help organization called the Alzheimer's Disease and Related Disorders Association. The "cumbersome tongue twisting name," as Lonnie Wollin described it, was the compromise over the difference in what should be the mission of the organization. It was a debate that would resonate throughout the association's history and the public response to the Alzheimer's crisis. Should we advocate for care for the millions of people with dementia and their families or a cure for the most common cause of dementia? Or a bit of both?

They departed with a decision to meet again in Chicago. Chicago, because Jerry Stone offered to host the meeting. In his cab ride to the airport, Stone had one fellow passenger: Anne Bashkiroff. That was his style: patient listening and perspective taking.

Stone set to work. He secured convenient space for a meeting, he did his research, and he brought in consultants: Bernd Brecher, an organizational expert on bylaws, and Leonard Borman, an anthropologist at Northwestern University. Borman was a kind of philosopher for the nascent group, an expert in self-help groups. These were groups of people who came together with a common and unmet need. He offered wisdom on why these lay organizations such as Alcoholics Anonymous and Mended Hearts stayed together and also why they fell apart.

On the morning of December 4, 1979, the board of the Alzheimer's Disease and Related Disorders Association held its first meeting at a conference room at the Hilton Chicago O'Hare Airport Hotel. By the close of the day, the voluntary health organization elected as president of the board public board member number one: Jerome Stone. They then elected directors and officers, created a medical and scientific advisory board chaired by Katzman, and established four committees: program services, education and public awareness, public policy and advocacy, and finance. They had no funds, but Stone promised that within three weeks he and the other board members would raise as much as $25,000.

"It was an interesting and rocky beginning," Stone recalled in an interview. A meeting two months later at a hotel near New York's LaGuardia Airport grew so contentious that some attendees thought the nascent association would collapse. They reopened the raw wounds of the discussion of what should be the name and purpose of the organization, and there were complaints that Stone was too independent in making decisions. Within a year, the San Francisco Family Survival Project chapter withdrew and transformed into the Family Caregiver Alliance, dedicated to providing information, support, and resources for caregivers of adults with chronic physical or cognitive conditions.

Stone, however, thought these meetings were successes.

"It showed people had passion for the cause," he reflected.

The proof that their cause was vast and important came nearly a year after the dinner at Germaine's, when Dear Abby answered "DESPERATE IN NY." Tens of thousands of other "Desperates" wrote for help. America needed a self-help group for Alzheimer's disease and related disorders, and the nascent association was ready to help. They had a hundred thousand names for a direct-mail fundraising campaign.

DESPERATE IN NY was also proof of Jerry Stone's influence, power, connections, and relentlessly strategic approach to address a problem. He called on a friend who was a friend of Abby's. The letter was staged.

Jerry Stone was DESPERATE IN NY.

13

A CRISIS IN THE FAMILY

People are afraid. I'm afraid. They are afraid of what will happen to them if they get this disease. They are even more afraid of how their families will cope.

—Hilda Pridgeon, Testimony at *Alzheimer's—
The Unmet Challenge for Research and Care*, a joint hearing of
the Select Committee on Aging, House of Representatives
and the Subcommittee on Aging of the Committee on Labor and
Human Resources, US Senate, April 3, 1990

As a society, we have always depended on family caregivers to provide the lion's share of long-term services and supports for our elders. Yet the need to recognize and support caregivers is among the most significant overlooked challenges facing the aging U.S. population, their families and society.

National Academy of Medicine,
Families Caring for an Aging America, 2016

JERRY STONE MUST have been proud as Thomas Ennis addressed the October 18, 1985, meeting of the board of directors of the Alzheimer's Disease and Related Disorders Association at O'Hare Airport's Hyatt Regency Hotel. In just five years, the association had grown into a well-funded, nationally recognized organization.

Ennis was the association's first executive director. Alzheimer's disease, he announced, was becoming a household word. He described a recent national public opinion poll that found Alzheimer's disease was the fifth most feared and serious disease in the United States.

"It is extremely doubtful," he explained, "if Alzheimer's disease would have been listed even just two years ago in such a poll."[1]

The association, he explained, could take credit for this progress.

Ennis led eleven staff working out of the Stone Container Building in downtown Chicago and reported to a board whose fifty-eight members included prominent, connected, and accomplished leaders from industry, law, science, and society. They worked hard and they were committed. An electricity sustained them at committee meetings that often lasted until past midnight. Jerry Stone oversaw them all. He moved from conference room to conference room, stopping in to assess each committee's progress.

The structure of the association was a Chicago-based national office that oversaw a nationwide confederation of chapters that adhered to standards for governance, finances, and the delivery of services to patients and families. The board's chapter committee vetted and approved chapters and, as the organization aged, removed chapters that failed to comply with the standards.

Chapters offered the kinds of services the founders such as Jerry Stone, Hilda Pridgeon, Bonnie Glaze, and Lonnie Wollin had desperately sought. They included a toll-free help line, a quarterly newsletter, registration in a "safe return program" to identify a patient who had wandered, support groups, and educational materials about Alzheimer's and how to cope with it.

As the 1980s unfolded, America began to listen to the association.

Congress held hearings with attention-getting titles such as *Endless Night, Endless Mourning: Living with Alzheimer's* (1982) and *Senility: The Last Stereotype* (1983). Congress also commissioned research reports. Its Office of Technology Assessment published four reports. The first, the 1987 *Losing a Million Minds*, estimated the annual cost of dementia to range between $24 billion and $48 billion, though it admitted large margins of uncertainty in all cost estimates.[2] Subsequent reports addressed the quality of care and special care units.[3]

The executive branch took action. In 1983, President Reagan declared November National Alzheimer's Month and, observing that "right now, research is the only hope for victims and families," he instructed Margaret Heckler, secretary of the Department of Health and Human Services, to create a task force to coordinate Alzheimer's disease research efforts.

With oversight of the NIH, Heckler assembled representatives from its multiple institutes, as well as the surgeon general, the Administration on Aging, and the Department of Veterans Affairs. The 1984 report *Alzheimer's*

Disease: Report of the Secretary's Task Force on Alzheimer's Disease was notably ambitious and comprehensive. It mapped out research needed "from intricacies of brain tissue changes to how best to assist the family support system."

At each board meeting, Dom Ruscio, from the Washington, DC, consulting firm Cavarocchi Associates, reported steady increases in funding to the NIH: $22 million in 1983 doubled to $44 million a year later. In 1989, funding crossed triple digits when Congress appropriated $129 million. The association complemented its persistent advocacy for NIH funding with its own research grants to academic investigators. At each board meeting, the chair of the Medical and Scientific Advisory Board reported a steady increase in applications and grants awarded.

A regular output of public service announcements, the first in 1982, performed by the actor Jack Lemmon, raised awareness and encouraged seeing a doctor. The "ten warning signs" campaign, launched in 1993 and still used, was among the most effective. It describes the signs of dementia caused by Alzheimer's disease beginning with "memory loss that disrupts daily life" and urges: "If you notice any of them, don't ignore them. Schedule an appointment with your doctor."

In 1988, the Bethesda compromise passed into history. Katzman persuaded the board that "Alzheimer's Disease and Related Disorders Association" was cumbersome and distracted from the mission of convincing Congress to fund research for a cure for Alzheimer's disease. The board renamed the organization the Alzheimer's Association and adopted the tagline: "Someone to Stand by You."

To publicize the name change, the American R&B singer Ben E. King allowed the association to use the lyrics and music of his hit song "Stand by Me." This renaming and publicity sent America a clear message. Chapters' services were for people with dementia and their families, but the focus of research was a cure for one—and only one—of the diseases that caused dementia: Alzheimer's disease.

All this work was sustained by rigorous fundraising. Board members who weren't health care professionals or academics were expected to either donate or raise funds. Stone set the example.

After he learned that the actor Rita Hayworth had Alzheimer's disease, he reached out to her daughter, Princess Yasmin Aga Khan, the only child of Hayworth's short marriage to Prince Aly Khan, a member of a family of spiritual leaders of Ismaili Muslims. The thirty-two-year-old princess demurred, explaining that she didn't do boards, speeches, committee work, or fundraising. Stone persisted. "Well, I know what you don't like to do. Do you ever like to have lunch?" She accepted an invitation to the Four Seasons.

Three years later, in 1985, in the Grand Ballroom of Manhattan's Pierre Hotel, Princess Yasmin Aga Khan chaired the first Rita Hayworth Gala. She raised $300,000 for the association. As of 2016, yearly Rita Hayworth Galas in New York, Chicago, and Palm Beach had raised $70 million.

By 1990, the tenth anniversary of the founding of the association, "the house that Jerry built" (Wollin's description he gave at a Rita Hayworth Gala) was a large and influential organization. One hundred staff worked out of the Chicago headquarters with a budget of $17.5 million. Alzheimer's was becoming recognized as a crisis and the association was leading the fight. At least half of the NIA's budget was directed to Alzheimer's research, celebrities were speaking up about their personal experiences with the disease, and the covers of *Newsweek*, *Fortune*, and other major print and television media featured it.

At the May 1990 board meeting at O'Hare's Westin Hotel, Hilda Pridgeon, chair of the chapter committee, reported that in the past year, four more chapters brought the total to 210, divided among ten regions covering forty-nine states (Alaska was the last to have a chapter, in 1992). Success in achieving the association's goals of providing patient and family services and caregiver training included 1,600 support groups, 30,000 volunteers, and the then-innovative use of video media to produce the *Alzheimer's Disease Orientation Kit* and the *Caregiver Kit*, containing plain-language explanations of the disease, its stages, and how to address common challenges when caring for someone with the disease.

Congressional hearings were media events with witnesses such as Princess Aga Khan, Hollywood actors and celebrities (actresses Shelley Fabares and Angie Dickinson spoke about their experiences caring for their mother and sister, respectively), and even patients. The April 1990 joint Senate-House hearing *Alzheimer's: The Unmet Challenge for Research and Care* was a notable success.[4]

Senator Mark Hatfield, Republican of Oregon, brought room 2322 of the Rayburn House Office Building to a hushed, compassionate silence as he opened the hearing: "My father was a third generation in our family of blacksmithing." He told his colleagues about a man of extraordinary physical strength who became so forgetful that he lived his last years in a nursing home, "a powerful man reduced to practically nothing—as almost a vegetable."

His disclosure was a first for a national politician. Should the sixty-eight-year-old Hatfield experience a "senior moment," he now risked colleagues' and constituents' worried reactions and the experience of a spillover of the stigma of his father's disease into his life. Hatfield was a member of the powerful Senate Appropriations Committee, responsible for reviewing and approving the federal budget. He became the committee's dedicated advocate for Alzheimer's disease.

Seven months after *Alzheimer's: The Unmet Challenge for Research and Care*, Stephen McConnell, the association's vice president for public policy, prepared a memo to the board of directors. He opened "Congressional Action on Behalf of AD Patients/Families" with enthusiasm: "It's been one helluva year!"[5]

Hatfield's CARE Act had led to a $100 million increase, a doubling in research funds to the NIH. The association thanked Hatfield with a Safe Return bracelet, engraved with his name (the association later convinced a reporter who found the bracelet after Hatfield had lost it at an event that the reporter didn't in fact have a front-page story that the senator had Alzheimer's disease).

Hilda Pridgeon undoubtedly agreed with McConnell. It had been one helluva year. This national voluntary self-help association was her vision, started out of her Bloomington home. Like Stone, she'd come to the cause out of a devastating personal experience. Unlike Stone, that experience nearly cast her family into ruinous poverty.

In 1974, Pridgeon's husband, Al, was diagnosed with Alzheimer's disease. At fifty, he was out of his job as a factory manager and unemployable. Her life as a housewife, secretary, and mother of three teenaged children was at risk for coming undone. It was her job, and hers alone, to keep the family together financially, emotionally, and spiritually. Beloved and respected by the other board members and staff, Pridgeon was known for a tireless work ethic, unyielding commitment to the association, and a quiet, no-nonsense demeanor. No doubt she was proud of the chapters she shepherded into existence. They gave women like her access to information, support, and skills to care for their relatives.

Pridgeon was also frustrated. In a 1989 interview with the Associated Press, she observed: "It's amazing that the richest country in the world can't take care of its older people without impoverishing their spouses. People are going through their resources very rapidly."[6]

She knew firsthand what she was talking about. After Al ceased working, she'd stared poverty in the face. There were two children's college tuition bills to pay and a third child in high school. She was determined to rise from the secretarial pool at Control Data Corporation into a better-paying position in management.

She enrolled in a college degree program. Rising at 4:00 a.m. gave her two hours to study before she helped Al get dressed, bathed, and fed. In time, leaving her husband home alone while she worked became too dangerous for him and too stressful for her. His lunch remained in the refrigerator uneaten. She couldn't quit work to take care of him and struggled to find care the family could afford.

She took him to the Courage Center, a day care program, in hope that they could provide him a safe and social environment while she worked. "Go home," said the doctor. "You don't have any problems." The center only cared for patients with physical disabilities. She finally found a place that would have him, the Sister Kenny Day Care Center.

But how to pay for it?

She wrote to Medicare, explaining that she needed to work during the day and yes, the Sister Kenny Day Care Center wasn't medicine, but it was the only prescription that would help her husband.

Years later in an interview, she recounted the response from Medicare. "I just wanted the man in charge of Medicare for the Twin Cities area to sit down and talk to me. But he wouldn't even talk to me. He sent a letter back that said, 'That's entertainment for your husband and a relief for you and it doesn't qualify.' The fact that I had to work and that I had to have some help didn't matter."[7]

Hilda Pridgeon was a witness to and victim of the US health care system's enduring failures. Medicare's statutory language strictly defines that the social insurance program paid for the "usual and customary medical care" doctors' prescribed out of their offices and hospitals. A prescription for adult day care was not "usual and customary" medical care. It was considered "custodial" or "long-term" care. Medicare didn't pay for that. The Pridgeon family was on their own.

A wealthy man like Jerry Stone could manage the costs of caring for a person with dementia. At one point, he paid a staff of fifteen caregivers to care for Evelyn in their home. But for a middle-class woman like Hilda Pridgeon, caregiving was a tragedy. Support from the state was only available if she spent their savings and, as a result, the family became impoverished. Then and only then not Medicare but Medicaid—state welfare—would pay for Al's care. Or she could divorce him and thus leave him to the care of the state.

The problem was a divided Congress. It agreed to fund the NIH to support research to discover a cure. It could not agree on how to care for persons with Alzheimer's disease. The idea of social insurance for long-term care, to support the costs of interventions such as an adult day care program and the time spent caregiving, exposed ideologically charged flash points.

Hilda Pridgeon and other caregivers needed Congress to think and feel differently about the time and effort she spent to bathe, dress, feed, and be present with her husband. This wasn't the private and freely given labor of family; this was caregiving. Congress needed to recognize that Hilda Pridgeon was offering skilled labor worthy of a wage paid either to her or to someone else while she worked at Control Data Corporation. Congress, however, couldn't agree that this new way of thinking and feeling about living with and caring for a person with dementia required revisions to Medicare to pay for long-term care for people like Al Pridgeon.

Hilda Pridgeon testified on behalf of the Alzheimer's Association at the same 1990 joint House and Senate hearing where Senator Hatfield told his colleagues of his father "reduced to practically nothing—as almost a vegetable."

She recounted her story of caring for Al and then she expanded her vision. She talked about "the national crisis" whose annual bill is $80 to $90 billion. She emphasized that this bill is paid for by families. Most of the billion-dollar cost of Alzheimer's disease was—and still is—the tally of the time caregivers spend to provide care instead of working or the money the caregiver pays to someone else to care for their relative.

"People are afraid. I'm afraid," Pridgeon told the Congress. "They are afraid of what will happen to them if they get this disease. They are even more afraid of how their families will cope."

Even more afraid.

It was as if she were back at the acrimonious October 1979 afternoon meeting in the NIH conference room, when the representatives of the seven families were caught up in the tense struggle to reconcile how to help all the many selves affected by Alzheimer's disease. Should their focus be dementia, Alzheimer's disease and other causes of dementia, or just Alzheimer's disease? Should they be advocating for a cure for the disease or care for patients and their families? Or both? On this April morning, some eleven years later, she was advocating for care.

"We cannot yet prevent the terrible emotional cost of Alzheimer's disease,"

she admitted. "But we can and must do something about the financial burden that is impoverishing all but the wealthiest families." She concluded with
the specifics of national legislation needed to provide social insurance for patients and their families who need long-term care.

Congress listened but did nothing.

Hilda Pridgeon died in 2016. She was ninety years old. In high school, she
was forced to cede the valedictorian spot to a male classmate. The school explained the honor was his because he was soon to be deployed overseas to
fight in the Second World War. Pridgeon couldn't fight that decision. She
couldn't even fight in the war.

After graduating high school, the only job for her was as a secretary, but
as the world around her changed, she worked her way out of the secretarial
pool and became an executive like Jerry Stone.

Hilda Pridgeon was a leader of a revolution in the right to exercise one's
liberty and self-determination. She and her colleagues at the Alzheimer's Association had picked up where Alois Alzheimer and his colleagues left off after the devastation of Germany's medical and social systems. They'd redrawn
the border between aging and disease and in so doing retired senility into an
insulting stereotype. They replaced it with a biological problem, a disease in
need of a diagnosis and treatment.

In the years that followed, she witnessed substantial progress. There was
wide recognition that this disease was legitimate. Advances such as MCI and
amyloid imaging, and tests of drugs were progress toward Katzman's goal
that Alzheimer's disease must be prevented. She herself even underwent an
amyloid scan (her result showed no amyloid).

She also witnessed a frustrating lack of progress. There was not wide recognition of the need for a plan to address the burden on the patient and the
American family. To the day she died, twenty-six years after her congressional testimony that called for a national long-term care system, that system
still didn't exist. The health care system that called care for Al entertainment
still offered care that was fragmented, uneven, and expensive. Families like
hers were still struggling.

Why this uneven progress happened is the story of how people like her
husband and caregivers like her and her children were among the last casualties of the Cold War.

14

THE LAST CASUALTIES
OF THE COLD WAR

The current Medicare fee-for-service system, designed in 1960 to address
the acute care problems that predominated at the time, regularly fails those
with Alzheimer's disease and their families.
> —Alzheimer's Study Group, *A National Alzheimer's Strategic Plan:*
> *The Report of the Alzheimer's Study Group*, 2009

Keep the law responsible where the good Lord put it, on the man to bear the
burdens of support and the woman to bear the children.
> —Senator Sam Ervin

THE OPPRESSIVE HEAT and humidity of a typical Washington, DC, summer day discourages an outdoor political ceremony, particularly one requiring a jacket and tie. The Friday of the eve of the Independence Day holiday
weekend of 1988 was, however, quite pleasant. The White House's sun-soaked
Rose Garden was the fitting place for a bill-signing ceremony. Behind President Ronald Reagan was Dr. Otis Bowen, a physician and the secretary of
the Department of Health and Human Services, and congressional leaders.

The president asked Americans to imagine the threat of an illness that could
wipe out the savings of an entire lifetime, leaving a family to have to skimp
on groceries. "And even for those never actually forced into this situation," he
said, "there's the gnawing worry, the fear, that someday it might just happen."

He explained how the bill he was about to sign would end this. "It would
replace worry and fear with peace of mind."

And with that, the president signed into law the Medicare Catastrophic

Coverage Act. The "intolerable choice, a choice between bankruptcy and death"—Reagan's words in his legislative message to Congress—would end.

Alzheimer's was very much on the mind of Congress as it passed the bill with notable bipartisan support (328–72 in the House and 86–11 in the Senate). A Government Accountability Office report commissioned by Congress singled out Alzheimer's disease as among the conditions whose catastrophic expenses the elderly and their families needed to be protected from.

At the same time that the Catastrophic Coverage Act became law, a presidential election was heating up. The 1988 election was in an auspicious year for Alzheimer's disease caregivers and patients. Reagan was coming to the close of his second and final term in office and the election for president was an open race. At one point, fifteen candidates were running. Another campaign was underway as well. One hundred and forty advocacy organization—including AARP, several labor unions, and the Alzheimer's Association—were united for a cause: Long Term Care 88.

The campaign, principally funded by AARP and the Villers Foundation, set an ambitious goal. Stephen McConnell, the Director of the Campaign, explained in an interview: "Our goal was to move long-term care from the style section, to the political section, to get the political writers to care about it and not just the people that write about family issues."[1] They sought to convince all fifteen candidates to agree on one policy: If I'm elected, America will have a long-term care social insurance program.

Long Term Care 88 asked all the presidential candidates to talk about their vision for such a program. The bipartisan pair of senators from Iowa (Charles Grassley, the Republican, and Tom Harkin, the Democrat) interviewed each candidate at public forums on long-term care. Each candidate's comments were edited into a three-minute ad broadcast before caucus and primary elections.

Long-Term Care 88 "was all about social insurance," McConnell recalled. "We'd done a lot of polling. The public supported it. They'd be willing to pay extra money in taxes. And we actually were quite critical of Medicaid because it was considered a welfare-type program." The goal was passage of a social insurance program like Medicare and Social Security, paid out of payroll taxes, that would provide long-term care for all Americans.

Long-Term Care 88, the Medicare Catastrophic Coverage Act—finally, the richest country in the world was going to do something about family impoverishment. Two years later though, Hilda Pridgeon testified before Congress that she was afraid.

She wasn't alone.

✦

On Thursday, August 17, 1989, Congressman Dan Rostenkowski of Chicago, Illinois, fled from an angry crowd. "You're a bum!" one man yelled. They booed him. They carried signs. As chair of the House Ways and Means Committee, Rostenkowski was among the congressional leaders who'd shepherded the Catastrophic Coverage Act into law. The crowd of mostly elderly Chicagoans were furious over an act that was intended to help people just like them.

The senior citizens were objecting to the increase in their Medicare premiums. Reagan insisted that the Catastrophic Coverage Act "pay for itself," and so the funds came not from a tax on all working Americans, that is, a payroll tax, but from a tax on Medicare beneficiaries. Within a year of Reagan's Rose Garden ceremony, Congress repealed the unpopular act.

Long-Term Care 88 also failed. On election night, McConnell was downcast. All the candidates had supported some form of social insurance program except for one. "Basically what he said was: 'I'll give it the attention it deserves.'" That candidate was George H. W. Bush, and on November 4, 1988, Bush won the presidential election in a landslide. "I think we see what attention he gave to it, which was zero," McConnell recalled.

Social insurance for long-term care was dead.

From the vantage point of history, these events make sense. The year 1976—the year that Alzheimer's disease was born as a social movement—could also be dated as the birth of another social countermovement.

In 1976, Ronald Reagan nearly defeated President Ford for the Republican Party nomination. Four years later, he won the presidency in a landslide and the Republican Party took control of the Senate, ending twenty-six continuous years of a Democratic majority.

Reagan and his allies in Congress did not advocate policies that opposed the care of patients with Alzheimer's disease. The ideological forces of the Reagan Revolution and the policies they did support together with the ones they opposed did, however, cripple any progress toward improving the care of patients and their families.

In the run-up to Reagan's victory, the United States was in a recession. Inflation and interest rates for loans to purchase a home or car were both in double digits. In his 1984 State of the Union address, Reagan described the seventies as: "Years of rising problems and failing confidence. There was a feeling government had grown beyond the consent of the governed. Families felt helpless in the face of mounting inflation and the indignity of taxes that reduced reward for hard work, thrift, and risk taking. All this was overlaid by an ever growing web of rules and regulations."[2]

Reagan's solution was to reduce the role of the federal government in Americans' lives through budget cuts, privatization of social services, and deregulation. He quipped at an August 1986 press conference that the nine most frightening words in the English language were: "I'm from the government, and I'm here to help."[3] He achieved budget and tax cuts and decentralization of federal authority back to the states. He argued that the Soviet Union's military power was surpassing America and achieved increases in defense spending that further eroded the political will to spend money on long-term care.

In his 1982 State of the Union address, Reagan singled out the Medicare and Medicaid social insurance programs as being among those in need of cutting. Medicare, he complained, was "rife with waste and fraud." He bemoaned how "in just ten years" its costs had increased from $11.2 billion to $60 billion. "The time has come to control the uncontrollable," he demanded.[4]

Budget cuts of billions of dollars ensued. Long-term care insurance was a political nonstarter. The chapter on long-term care financing was excised from Department of Health and Human Services secretary Heckler's report on Alzheimer's disease, and following the secretary's expressed concern over cuts to Medicare and Medicaid, she was eased out of leading the department with a "promotion" to the ambassadorship to Ireland.

In the face of these policies, the Catastrophic Coverage Act stood out as aberrant, even bizarre. In fact, it was. Reagan wanted to veto it, but Bush, then his vice president and running for president, persuaded Reagan that a veto would harm his chances of election.

It is no wonder that the minutes of Alzheimer's Association board meetings routinely refer to the "enormous pressures" to reduce federal spending and thus the board should take solace that Congress continued to increase funding to the NIH. No one in Congress questioned whether Alzheimer's disease was a problem. They disagreed over what to do about it.

On the same April day as the 1990 hearing when Senator Hatfield spoke of his father being reduced to a vegetable and Hilda Pridgeon pled with Congress to create a long-term care social insurance program, volunteer Alzheimer's disease advocates visited the offices of their senators and representatives. A reporter covering the visit to Texas representative Tom DeLay's office captured the problem of improving care.

"Though DeLay greeted the volunteers warmly and assured them that their issue was 'dear to my heart,' he cooled when the talk turned to the need for a federal long-term care program." After the volunteers left his office, he explained, "That's where we may break ranks. No one has yet told me how we're going to pay for this."[5] He refused to raise taxes.

For Reagan and his allies like Congressman DeLay (who, five years later, became the House majority whip), opposition to raising taxes for social insurance programs was an ideological position staked out in a determined and ongoing fight against an enemy they said was attacking America not only from abroad but also from within—Socialism.

On April 15, 1961, the American Medical Association's Woman's Auxiliary sent an urgent letter to its members. "Physicians have asked doctors' wives to assume full responsibility for Operation Coffee Cup, an all-out effort to stimulate as many letters as possible to Congress opposing socialized medicine and its menace as proposed in the King bill."[6] The King bill was Representative Cecil King's proposal to create social insurance for older adults' medical care. The letter was signed by Mrs. William Mackersie, Mrs. Leo Smith, and Mrs. James Morrison, president, legislative chairman, and vice chairman, respectively, of the American Medical Association's Woman's Auxiliary.

With a name that sounds like an idea cooked up at CIA headquarters in Langley, Virginia, Operation Coffee Cup resonated with the times. The Cold War was on. A metaphorical Iron Curtain divided Europe into the communist East and the democratic West. The United States and the Soviet Union were in a constant give-and-take to gain the upper hand in a perilous balance of power. Armed with nuclear weapons, bombers cruised the skies and submarines prowled the depths of the oceans. Each side possessed sufficient weapons to destroy the world several times over.

The Cold War also shaped domestic policies. The charge that a policy such as the King bill would lead to socialism was a crippling blow to legislative consensus and adoption because socialism was typically considered synonymous with communism.

The campaign for Operation Coffee Cup included ten suggestions to persuade senators and congressmen to oppose ("#5—Be polite—members of congress deserve respectful treatment"), a written summary of the issues, and, for its time, an innovative means of direct communication: a phonograph record. The "Coffee Cuppers" were instructed to invite their friends and neighbors over for coffee: "Put on the coffee pot. That's simple." And then they were to play the record to galvanize their guests to write to their representatives and senators. The record's title was *Ronald Reagan Speaks Out Against Socialized Medicine*.

The actor turned political activist explained that the King bill—that is, social insurance for the health care of all adults sixty-five years and older—was the first step to government control of medicine. Reagan "used the enemy's own words" to close his argument when he quoted the American socialist Norman Thomas: "The American people will never knowingly adopt socialism. But under the name of 'liberalism' they will adopt every fragment of the socialist program, until one day America will be a Socialist nation, without knowing how it happened."

Ronald Reagan and the AMA and its Woman's Auxiliary lost this Cold War battle. Medicare became law in 1965. But they won the war. As a result of AMA lobbying, President Johnson signed into law a Medicare program that simply reimbursed physicians for their medical practice, what came to be referred to as "usual and customary care." Medicare did not cover all the health care older adults needed.

In the law's list of exclusions from coverage—between item #8 ("orthopedic shoes") and #10 ("cosmetic surgery")—was item #9: "custodial care."[7] This dehumanizing term, suggesting the work of janitors to clean a building, describes the daily work Hilda Pridgeon and other caregivers did—or paid someone else to do—not simply to keep their husbands bathed, dressed, and fed but also to keep them alive and happy. The law further provided no guidance to Medicare to develop care programs for the medical problems the elderly faced, problems such as Alzheimer's disease or what was then called senile dementia.

True, it was not until 1976 that senility was recast as a disease, but even in 1961, people in the medical community were aware of the growing numbers of older adults and the problems of aging. At the same time the AMA was rallying doctors' wives to oppose Medicare as socialized medicine, the *Journal of the American Medical Association*—widely known as *JAMA* and among the leading medical journals—published scientific articles examining how best to care for the increasing numbers of older adults, particularly those with multiple geriatric syndromes.

Dr. Louis Friedfeld summarized the results of his geriatric medicine clinic at New York City's Beth Israel Hospital where "medical, psychiatric and psychosocial studies were integrated to determine needs and to provide broad, centrally coordinated services."[8] Dr. Michael Dacso's article "Maintenance of Functional Capacity"—in other words, "custodial care"—presented a litany of statistics on the rising numbers of older adults and the disabilities they face to argue for long-term care.

"The prevention of superimposed crippling conditions and maintenance of functional capacity in the disabled and infirm elderly patients is one of the primary responsibilities of physicians in a society which is faced with the problems of the continued accumulation of such persons," Dacso wrote.[9] He summarized a set of "comprehensive medical services" to address problems like osteoporosis, contractures, and atrophy and to preserve physical and intellectual function.

Doctors committed to using science to improve the lives of their elderly patients knew they could provide better care for their patients, but they were practicing in a country that had adopted the cruel belief that federal support for "centrally coordinated" and "comprehensive" medical services for the elderly would cause us to surrender to the enemy.

Reagan kept on fighting. In 1962, he switched from the Democratic to the Republican Party and in 1967 won his first race for office as the governor of California.

In name, design, audience, and rhetoric, Operation Coffee Cup is risible (the AMA Woman's Auxiliary members were reminded "not to confuse a senator with a representative"). It's a historical moment, however, that encapsulates how culture and political ideologies affect the ways we think about care for older adults.

America in 1961 was so afraid of communist takeover that it worried that paying doctors to care for older adults could lead to one. A married doctor was assumed to be a man whose wife took his name—Mrs. William Mackersie, Mrs. Leo Smith, and Mrs. James Morrison—and served him. Implicit in that role was the role of caregiver (and roles she was discouraged from taking, like being a doctor). Within a decade, however, culture began to change and what ensued was a fierce battle over the American family that left as casualties persons with Alzheimer's and their caregivers.

In November 1977 in Houston, Texas, at the same time that *Feminine Mystique* author Betty Friedan and tens of thousands of other Americans attended the National Women's Conference, across town at the Astro Arena some ten to fifteen thousand people gathered in counterprotest. The Pro-Life, Pro-Family Rally led by Phyllis Schlafly, who had transitioned from fighting liberalism and communism to leading the anti-feminist movement, decisively rejected the conference and its recommendations.

"Solidarity among feminists was not the same as solidarity among American women," writes the historian Marjorie Spruill in her study of those four days that changed the world.[10] Both sides left Houston energized to achieve their causes. Each side bundled together a set of positions and policies. Each was a mirror opposite of the other's positions and policies. None of them were negotiable.

The conference, for example, called for passage of the ERA amendment. The rally championed STOP ERA (Stop Taking Our Privileges). Schlafly warned that passage of the ERA would lead to women serving in combat.

Her "pro-family movement" argued for "family values" over "women's rights." Its positions included firm opposition to the expansion of social insurance programs that would cover the costs of so-called custodial or long-term care. These were labeled "welfare programs." They, like abortion and gay rights, were called a threat to the American family. Schlafly's success was notable. By the 1980s, "family values" was an organizing ideology for the Republican Party.

Democrat Bill Clinton's 1992 presidential victory opened a window of opportunity to achieving the long-term care social insurance program Hilda Pridgeon called for in her 1990 congressional testimony. Clinton's promise of "health care reform" included comprehensive long-term care social insurance.

The 1994 midterms smartly shut that window. The Republicans took decisive control of the House, nearly one-quarter of the Congress was replaced, committees had new chairs, and the Office of Technology Assessment was shuttered, leaving unfinished a report on how the federal government needed to address the problems of fractured and uncoordinated care for older adults with chronic disease. The Advisory Council on Alzheimer's Disease was disbanded. Health care reform was dead.

At the January 22, 1995, meeting of the board of directors at Le Méridien New Orleans Hotel, Stephen McConnell, who after Long Term Care 88 had become the Alzheimer's Association's first vice president for public policy in 1989, summarized the 1994 elections' implications for the association.

There is also a changing philosophy that stresses a balanced budget, smaller government, lower taxes, less "entitlement" spending [the scare quotes are original], a shift from federal to state government, and an emphasis on personal responsibility.[11]

The association, he concluded, faced a new environment with new challenges and opportunities. It needed to educate these newly elected congresspersons about Alzheimer's disease and the association's central issues—research and long-term care—and to develop strategies to advance those issues.

A dark narrative about America's senior citizens had seeped into policy-making discussions. The elderly were entitled "greedy geezers" riding about in golf carts at resorts, living off the largess of federal benefits.[12] They were a burden who needed to pay their own way. Such messaging challenged the association's efforts to rally congressional support for comprehensive long-term care.

As the nineties wore on, the association found itself in a kind of political trench warfare, devoting its efforts to protecting—not expanding—programs and settling for small victories instead of a massive and sustained increase to funding to the NIH for research and fundamental improvements to the delivery of health care to older adults with dementia.

Clear and consistent messaging was of utmost importance, and one key message was the answer to a simple question: how many people in the United States have Alzheimer's disease? This one number—what epidemiologists call prevalence—is the answer to: how big is the problem? It is *the* starting point for making the case for federal funding for research and care.

This one number is the denominator upon which federal dollars are divided. From the 1980s onward, the ratio of dollars per Alzheimer's patient showed how little was spent compared to the funds for research on cancer and cardiovascular disease. The prevalence number was the starting number to calculate the number of caregivers who desperately needed help. Their hours spent caregiving would show the cost of the disease and its billion-dollar impact on families and America. This one number was the fact to make the case to Congress and to America to spend millions if not billions of dollars more on Alzheimer's disease.

How many people have Alzheimer's disease? In a 1990 Alzheimer's Association public service announcement, the nation's most trusted reporter delivered the answer. Walter Cronkite reported: "Today, there are at least four million victims of Alzheimer's disease. But for almost every one of those victims, there is another, a husband or wife . . . a son or daughter . . . whose entire life changes with the demands of caregiving." This astonishing number, the result of a 1989 study funded by the NIA, doubled prior counts.

Unfortunately, this powerful message soon became not just scientifically but also politically contentious. "The Selling of Alzheimer's" was the cover title of the April 28, 1990, issue of the *National Journal*, a weekly newsmagazine that catered to Congress and Washington insiders. A sidebar story, "How Many Victims of Alzheimer's? . . . Numbers Are Subject to Dispute," reported how experts were debating the methods the investigators used to arrive at their count of 4 million victims.[13]

The number came from the results of a study of the population of East Boston, Massachusetts, published in *JAMA*.[14] For the association and the NIA this was very bad press. They struggled to explain to nonscientists the nuances of epidemiology and demography. Counting the number of people with Alzheimer's disease in fact wasn't as simple as adding up all the diagnoses that doctors made. Doctors notoriously under- or misdiagnosed it. Counting Alzheimer's prevalence required the work of researchers. Their methods were fraught with assumptions and their results subject to a variety of interpretations.

The 1984 diagnostic criteria for Alzheimer's disease closely linked the disease label to a diagnosis of dementia. The researchers' methods, however, didn't use a clinical diagnosis based on interviews with both an older adult and someone who knows the person well to determine that he or she had dementia and that the cause of the dementia was Alzheimer's disease. Instead, they used the results of surveys the older adult filled out and relatively brief in-home tests of the adult's cognition. Reliance on the scores on cognitive tests could label an older adult with "Alzheimer's disease" when in fact all she had was mild memory problems or just a bad day of cognitive testing. Remember, this was the era when Alzheimer's disease and dementia were tightly linked (no dementia, no Alzheimer's disease) and MCI hadn't yet been discovered. The study's result was therefore contested for misrepresenting the size of the Alzheimer's problem. Other NIA-funded studies used different methods and arrived at still large but notably lower prevalence estimates.

It is important to recognize that at the time of this heated dispute over how best to measure the prevalence of Alzheimer's disease, the disease was still quite young. If its recognition as common and life threatening is dated to Dr. Katzman's 1976 essay, it wasn't even twenty years old. The task before the Alzheimer's Association and the researchers at the NIA was to make the case to America—and especially to Congress—that funding for this common disease should be proportionate to its size and burden on the country, proportionate, for example, to other common and life-threatening diseases like cancer and heart disease. Disputes over prevalence were therefore politically devastating. There was also a need to keep America's attention, and Alzheimer's disease had notable competition.

At the same time that Alzheimer's was coming of age, so, too, was another equally young and frightening disease: the human immunodeficiency virus, or HIV, the cause of the deadly acquired immune deficiency syndrome, or AIDS. The first cases were reported in 1981.

Much like Alzheimer's disease, HIV/AIDS was slow to be recognized as a public health crisis that needed massive and sustained increases in funding for research and care, and, as it was recognized, the patients experienced notable, crushing stigmas. As the 1980s unfolded, however, the two diseases' stories radically diverged.

By the early 1990s, despite frustrating indifference on the part of the Reagan administration, HIV/AIDS gained great public attention. The infectious virus was an epidemic like the 1918–1919 influenza pandemic that had infected 500 million and killed 50 million people worldwide. In 1980, there were zero cases. Ten years later, the World Health Organization estimated that 8 to 10 million people were infected with HIV and 283,000 had developed AIDS.[15] Like influenza, young, previously healthy people were getting very sick, very quickly, and they were dying. They spoke up and demanded national action. America needed to immediately and massively increase federal research to discover ways to diagnose, treat, and prevent HIV/AIDS.

Alzheimer's advocates, in contrast, struggled to secure America's attention. The call to action that Alzheimer's disease is a common, deadly, and costly disease that America needs to massively increase research funding for got caught up in a tangle of vexing questions. Isn't it senility or just normal aging? What's the difference between Alzheimer's and dementia? How many people have it? Caregiving is just what families do, right?

The year 1993 marked an inflection point for HIV/AIDS. In that year, Congress authorized the NIH's Office of AIDS Research, established in 1988, to create a yearly trans-NIH research plan and to request directly from the president the amount of money needed to achieve the plan.

NIH researchers and advocates for persons with HIV/AIDS had been granted enormous fiscal discretion and authority. They were empowered to make a plan and then receive exactly as much money as they needed to execute it—and they used this power. Cancer researchers, as a result of the National Cancer Act of 1971, had similar authority to "bypass" the usual back-and-forth politics of congressional appropriations. These so-called bypass budgets were two notable exceptions to the dictum that Congress doesn't do "disease-of-the-month funding." By 1999, NIH funding for HIV/AIDS and cancer research was $1.8 billion and $3 billion, respectively.

In that same year, Alzheimer's research funding was $400 million. It was just one among the many diseases that received a slice of the congressional budget given to the NIH. Alzheimer's research funding followed the ups and downs of the overall NIH budget. It rose and fell as the economy rose and fell, administrations and Congress debated spending priorities, or an anguished and powerful congressperson such as Senator Hatfield pushed forward a one-time, earmarked appropriation.

As the twentieth century ended, the disease of the century remained a crisis without a national plan to address it. There were frustrating ironies. All agreed that Alzheimer's disease was a disease of the family, but an ideology of family values and a distaste for federal programs decisively thwarted progress to deliver care to the millions of patients and their families. They were collateral casualties in enduring Cold War battles that continued even after the Soviet empire collapsed in 1991. And one of those patients was President Ronald Reagan, who in November 1995 announced he had been diagnosed with Alzheimer's disease.

All agreed the disease was common, that Reagan and his wife, Nancy, were two among millions of patients and caregivers, but the question of how common people like them were was an elusive and indeterminate estimate. A 1996 United States General Accounting Office report added to the unease over a definitive answer of how many Americans had the disease. *Alzheimer's Disease: Estimates of the Prevalence in the United States* estimated there were not 4 million but instead 1.9 million people with Alzheimers disease. Even decades later, the NIA's 2019 answer to "how many Americans have Alzheimer's disease?" is qualified: "Estimates vary, but experts suggest that as many as 5.5 million Americans age 65 and older may have Alzheimer's."[16]

Hilda Pridgeon was at the board meeting in New Orleans where Steve McConnell presented his sobering analysis of the 1994 election. She also learned that since President Reagan's announcement, calls to the association's toll-free help line had increased by 200 percent. These calls were simple proof. Families like hers—the middle class, the neither rich nor poor—*still* needed help, but McConnell's analysis said their country was changing. It would be hard for families like hers to get help. Hilda had also changed. Like Reagan, who'd started out as a Democrat and then become a Republican, she, too, had switched her political affiliation. The lifelong Republican had become a Democrat.

15

HOPE IN A PILL

If these interventions were drugs, it is hard to believe that they would not be on the fast track to approval.
—Kenneth Covinsky and C. Bree Johnson,
"Envisioning Better Approaches for Dementia Care,"
Annals of Internal Medicine, 2006

ON TUESDAY, JULY 15, 1980, at half past ten in the morning, in room 4232 of the Dirksen Senate Office Building, the people of the United States of America met an Alzheimer's disease caregiver for the first time. The occasion was the joint hearing *Impact of Alzheimer's Disease on the Nation's Elderly*, before the Subcommittee on Aging of the US Senate's Committee on Labor and Human Resources and the Subcommittee on Labor, Health, Education, and Welfare of the House Committee on Appropriations.[1] The host, and the only congressperson present at the hearing, was the chair of the subcommittee on aging, Senator Thomas Eagleton of Missouri.

He explained that the hearing was intended "to analyze and take testimony on the impact of Alzheimer's disease and other dementias of aging on our society." He cited the "alarming statistics" of prevalence and cost (some 1.5 to 2.5 million Americans costing $60 billion annually), and then he invoked "the true cost of this silent epidemic. The loss of productive members of society, disruption of families, and loss of human dignity are incalculable drains on our society as a whole."

His opening remarks ended, he introduced the first witness, the first American to speak to her fellow Americans about living with Alzheimer's disease. She was Bobbie Glaze, one of the founding members of the Alzheimer's Disease and Related Disorders Association and the Minnesota-based self-help group Association for Alzheimer's and Related Diseases.

Glaze told a horror story. Life with the disease was "a funeral that never ends." Her husband was once "a handsome, vital, athletic man, a civic leader, a public speaker, a highly respected businessman." Now, she explained, he was "a statistic." It had been four years since he had spoken or recognized her. She, too, felt stripped of identity.

"I have a husband, but I speak of him in the past tense. I am not a divorcee; I am not a widow; but where do I fit?" she asked her fellow Americans.

Then she started at the beginning. She narrated their yearslong decline. It was their decline because, as he became more and more disabled, agitated, and withdrawn, they became impoverished and she, isolated.

Along the way were unremitting indignities. The neurologist delivered his diagnosis in the waiting room. *Diagnosis and adiosis.* Ignorance and indifference were the norm. "I was given no explanation of what Alzheimer's disease is, what to expect, how I might learn to cope, nor was I directed to someone who might be able to direct me in the monumental problems ahead."

They moved multiple times to increasingly smaller and simpler quarters. She was alone and wandering in a surreal world. "I felt no sense of belonging." She explained that she had become a "nonperson."

Slowly, though, as he lay dying in a VA hospital, she found meaning in the self-help group she formed with Hilda Pridgeon and the other women. She ended her testimony invoking their efforts. "Our families have lost, but we choose to continue. Perhaps our greatest loss is our spirit, for we have been degraded to a point of 'begging for help' when we are already shattered."

It was the saddest story.

When she finished, Senator Eagleton began what reads like a cross-examination. The former attorney general of Missouri asked her to explain the early telltale signs: How old was he? Had he been a golfer? He had. She'd given away boxes of trophies, she explained. He asked about periods of depression before the start of his first symptoms and the pace of his decline. Did he acknowledge his symptoms? And so on. Question after question. At times, the back-and-forth of question and answer—the pressing for dates and details—reads like a prosecutor trying to catch up a witness. Glaze was consistently forthcoming, replying with intimate details—"I was becoming very lonely . . . there was no communication between us"—and she was polite, addressing the senator as "sir."

The senator's twenty minutes of questioning had laid plain the horror of life with Alzheimer's disease. Glaze's husband—she neither spoke his name nor was asked it by the senator—was "like an infant." A nameless, mute, bedfast man.

For Eagleton, this must have been personal and painful. He knew the pain of life with a stigmatizing illness. In 1972, he'd withdrawn as the Democratic nominee for vice president after his diagnosis of major depression and treatment with electroconvulsive therapy became public.

The senator concluded his questioning.

"My final question," he announced. "If you knew back in 1968, what, through experience and personal, diligent effort, you have learned since 1968 to date—if you knew back in 1968 that which you now know today—what would you or should you have done with respect to your husband back in 1968?"

This was Bobbie Glaze's moment. The senator had set her up. He'd given her a national platform to make sense of her and her husband's sufferings. She could tell America what everyone should or shouldn't do. And so she spoke.

"I am sure I would have sought help quicker, but I cannot believe that that would have been any help at this point, because," she explained, "there is no treatment." There was, in short, nothing she would do differently. Her message was pure hopelessness.

The witness who followed repeated her loud, reverberating lamentation. Jerry Stone described how the personality deteriorates before body and then body deteriorates in "mysterious but ineluctable ways." Only then was treatment available. He described his "hospital at home" staffed by full-time nurses and housekeepers who tended to his wife's physical needs.

The rich and the poor together shared the same despair. These two caregivers only had treatments for "the physical aspects of the disease," such as antibiotics for lung and urinary infections, diapers for "double incontinence," blenders to puree food, and suction to clear a mouth full of secretions. What they desperately wanted was a treatment for the mind, a pill that would preserve the person—or even better—bring back the person who was lost. This would be a reason to seek a diagnosis. After Glaze spoke of her helplessness, she did invoke hope. "I am very thrilled and excited about what is being done in research, though, for the future."

Six years later, in November 1986, the future was now. Researchers announced a breakthrough discovery.

Thanksgiving 1986 came early. The lead article of the November 13 *New England Journal of Medicine* was "Oral Tetrahydroaminoacridine in Long-Term Treatment of Senile Dementia, Alzheimer Type," a study of the effects of treatment with the drug tetrahydroaminoacridine, or tacrine for short, on seventeen people in "the middle and late stages of suspected Alzheimer's disease."[2] William Summers and colleagues described their results as "dramatic." "One subject was able to resume more of her homemaking tasks, one was able to resume employment on a part-time basis, and one retired subject was able to resume playing daily golf." An accompanying editorial described the study as "a triumph for the scientific method" and praised it and the "rational path" of studies that led up to it as "a positive reflection of our nation's investment in science." Tacrine was exhilarating news. It was the pill Bobbie Glaze was hoping for, the treatment that might restore her husband. She could, once again, speak of him in the present tense.

Seven more years of research and three FDA reviews would pass before tacrine became Cognex, sold by Parke-Davis. It was a challenging medication to take, requiring four-times-a-day dosing of increasingly higher doses and careful monitoring for liver toxicity and tolerance of side effects of nausea and diarrhea.

In 1996, however, these challenges largely vanished. The FDA approved a new cholinesterase inhibitor called donepezil. Pfizer and Eisai, joint owners of the medication, named it Aricept and trademarked it: "Therapy to remember." The once-a-day pill required no blood tests and caused fewer upsetting side effects. Advertisements in medical journals showed an elderly man and woman standing arm in arm on a sun-dappled pebble-paved lane. "Help their walk down memory lane last a little longer. Enhance cognitive function."

Cognex, Aricept, and later Exelon and Razadyne were all members of a class of drugs called cholinesterase inhibitors. Their effect was to increase levels of a protein called acetylcholine in the brain.

Their discovery as treatments for Alzheimer's disease was the convergence of two lines of research. The first was the finding that an anticholinergic drug, that is, a drug that blocked brain acetylcholine, caused a person to experience memory loss. Anesthesiologists, for example, exploited this effect when they administered the anticholinergic scopolamine to women during labor and delivery. Researchers who gave the drug to cognitively unimpaired older adults reported declines in memory tests that resembled the impaired performance of patients with Alzheimer's disease dementia. The second finding was the work of neuropathologists. Several of the regions of the brain affected by Alzheimer's disease were dependent on acetylcholine for cell-to-cell communication.

Together, these findings and the results of studies of Cognex, Aricept, and similar drugs supported what came to be called the cholinergic hypothesis of Alzheimer's disease, or more simply the statement at medical conferences that Alzheimer's disease was a disease of cholinergic neurotransmission. Experts used the analogy of how Parkinson's disease was a disorder of dopamine. After taking a dopamine pill, the patient's tremor ceased and gait once again was smooth and steady. Similarly, after taking Cognex or Aricept a patient with Alzheimer's disease showed improvements in her memory and other cognitive abilities. Six years after the founding of the national Alzheimer's Association and the NIA's commitment to Alzheimer's disease, researchers had discovered a treatment for the disease.

Aricept was a reason to go to the doctor. It was hope in a pill.

Or was it?

On January 11, 2015, Dr. Bruno Dubois was caught on a hot mic.[3] Dubois, a professor of neurology at the University Salpêtrière Hospital in Paris and director of its Memory and Alzheimer's Disease Institute, was being interviewed by a reporter from the radio station France Inter for a story on Alzheimer's disease. Dubois was an internationally recognized Alzheimer's researcher. His work included studies of cholinesterase inhibitors and developing diagnostic guidelines for Alzheimer's disease that have come to be known as the "Dubois criteria."

Toward the end of the interview, thinking the reporter had turned off the microphone, he opened up.

In translation from the French, DuBois told the interviewer, "It's a pity that we are . . . There are so many things more important than talking about medications that are useless. I know well that they're useless, but . . . but not only do I know that they're useless, but I'm obliged to say that they are a little useful because otherwise it loses the trust of the patients who take them."

"*Ils ne servent à rien.*" Translation: "They're useless."

These words were broadcast throughout France.

The drugs he'd studied and prescribed, that millions of patients had been prescribed since 1993, were in large part clinically useless. His candor was unusual, but his message, while exaggerated, was not. In 2016, the NIA issued a call for researchers to apply for funds to set up a national consortium of clinical trial centers to study treatments for Alzheimer's disease. In the preamble, the NIA summed up that current treatments "have demonstrated only modest effect in modifying the clinical symptoms for relatively short periods. None has shown a clear therapeutic effect on disease progression."[4]

In fact, from its beginning, controversy vexed the cholinergic hypothesis. A lot more went on in the brain of a person with Alzheimer's disease than the loss of cholinergic neurons, and the hypothesis offered no explanation for the fundamental problem. Brain cells are dying.

In the years after the 1986 Summers study, multiple clinical trials of tacrine failed to replicate his dramatic findings. Instead, they showed modest improvements on measures of cognition. The effects on measures of daily life, such a homemaking or playing golf, were difficult to demonstrate and, in some studies, not detected. Clinicians and researchers debated the medication's benefits.

These debates flared at FDA hearings over Parke-Davis's application to approve tacrine. Twice, the FDA rejected the drug. At the third hearing, the one that resulted in approval, one of the advisory board members, the neurologist Leonard Berg of Washington University in Saint Louis, summed up the field's ambivalence over the drugs.[5]

Berg engaged in an imaginary clinical encounter with a patient and a family over whether to take tacrine. "You can't expect it to do very much for you. There is a very small chance that it will help you a good deal; there is a little better chance that there will be some measurable improvement that some people might say is clinically significant. How important that degree of improvement is depends on your perception, not on my perception, and we know there are many people who will be delighted and see as very important something that many of us around the table would consider of little or no impact."

"*Some measurable improvement that some people might say is clinically significant . . . depends on your perception, not on my perception.*" Berg's words reveal the problem.

If the topic was a drug to treat Parkinson's disease, he would've been more plainspoken. He would've discussed faster walking, fewer falls, and less shaking. Each of these is easy to measure and to explain to a patient and family. Talking about Alzheimer's disease is not as clear and coherent.

Alzheimer's experts like him had figured out a scientifically valid language to talk to each other about the benefit of the drugs. Their vocabulary was the result of cognitive testing, the Alzheimer's Disease Assessment Scale, or ADAS, a complicated measure of cognition that took some thirty minutes to administer and so was not used in clinical practice. The problem was how to translate scores on this cognitive test into the day-to-day lives of patients. The controversy was about a complex and nuanced matter.

Summers's short narratives displayed the challenge. The patients' stories were deeply personal and captured in diverse activities like housekeeping, golf, and part-time work. They revealed the complexity of measuring the extent to which a drug has allowed a person to self-determine her life, to exercise her autonomy. The field settled on a semistructured interview that would capture the personal and particular aspects of each patient's life. When performed over time, the interview produced a short narrative that enabled the clinician to judge whether it showed overall improvement, no change, or decline. The interview came to be called the clinician's global impression of change, or more simply, the global.

But whom should the clinician interview for these narratives? The disputes over the answer to this question reveal why, for as common as Alzheimer's disease is, it remains an enigmatic disease. There was great skepticism, for example, about interviewing the patient. Their minimization of functional problems risked not detecting an effect. Or, if the drug did work and the patient improved, she might become more frustrated with her milder but now more annoying cognitive problems. As a consequence, while her cognitive scores improved, her global would get worse. The caregiver, people like Bobbie Glaze, seemed the obvious person to talk to, but a caregiver like her would bring into the interview problems such as side effects, her own distress, and perhaps exaggerated reports of improvement. Hope in a pill—that is, the placebo effect—risked showing improvement when in fact no improvement was happening.

The field settled on a strategy. A drug to treat Alzheimer's disease was effective if a study showed two results: it improved both cognition measured using the ADAS and a clinician's global rating with caregiver input. That second result was what Berg was trying to explain when he talked about "some measurable improvement that some people might say is clinically significant . . . depends on your perception, not on my perception."

Most clinical researchers agreed that studies using the dual endpoints of cognition and a global showed that cholinesterase inhibitors had a benefit over and above taking a placebo. The debate that would dominate the field, and the debate that Dubois was tipping his hand to twenty-two years after the FDA approved Cognex, was whether these benefits were worth the resources being spent to achieve them.

Among researchers, the answer was an enthusiastic yes. The cholinergic hypothesis made Alzheimer's disease a disease that could be studied not just in brains preserved in the labs of neuropathologists but also in the living. It was a disease that neurologists and psychiatrists, clinicians and investigators like Dubois, could make into a career. Grants and, for some researchers, lucrative corporate consulting followed.

For clinicians, patients, and society, a favorable balance of benefits to risks and costs wasn't as evident. Many patients and caregivers experienced an upsetting oddity. They received their diagnosis at the pharmacy because the physician hadn't told them what the drug was intended to treat. Most physicians simply lacked the skills and time to properly disclose a diagnosis. Diagnostic disclosure occurred instead when the pharmacist provided the patient and family information about the drug. Most significantly, many caregivers reported that their relative experienced minimal if any improvement on the drugs.

In countries such as Australia, Canada, the United Kingdom, and France, where a drug's cost is included in decisions about drug approval or whether to include the drug in a national formulary, the cholinesterase inhibitors were a policy maker's nightmare. The United Kingdom's independent institute responsible for providing evidence-based guidance on the value of health and social care got caught up in years of controversy and even litigation over its decisions to limit the drugs to patients whose dementia fit within a certain range of severity and showed response to the treatment. France essentially gave up paying for them, announcing in May 2018 that the funds spent on them were better used to provide care interventions.[6]

There's a coda to hope in a pill. The Summers study was invalid. Five years after its publication, the *New England Journal of Medicine* published the results of an FDA investigation of his study. The agency found significant errors in the design and conduct of the study. It appeared that the paper was not so much a scientific report as merely a series of anecdotes.

Arnold Relman, the journal's editor, explained in an editorial that reviewers in fact did express concerns about the study's design, but he defended the decision to publish the report, quoting one of the reviewers: "The author's results should encourage further studies, which in itself is reason for publication."[7] Like Dubois's candid admission, this was an unusual display of what scientists were truly thinking *and* feeling.

The "triumph of the scientific method" in fact was the desire for a treatment for an untreatable disease. The editors and the peer reviewers had in effect relaxed the standards for review and critique of the study. They were as human, flawed, and desperate as the patients and families they served. Dr. Relman concluded his editorial: "We can only hope that out of this controversy will come some real advances in the management of a common and dreadful disease." He offered hope not in a pill but in controversy.

So then why did the drugs Dr. Dubois described as "useless" continue to be studied and prescribed? The answer to this question comes from the system that branded the results and then marketed them to clinicians, patients, and caregivers. For a time, the cholinesterase inhibitors had a robust business model that began with both private and public funding for research to discover and test them, followed by regulatory review of their benefits and harms. Most important was a highly coordinated and organized system to promote their prescription.

I recall frequent visits from pharmaceutical representatives asking me about "my experiences" with the drug the salesperson was promoting and whether I needed any support or funds for educational events. The sales representative for Razadyne gave me a package of Razzles, a candy that once chewed transforms into gum ("Razzles for Razadyne!!!" was her note to me). I received (but declined) invitations to advisory boards such as the one Dr. Dubois served on.

By 2002, the ads for Aricept showed an elderly woman reading a book to a young child. "You see it as maintaining cognitive function. She sees it as a bedtime story." The message was a pivot from the earlier messages of improvement. The new message was that these drugs slow the disease and so should be started early and not discontinued. Liquid and patch forms ensured dosing to patients who either refused to take pills or were so impaired they could no longer coordinate a swallow. Private insurance and, starting in 2003, Medicare, paid for these.

In 2006, the *Annals of Internal Medicine* published the results of two Alzheimer's disease intervention studies.[8,9] Their results were notably impressive.

Not only patients but also their caregivers showed improvements in measures of health, well-being, and satisfaction. Burden was decreased. Social support increased.

Both tested what are called behavioral interventions. One assessed if a health care professional, typically a social worker, could help a patient and family manage and organize a typical day. The social worker would help the caregiver identify activities the patient enjoys and that could be done together with the patient, such as cooking or going for a walk or how to set up alerts on financial accounts the person has access to. The other tested an intervention to train caregivers to identify and address common behavioral and functional problems, for example, to know what is apathy (a lack of initiative), how it differs from depression (a low mood), and how to address it by asking the person not to choose whether to do an activity but instead to pick between one of two activities or simply to state that it's time to do an activity rather than ask the person if she wants to do it.

Bobbie Glaze lamented in her testimony to the people of the United States that "I was given no explanation of what Alzheimer's disease is, what to expect, how I might learn to cope, nor was I directed to someone who might be able to direct me in the monumental problems ahead." These were precisely the interventions she needed. And yet, twenty-six years later, even after these studies were published, caregivers like her were still not receiving them.

An accompanying editorial summed up the problem: "If these interventions were drugs, it is hard to believe that they would not be on the fast track to approval. The magnitude of benefit and quality of evidence supporting these interventions considerably exceed those of currently approved pharmacologic therapies for dementia."[10] The "approved pharmacologic therapies" were the cholinesterase inhibitors. The problem then and still today in America is that an effective intervention is not a treatment unless it has a business model.

Behavioral interventions, however, aside from grant support from the NIA, foundations, and state agencies, were without a system to disseminate, brand, promote, or sustain them. It is this disparity between the two systems—one financially robust, the other fragmented and uncoordinated—that is at the heart of the Alzheimer's crisis.

This disparity leads to a perverse competition that pits cure against care. From the beginning of the founding of the Alzheimer's movement, researchers, NIA officials, and the Alzheimer's Association would compare Alzheimer's disease to polio. It was an epidemic that without a cure will leave America caring for millions of disabled older adults. We didn't fight polio by building iron lungs, they argued. We discovered a vaccine. So, too, with Alzheimer's disease. We could build more nursing homes or we could discover a cure.

Forty years later, there is no cure. Caregivers are in similar positions that Bobbie Glaze and Hilda Pridgeon were in, and they still complain they receive no explanation of what Alzheimer's disease is, how it differs from dementia, what to expect, and how to cope with the monumental problems that lie ahead.

There is a historical irony to the tension we create between care and cure. For a time, Parke-Davis tried to settle it. They created "Alzheimer's Family Care."

The cover of the program's brochure explained "free enrollment" for patients taking four-times-a-day Cognex. Beneath the toll-free number to call to enroll the brochure explained: "You will be assigned a personal Nurse Counselor, available by telephone, and have access to educational and support services." Care and cure were, for a time, united, but when Cognex faded from the market, so, too, did family care.

PART 3

· · · · · · · · · · ·

LIVING WELL IN

THE HOUSE OF ALZHEIMER'S

Every time a physician sees a patient and asks, "What can I do for you, what is wrong, what is the problem?" he or she is professing to two things: one is competence and the other is to use that competence in the best interests of the patient.
—Edmund Pellegrino, "Professionalism, Profession and the Virtues of the Good Physician," *Mount Sinai Journal of Medicine*, 2002

Just as we lower elevated cholesterol levels to reduce the risk of myocardial infarction, the hope is that one day we might be able to treat asymptomatic individuals with brain amyloidosis to delay or even to prevent further A-beta [amyloid] accumulation and clinical symptoms of Alzheimer's disease.
—Pascual Sánchez-Juan and Sudha Seshardi, "Dynamic Measurements of β-amyloid Accumulation: The Early Effect of APOE," *Neurology*, 2017

16

THE EXTRAORDINARY
ORDINARY

To everything there is a season, and a time to every purpose under the
heaven.

—Ecclesiastes 3:1

IN THE MONTHS after her husband Darren's death, as Beverly was starting her
new life alone in a new and smaller home, she arrived at an understanding. The
moment when their life as a couple began to become untethered from its ordinary cycles, from the fifty-five years of ups and downs, was during the drive
home to their house in Scranton, Pennsylvania. They were returning from the
appointment with his primary care doctor. Darren insisted that Beverly swear
not to tell anyone about "it." "Not the kids, not the gang at the club. Nobody."

They stared ahead. The gray road was better company than each other.

"Why?" she asked.

After a while he spoke. "Because, it's nothing. I'm fine."

And for a few weeks, he might have been right. Some days felt like they
were back to their usual ordinary life. She slept better. He tinkered in his
workshop. The visit to the doctor was quick—Darren said they always were—
but the news helped her. The "it" she'd raised with the doctor, Darren's
withdrawal—the silent suppers, the lack of affection, his indifference to the
pieces she brought home from the clay studio—were not what she had feared.
What she had feared was that he was depressed or had a brain tumor or was
having an affair. But the doctor had simply called it a mild memory problem.

The doctor prescribed Aricept and for a few months, maybe—it was hard to tell—it seemed to help, but then she wasn't so sure. Her days became over-whelming with chores and she felt entirely responsible for keeping the house in order. Darren insisted on managing his medications and their bills, and she wasn't sure the bills were being paid correctly or that he was remember-ing to take his pills. Talking with him about these—or any of the other prob-lems she was noticing—was a fight about things he didn't seem to accept as true. He just jumped to conclusions.

At the one-year follow-up visit with his doctor, she felt uncomfortable talking about these problems in front of Darren, and so she kept them to herself. All that she could say in the little time with the doctor was that Dar-ren's memory didn't seem any better on the pill. The doctor recommended he start using a brain game.

"What about these?" Darren shook a paper bag. The bottles of pills rattled. Their labels were icons of hope: Brain Pill, Lumonol, OptiMind, and Focus Factor. The monthly expense was near $200.

The doctor shrugged. "Couldn't hurt. See you in six months."

She didn't tell the doctor that she felt isolated and Darren's repetitious questions were maddening or that her hope for travels to visit family was put on hold indefinitely and her life was turning into a lonely, homebound, cash-strapped nightmare.

How could she tell him? The doctor only saw them together, spoke only to Darren, and essentially ignored her. She'd given up the clay studio. Most of their friends at the club had drifted away. Her life seemed reduced to fight or flight. Sometimes, in her darkest moods, she dreamed that her husband, the father of their three children—none of whom talked about Dad's memory problems because no one was allowed to talk about them, he'd made that clear on the car trip—would die.

When I saw Darren and Beverly Johnson at his new patient visit at the Penn Memory Center, they were both suffering. Instead of the six-month visit with his doctor, they came to see me (having waited some eight months for the appointment). Her answer to my opening question, "What's the problem? How can I help you?" went on for some five minutes. The essence of the prob-lem, though, was in her first words. "His doctor said it was a memory prob-lem, possibly dementia, but a mild form, possibly aging, but I'm wondering if it isn't Alzheimer's. I really don't know what it is. But whatever it is, the doc-tor keeps saying its mild, but it seems more severe to me."

It was her answer to my follow-up question—"So what's the goal of this visit?"—that got to the heart of the matter.

"What's wrong with him and what can we do about it?"

The Johnsons' new patient visit lasted one and a half hours. The center grants me time and space to separate the patient and family into different rooms and then effortlessly bring them back together. I also worked with essential staff. In a quiet windowless room, a technician performed thirty minutes of cognitive testing on Mr. Johnson before I met with him. I used these test results and his history to conclude that he did have dementia and my leading diagnosis of the cause was the common "amnestic form" of Alzheimer's disease, meaning the form that has early and notable problems with memory and executive function with, for now, a relative sparing of his language and spatial abilities.

To deliver this diagnosis and formulate his treatment plan, I measured one of the most important of his cognitive abilities, his insight, or awareness of his cognitive and functional problems. My goal was to discover an essential part of his identity. How aware is he that he is in fact a patient?

I began measuring this right from the start of my private time with him. "I'm Dr. Karlawish. Welcome to the Penn Memory Center. How can I help you? Why are you here?"

"Memory." He shrugged. "It's shot."

"Thank God," I thought. These two have a chance. I was thankful because the more he was aware of his problem, the more he perceived something was wrong with his memory and at least accepted that it was causing troubles with daily activities, the better my colleagues and I could help him and his wife live as ordinary a life as possible. He'd be more open to talking about his problems and taking up suggestions on how he and his wife should manage them. In contrast, I knew that the more he perceived himself as "fine" or "doing OK for my age," the more my colleagues and I would need to help his family orchestrate a world that simultaneously conformed to this reality and gave him the interventions he needed, sometimes to the degree that caregivers engage in elaborate loving deceptions to provide care. Most patients reside somewhere along a continuum defined on the one end by complete awareness (I once knew a couple who kept a notebook detailing her problems; they lived by the motto "we live in the facts") and, on the other, complete indifference or denial.

My goal was to arrive at a common understanding of the facts. This begins at the close of the new patient visit when we are finally together again: patient, family, and I reunited in one room. With my clipboard before me, I paraphrased back what Mr. Johnson told me about why he was here.

Beverly looked at him. "Really?"

"Yeah," he said.

I continued. "And you said that this memory problem's not really getting in the way of your life, that you're still in your wood shop." Beverly nodded. "And doing OK with the bills." Beverly shook her head. "I know your wife agrees with you about the memory problem. She told me that you've been having memory problems, but I think she sees them a bit differently than you. I don't mean to cause dissension here, but she's noticed you've missed some bills."

"I have?" he asked her.

"You have," she replied.

"Maybe I forgot." And then he laughed.

The visit ended with Mr. Johnson agreeing that he wanted to look into what was causing these problems. I ordered an MRI of his brain and concluded that I'd see them back in a few weeks for the diagnostic follow-up visit. "We'll go over what's going on and come up with a plan to take care of the problems you all have told me about."

They thanked me. And then they departed for the long drive home to Scranton.

It was at the diagnostic follow-up visit that my colleagues and I began our interventions. Beverly and Darren Johnson, Felicia Greenfield, the social worker, and I gathered in an exam room. I introduced Felicia and reminded them that after our time together, they would meet with her. Our goal was to help the Johnsons do whatever extraordinary things they needed to do to live as ordinary lives as they could. And then I started where I'd left off four weeks earlier. I summarized the problems and then I asked Mr. Johnson the question. "Would you like to find out what is causing these problems?"

This was his last chance. This was his last opportunity to remain ignorant, to keep the problem hidden, to never talk about "it."

"Yeah, doc, that's why we're here."

"Well, what do you think is causing these problems?"

This question bothers some patients. They come to me for answers, not reflective questions. I offer the question, though, as a kind of probe, to assess what they know or don't know about what might be causing their cognitive problems.

"Aging?" he said.

"Aging can cause memory problems, troubles finding words, but this, I think, this isn't aging but a disease. Do you have any thoughts of the disease that might be causing this?"

He shook his head.

"Have you ever heard of Alzheimer's disease?"

I was of course leading him to the truth as best as I know it, leading him to the simple statement that I would also write down on the discharge instruction sheet and the billing form. At the end of the visit, I would swap out the diagnosis I entered at his new patient visit—memory loss—with his new diagnosis: Alzheimer's disease.

He told me he'd heard of it.

"That's what you have."

What followed was a discussion of the diagnosis and the stage of the disease. I'd give them the prognosis—that is, what to expect in the future—if they asked. They didn't, and so I reserved that topic for later visits, after they'd learned more about the diagnosis, the stage, and how to care for each other.

They asked about treatments. He was already on Aricept. For some physicians, drugs are the end of the conversation. For me, they're just the beginning. I needed to prescribe ways of living. I framed this with a message: "You want to put together a day that is safe, social, and engaged," and I explained how this required a balancing. A typical day cannot be completely safe and also entirely social and fully engaged. Each has to yield a bit to the others. With that framing, I pressed them on his typical day, on the problem of his managing the money and his medications. "With a diagnosis of Alzheimer's disease, I have to urge you to set up a system to make sure you're not having problems doing these. It's simply not safe to do them alone."

He seemed to agree but also stated, yet again, that he was doing OK.

I wasn't going to challenge him directly but neither was I going to give in. "Maybe you forgot you made a mistake."

He smiled.

"What about these?" he asked. He rattled the bag full of Brain Pill, Lumonol, OptiMind, and Focus Factor.

As I inspected each bottle, I explained how some of these brain supplements have been studied, most not, to discover if they help patients with Alzheimer's disease. The bottom line was the data just aren't there to show that they slow the disease. So, too, I explained about the brain game he was trying to play.

They weren't alone. In 2016, Lumos Labs paid a $2 million fine to the Federal Trade Commission and agreed to cease advertising that regular use of

Lumosity, their online brain-training program, delays age-related declines in memory and protects against mild cognitive impairment, dementia, and Alzheimer's disease until it had reliable scientific evidence to support such claims. Brain games, like supplements, are a big business with annual revenues of billions of dollars. Scant evidence, however, supported the manufacturers' claims of inspiring benefits for brain health. It was time to put the brakes on the hype. But the hype was saying something. People—people like Beverly and Darren Johnson and their children at risk of dementia or caregiving—were desperate.

"How much do you pay a month?"

"A hundred or so. . . ."

"That's money better spent on things you two can do together. Like a nice meal out."

Much of what I was doing was setting them up for their meeting with Felicia, the social worker, a meeting without me, where the discussion would be what might constitute an ordinary, safe, social, and engaged day.

At the new patient visit, Beverly filled out a questionnaire about her experiences with the common challenges in caring for a person with dementia—such as repetitious questions, too many jobs and chores, feeling alone, and troubles communicating—and with each challenge, the degree of distress she was experiencing. Her answers allowed Felicia to tailor her conversation with them—and later a private conversation with Beverly—about their plan of care. Within a few weeks, the Johnsons were executing this plan.

Once a week, they did the laundry and set up his pillbox, and once a month they reviewed the bills. Within a few months, Darren lost interest in these activities and so Beverly took them over. The same happened with the driving. For nearly a year, he helped her in the kitchen. A retired machinist, his skills with a chopping knife and dish washing remained well intact. They started to go to concerts and to a coffee shop at a bookstore, him to look at people, she to read.

These activities were intentional. They were the results of her caregiver training class at the Memory Center. For two hours a week for six weeks, she learned how to be a better caregiver. Like most caregivers, she needed to learn how to do things together with the patient. She was given a paper and pencil. "Make a list of activities you and Darren can do together, even the simplest, like making lunch or taking a walk." That done, she was assigned homework: pick one, do it for one week, and then pick another one.

She learned skills. We taught her how to ask family or friends for help and how to cope if they declined, how to use meditation to calm her racing thoughts about the future. She learned how to manage his repetitious questions. The trick was to balance properly his abilities and disabilities. He had problems with memory, attention, and concentration, but his ability to feel emotions of fear and joy was intact. So, too, was his ability to imagine.

He was therefore likely to remember fragments of emotionally charged events, like an upcoming visit to see me. The more she delayed telling him about those kinds of events, the fewer would be the number of days when he asked over and over about the event. And when he did repeat the question—"When are we going to see Dr. Karlawish?"—we taught her to tap into his creativity and ask him a question to prompt his imagination. "What would make for an entertaining visit to Dr. Karlawish?"

She was learning how to manage time, task, and truth, to negotiate how to do everything she possibly could for him while at the same time living her life.

The class, the brochures and web pages, the visits, emails, and telephone conversations with the Memory Center collectively gave Beverly and Darren Johnson knowledge and skills, and for about three years, our prescriptions of ways of living maintained their day-to-day well-being. But in time things began to fall apart. He could no longer read the newspaper. Television programs and his wood shop were confusing. He stuck to Beverly like a pet. She found this maddening. And then he became frightening. At the end of the day, he left her side to pace up and down the stairs and close the drapes. Home wasn't working for Mr. Johnson.

She called me panicked. "He needs something to calm him. A tranquilizer of some sort."

I agreed. He did need a new treatment, and so I drew up a prescription: not for a tranquilizer but for adult day care.

Of all the treatments for dementia, this is the most misunderstood. The confusion starts with the name. In Pennsylvania, where I practice, the state refers to the service as "older adult daily living centers." The trade association that represents the providers of the treatment calls it adult day services. The recipients of the care are called clients, participants, or members.

The center I prescribed, Main Line Adult Day Center, describes itself as an "adult day care center" and the twenty-six people who attend it are "members." That center is a two-story house set along a suburban street. The front lawn leads up to a porch and a side driveway to the back entrance. It is all quite homelike, but inside is a lobby with a chest-high counter that resembles a physician's waiting room and a room equipped with basic medical equipment. And yet the space is neither a medical nor a rehabilitation facility. The multiple names for the place, the people who attend it, and the hybridized architecture denote something distinct, a therapeutic activity program for adults with cognitive and behavioral impairments.

Families often react to my calling it a treatment as though I'm kidding them, that I'm playing with the idea of treatment. I'm insistent, however. I'm not joking. For many patients, a therapeutic activity program is a far more effective and safer treatment than the medications prescribed for agitation. It reduces agitation and stress not only in the people who attend it but also in the family members I persuade to try it.[1]

I insist that before they reject the idea, they at least visit a center. In these places, I explain, every activity has a purpose and the staff are mission driven to achieve that purpose. They're typically trained in occupational or recreation therapy and how to communicate with persons with dementia, a skill that relies on listening to emotions more so than exact words. They're not in it for the money.

The days are a scheduled succession of activities beginning with breakfast and then exercise, word games such as using the letters of a long word ("astrophysics") to spell shorter ones ("chat," "sit," "spot," etc.), singing, and trivia. Volunteers play music or bring in pets. Among all the activities, one stands out. It is the activity that captures all of what is intended at an adult day program.

Beanbag toss.

Pam Barton, the director of Main Line Adult Day Center, explained why.[2] All who can stand, stand up and, one at a time, take position at a spot on the floor. A few feet before them is a target like a giant dartboard. Bags in hand, the person tosses one at a time, aiming for the high-scoring bull's-eye and earning fewer points when a bag lands elsewhere on the target. Score is kept, sometimes by a member who volunteers.

"We need to encourage some more than others to get up out of the chair and move to that spot. We want to get people moving, which helps to focus them on the activity. It works on balance, endurance, muscle strength, and coordination."

It is an activity that incorporates all of what the center intends to treat their members: physical, cognitive, and social engagement. "It might look like a very simple activity, but it helps get people up and moving again. We give out points and write them on a board so they pay attention and follow the score. They cheer on the winners and encourage each other. They have a lot of fun with it."

Beanbag toss, the most effective intervention, the one the participants enjoy the most, that even the most amnestic members remember and tell their families, is also the most stigmatized. Barton explains, "The families think, 'Oh my gosh, that's so juvenile.'"

I addressed this stigma in my prescription for Mr. Johnson. He was a different person who therefore needed different kinds of activities. Once again, I made the case for the extraordinary ordinary. I prompted Mrs. Johnson to reflect on their past ways of living. Surely they didn't spend each and every hour of every single day of the week together? He was at work while she was at home. Why should life be any different now? Give it a try for at least two days a week for at least a three-week trial. I appealed that it was far safer than the tranquilizers she'd asked me to prescribe.

Why should life be any different now?

Did I really mean that? Was I using cruel irony? Life was very different for the Johnsons. Out of Mrs. Johnson's caregiver class, a support group had developed. The members were all women. They met monthly, and as their relationships with their husbands fragmented—one day Darren asked Beverly if they were married—the women developed bonds that filled the gaps in their relationships. At Darren's funeral, when she spoke of him, she didn't cry. She'd done that years before. When she spoke of her "support sisters," she wept.

I learned of Mr. Johnson's death from a letter Mrs. Johnson sent me several weeks after he died. I had last seen them two and a half years before. The travel from Scranton to Philadelphia was too much and besides, we'd done all we could. She'd learned how to care for him and had assembled a network of support. I promised them that they'd hear from us should a new medication be discovered, but in the years to follow, several of the promising drugs under study, drugs that targeted amyloid and therefore articulated the hope of slowing the disease, would fail. There were no new medications to prescribe. She had skills and a plan for what to expect in the future.

At least she thought she did.

One Friday afternoon, while stepping off a curb, Mr. Johnson fell. The emergency room diagnosed a hip fracture and he was admitted to the orthopedic surgery service. Three days later (it was the weekend and so he waited until Monday), his fractured right hip joint was repaired with a chrome and cobalt implant. One year later, that implant lay among his ashes. The days in between were a story of extraordinary but sadly all too ordinary disasters: the best of care and the worst of care.

Within a day of his hospitalization in his semiprivate room, he developed confusion, asking over and over where he was and crying out for help to the people he heard from his roommate's television broadcast. An antipsychotic was prescribed. The chemical restraint worked, of course. His crying out ceased, but he couldn't stand. He grew weak. Urinary retention developed and so a catheter was inserted. He yanked at it. He developed a fever and a drop in blood pressure that sent him to the ICU for a day. Broadspectrum antibiotics were prescribed. He developed diarrhea. He had trouble swallowing and was observed coughing while eating the scant amount he did eat. A speech therapist judged him an "aspiration risk," and so his food was switched to "honey-thickened liquids." His mouth grew pasty and dry. He ate even less. His skinny purple arms looked like he'd been beaten. After two weeks, the husk of a man was ready to leave the hospital.

A rehabilitation unit accepted him for "subacute rehab," but within three days he developed a fever and became restless so was sent back to hospital, though to a different one than where he had his surgery. His bladder was unable to drain urine. The cycle repeated itself: confusion, agitation, sedation, fever, cough, thickened liquids, diarrhea. New problems burst forth like thunderstorms. A knee became red and swollen. The skin around his lower back broke down into an ulcer. Mrs. Johnson lost count of the names and kinds of doctors.

In time, he returned to a rearranged home. The living room was now his bedroom and toilet. There, he slept in a battleship-gray hospital bed with a matching metal commode chair. His medications, the list one page long, were arranged on the coffee table. But then he went back to hospital. And then home again. In the thirty days after each hospital stay, they were overrun with care, visiting nurses, a social worker, and physical and occupational therapists, but then on the thirty-first day, the last day of care covered by Medicare, his care became custodial. She was on her own to manage his mismanaged care.

One afternoon, at what would be the last hospitalization, one of the too-numerous-to-count and ever-changing cast of doctors asked her, what were her husband's "goals of care"? Would she like him to be kept comfortable? Of course, she replied. She'd wanted him to be comfortable since the afternoon when they drove home from the primary care doctor with the prescription for Aricept.

The cause of death on his death certificate lists pneumonia secondary to hip fracture. His Alzheimer's disease was forgotten.

The Johnsons' experiences with the health care system—from his nondiagnosis and undertreatment in the community to the spectacularly disorganized treatment assaults in the hospital—have been compared by one researcher who studies the delivery of care to older adults to a drive-by shooting.[3] How could this have turned out differently?

The well-known answer to this simple question is as old as the Alzheimer's movement itself: the care that the seven families were hoping for and expecting in the coming decade after they founded the Alzheimer's Association in 1980 but didn't receive. Progress to achieving that has been slow, and part 2 explained why. This part examines what needs to be done to improve care.

I'm reluctant to claim that the story of how Alzheimer's transformed from an unusual disease into a crisis has "lessons to be learned" because this story is laden with nuance and interpretations. But if there is a lesson, it is this. Short of a cure, short of a cure for each and every cause of dementia, we will have to learn to live with the disease so as to improve the lives of persons like the Johnsons. We will have to provide the care they needed to live well at home and repair the broken system that slowly killed Darren Johnson. That is the focus of the remainder of this book.

17

A CORRECTION

Dr. Johnson and I do have dreams of ways that the clinic could be more
comprehensive (addition of a social worker and mid-level practitioner, physician home care division, increased community education and training of
caregiver, development of a resources center), but all of these dreams have
been on hold as we've realized how much they cost.

Margaret (Peggy) Noel, MD, Director, Center on Aging,
in a letter to Char Norvell, President, Community Care Partners,
Asheville, North Carolina, June 21, 1999

IN PART 2, I made the case that in the last quarter of the twentieth century, two events recast senility as a disease. The first was scientific advances
in electron microscopy and biochemistry. These allowed physicians to point
to specific and visible things—such as proteinopathies of amyloid and tau—
rather than aging as the cause of older adults' progressive and disabling cognitive impairments.

The second was advances in ethics. The twentieth century began with
whole classes of people kept under the bondage of culture. In America, for
example, women could not vote, and persons of color were routinely denied
equal access to public goods such as education, housing, loans, and employment. By century's end, autonomy—the right to self-determination—had
burst forth and demanded respect. The more the right to live as we choose to
has become the core value all adults must have as well as respect in others,
the more the pain of dementia has become unacceptable suffering. The stuff
of autonomy—independence, capacity, identity, and privacy—all are under
attack by amyloid plaques and tau tangles as they turn people into patients

with dementia and family into knowledgeable informants and caregivers. Alzheimer's is a disease because of this value. Alzheimer's disease is a disease of autonomy.

Pushing against this progress was a tangled knot of social, cultural, and political events that transformed the disease into a crisis. They include: the early twentieth-century collapse of German society occasioned by two world wars, anti-Semitism, and fascism; the triumph of Freudianism, that is, psychodynamic theories of brain diseases; the collapse of the asylum as a site for research and care; and increasing numbers of older adults and declining numbers of younger adults to care for them. Of peculiar distinction to the United States, Alzheimer's has been caught up in deeply partisan battles over the proper role of the state to support the lives of Americans, the role of women, the responsibilities of the family, and the politics of welfare. Cold War fears of communism created a health care system that is unable to either correctly diagnose or adequately treat patients. Our system was explicitly designed not to support care in the community, or so-called long-term or custodial care. The problem isn't just bad long-term care, however. It's bad acute care, too.

Imagine a health care system incapable of diagnosing whether increasing numbers of older adults with weight loss, vague pains, and anemia have cancer, and, if they did, incapable of treating their cancer and caring for their common complications such as pain and fatigue. That's the problem confronting older adults with memory loss. The system is broken, and a correction is needed to remedy this.

It begins with creating a workforce. Simply put, there are millions of patients with Alzheimer's disease but not enough doctors to take care of them. I'm one of those unusual doctors.

I didn't start out as an Alzheimer's doctor. After my residency in internal medicine, I was a fellow at a prestigious critical care medicine training program, but after a year, I dropped out and switched to geriatric medicine. For three years, I was the only fellow in the geriatric medicine fellowship program. Critical care, in contrast, trained a full cadre of fellows, selected on the basis of a highly competitive, computer-run match.

"What . . . *happened*?" friends from medical school and residency asked. Their tone suggested suspicions that I'd been kicked out or committed some egregious misstep.

What happened was the health care system killed my grandfather.

✦

My grandfather was a reasonably healthy ninety-year-old man save for dementia. His internist never offered a clear diagnosis of the cause. The family managed as best we could, making sure he was cooking meals and helping him to take care of his bills. No question, his daughter living on the other side of town kept him going. But then he fell in his kitchen and fractured his right hip.

The ambulance took him to one of the nation's leading academic medical centers. There, he was cared for by a retinue of clinicians at the top of their training and equipped with the best technologies. Everyone did what they were supposed to do. Sure, there were a few missteps or near missteps, such as the surgeon who strode into the room to announce he wasn't eating and so needed a nasal-gastric feeding tube.

She held the skinny rubber tube before my father, who explained that he'd just fed my grandfather his lunch. With assistance he could eat. She turned and fled. Never to be seen again.

Everyone was doing what she thought she should do, but no one was working together. It was the best of care and the worst of care. It was uncoordinated care. It was a medical fun house run by madmen.

That's when I started to remember the old woman in the tower. She was the first patient I saw with dementia, probably caused by Alzheimer's disease. I was ashamed at what we did and what we failed to do. I was embarrassed for my profession. I was angry at myself.

Something was really wrong. I needed to change my profession.

That was 1994. Alzheimer's wasn't yet widely recognized as a national crisis, but the hospitals were full of elderly men and women like Mr. Johnson and my grandfather, with families at wits' end. And yet, it was hard to assign a cause for this spectacle of well-funded disorganization and deprivation. We were citizens of the richest nation in the world being cared for in some of the finest medical centers.

Something was very wrong, but what was it?

The director of the critical care fellowship's candid remark to my news I was dropping out holds a clue. He plainly and simply said to me: "I don't know what geriatricians do."

Few knew what a geriatrician did in part because there were few geriatricians or other doctors dedicated to the care of older adults, especially older adults with Alzheimer's disease. The places geriatricians practiced were either out of the way, such as nursing homes, or places that struggled to financially survive. In my career so far, I've witnessed two inpatient hospital units for older adults close and a third moved to one of the hospital complex's outer buildings so that the original space could be remodeled to care for patients receiving well-reimbursed joint replacements.

Doctors whose focus is the care of older adults, especially older adults with Alzheimer's disease—whether as geriatricians, neurologists, or psychiatrists—are hard to define. In fields such as oncology, endocrinology, or cardiology, training ensures expertise in caring for cancer, diabetes, or heart failure, respectively. Training in neurology, psychiatry, or geriatric medicine does not in fact ensure expertise in caring for patients with Alzheimer's disease. Most neurologists, psychiatrists, and geriatricians have some exposure to some aspects of diagnosis and treatment of the disease, but their training does not guarantee an expertise to run a memory center or to care for patients from diagnosis to death.

A panel charged with developing best practices for the prescription of brain amyloid imaging settled on a definition of an Alzheimer's expert that is based on volume: an Alzheimer's disease expert is a geriatrician, neurologist, or psychiatrist with at least 25 percent of patients who have Alzheimer's disease.[1] Volume—not skill—defined an expert.

There are very few of these doctors or other health care professionals committed to diagnose and treat persons with mild cognitive impairment or dementia. The reasons why include the stigma of dementia (laypeople often lean away from me when I tell them what I do). They also include the nature of the doctoring. Diagnosis is interesting. Treatment is satisfying. Alzheimer's disease doctors however don't have the armamentarium of treatments that cardiologists and oncologists have. Which leads to the crux of the problem: money.

In the United States, funds to care for patients are driven by payments for prescriptions for surgical and drug treatments. Alzheimer's care is in the awkward position of not having a comparable business model. The richest nation in the world does not have a viable market to support this care. Simply put, a clinician can't make a living as an Alzheimer's doctor because the reimbursement from insurance cannot support a physician's most essential resource: time. To be able to ask: "What's the problem? How can I help you?" and then take the time to listen.

In 1999, Dr. Peggy Noel learned this painful truth.[2] The first geriatrician in Asheville, North Carolina, she was ten years into running the Center for Older Adults at Thoms Rehabilitation Hospital when she received very bad news. The center was closing. She had one year to find a new job. Twenty years later, I interviewed her about the events leading up to the closure of the center and the wild risks she took in response to this near collapse of her career.

Her center saw older adults whose multiple illnesses were a complex web of social, medical, and financial problems. Her practice used the principles of geriatric medicine to solve these problems. This involved, for example, assessing the patient's typical day. The visits, as a result, routinely involved not only a patient but also a family member. And they took time—as long as one hour or more—nearly triple the time for a typical new patient visit with a general internist.

As she and her colleagues set to work, something started to happen. "While I thought I'd be taking care of all types of geriatric problems, about nine out of ten of the people who came to see me came with dementia." The Center for Older Adults was transforming into a memory center with a model of care much like the memory center where I practice.

The problem was her business model. Most memory centers are run by researchers based at an academic medical center. They rely on cross subsidies from generous philanthropy and research funds. We divide our attention between research and care. Hers, in contrast, was run by clinicians based in a community hospital and dedicated to taking care of patients. They relied on the revenue from clinical care, which meant the funds collected from billing Medicare.

"The hospital had been cost shifting the income coming in for the nursing home care and hospital consults to cover the center but then there was one of the Medicare budget acts. It took away the ability to cost shift." The accounting that allowed the hospital to cover the losses of her clinic ended. She hunted for cost savings. She offered to take a pay cut, to fundraise. Her colleagues saw more patients, but this poorly reimbursed care only worsened the center's losses.

The center closed.

Dr. Noel could have given up on her commitment to caring for persons with dementia. She could have taken a job doing general medicine with just a sprinkling of geriatrics. With this "patient mix," the care of a high volume of relatively healthy adults (the leaders of clinical operations describe this volume as "the churn") generates revenue that then offsets the losses from the time needed to care for the more complicated older adults. But her passion was dementia. She was committed to the model of separate interviews with the caregiver and patient, time with a social worker to create a plan of care, and telephone follow-up to assess how that plan is unfolding.

And so she took a big risk. She created Memory Care and eighteen years later, when I was on a panel at the international Alzheimer's meeting in Chicago and remarked that Alzheimer's disease won't fully be a disease in the American medical system until it has a business model, she stood up.

"I founded Memory Care in Asheville, North Carolina. We have a business model that works, and you are all invited to come to Asheville and see what we've done."

What she and her colleagues did is exactly what patients and their physicians need. The story of how they did this is inspiring. A community in need came together. Asheville is an isolated, small city (seventy thousand residents in 1999) in western North Carolina with a small-town feel that mixes a hipster culture with a popular retirement destination. A robust medical marketplace was available to serve those retirees and act as the region's medical center. It included an array of specialists and ample primary care. Dementia, though, was not addressed.

"It was," Dr. Noel recalls, "just beyond them."

She recalls families frustrated over how matters of patient privacy, time, and reimbursement all got in the way of their ability to have a candid conversation alone with the physician. After a visit to the Center for Older Adults, "I could feel their sigh of relief, literally from both patients and caregivers, when they were cared for this way."

After the Center for Older Adults closed, everyone agreed that a memory center was needed, but no medical practice or hospital was willing to take one on.

"We went all over town to see if we could find someone who would adopt the program because for one thing, I know the people who came there needed it. And there was such a really gratified sense of being useful to their needs."

Friends pushed her. Take a risk, Peggy. Do it yourself. She decided to form a not-for-profit, freestanding memory center.

Asheville came together. A retirement community donated space, a law firm donated its attorneys to prepare the documents for not-for-profit incorporation, and a foundation made a grant to pay the nurse and that nurse learned how to organize the billing. Still, it was a big gamble. After the grant ran out, she'd be short by about 75 percent because Medicare—the insurer for all the patients—would cover only about one-quarter of the memory center's costs.

Her 75 percent problem was particularly vexing because she needed to pay for the private time with the caregiver—the separate interview with the clinician and the meeting with the social worker. Medicare reimbursement could not be used to cover this.

"We talked to our caregivers, and they said, 'We'll help you.' And I said, 'OK. Help me then. I will need to charge you as a caregiver, a caregiver fee." The fee, which started at $250 a year, covers the training, support, and counseling for the caregiver. "It is paid by the caregiver. Not by the patient," Dr. Noel explained. "We were really strict about that because of Medicare guidelines."

Still, she was short by half. She was down to one option. She sent out a fundraising letter, and the donations came.

Twenty years later, the center has six physicians, three social workers, and a nurse working in teams. One team makes home visits. They've expanded into two rural satellites.

Dr. Noel's story is inspiring. She took a big risk and she succeeded. She beat the odds. But her story is also sad. Over the years, health care institutions have come to her to learn about her model, and among the few who have tried it, most have failed. It's simply too hard to make budget.

"They set up programs, but as soon as the funding that came in from the outside ran out, they pretty much killed them. Or they decide: we have to change the model, so you need to see patients every thirty minutes." The experience of running the memory center has transformed her. "One of the things about going through what I went through is a thoroughly profound sense of independence from any one system."

Which is the crux of the crisis. We are bound up in a health care system that cannot (or will not) care for persons with Alzheimer's disease. For decades, it hasn't paid for the hour-long work-up in the doctor's office that ensures an accurate diagnosis and plan of care or care in the community to ensure well-being from day to day. The adult day activity program—the treatment I prescribed the Johnsons—is the exact same treatment Hilda Pridgeon was struggling to find for her husband, Al.

Today, there are many more adult day programs available, programs designed for people like Al, but this prescription is not covered by Medicare. The treatment the man from Medicare in the Twin Cities called "entertainment for your husband and a vacation for her" remains an out-of-pocket cost, meaning Mrs. Johnson, like Hilda Pridgeon some fifty years ago, paid out of her and her husband's savings. Unlike other developed nations, the United States only supports long-term care for chronically ill and disabled citizens who can prove they are impoverished and so qualify for Medicaid. The middle class—the Pridgeons and the Johnsons—are for the most part on their own.

Slowly, though, the system has begun to correct itself.

In 2010, the Affordable Care Act squeaked into law (in both the House of Representatives and the Senate, the bill received no Republican votes). In the ensuing years, so-called Obamacare would become ground zero for partisan warfare. Among President Trump's earliest legislative acts following his 2017 inauguration was to push for the repeal of the entire act. For persons with Alzheimer's disease, repeal might seem an event with little impact on their care. Obamacare's central policy was to provide insurance for adults under sixty-five who lacked health insurance. Most persons with Alzheimer's are over seventy. But the ways the ACA has impacted their lives suggests it could be renamed the Alzheimer's Care Act. It has been the legislative engine transforming Alzheimer's care.

The Affordable Care Act created the Center for Medicare and Medicaid Innovation. The center developed the comprehensive primary care program to support physician practice groups to coordinate the care of older adults so that they don't suffer the chaos the Johnsons and my family experienced, the harmful readmissions to hospital, unnecessary medications, and subsequent declines in health. In the program, Alzheimer's disease is among the diagnoses that designate a patient at the highest tier of risk. Other innovations include reimbursement for creating a care plan.

Caregivers, particularly the daughters and daughters-in-law who are the majority of the caregiving workforce, also benefit. Persons with dementia need, on average, 171 hours of care a month or about 6 hours a day, compared to 2 hours per day for older adults who are cognitively unimpaired. A working, middle-aged mother doesn't have the time to add 6 more hours of work to each day. She faces a dilemma: either pay someone else to do the caregiving or limit her hours at her job, fail to advance at her job, or simply quit her job and do it herself. The choices are diverse but the result is the same: lost wages and lost health insurance as she suffers the physical and mental health effects of caregiving. The ACA prevents this. Assuming she lives in a state that has adopted a state-run insurance exchange, it allows her to obtain health care for herself that she might otherwise be unable to afford.

More money—a correction in the medical marketplace—will create a business model for clinicians to follow the money and practice like Dr. Noel.

Money, however, isn't the only correction needed. The hospital care received by patients like the Johnsons and my grandfather has been well reimbursed, but it's a mess. The system needs to do what I did when I dropped out of critical care. It needs to discern how it's part of the problem that sustains the Alzheimer's crisis. That done, it has to exercise its tremendous creative powers to transform and become something different.

18

DISCERNMENT

Discernment (n): the faculty or power of discerning or understanding clearly . . . good judgement.

—*Oxford English Dictionary*

A HIP FRACTURE complicated by delirium killed my grandfather.

Delirium describes an acute onset of confusion and disordered thinking, a kind of acute brain failure. The victim's alertness waxes and wanes. Some are lethargic. Others, like my grandfather, become fiercely agitated, tearing away at their catheters and intravenous lines. Delirium, whether lethargic or agitated, has a core feature. People who know the person well insist the person is really different.

A fall and fracture can of course happen for reasons other than the frailty caused by Alzheimer's disease. A bicycle accident could do it. And delirium isn't unique to patients with dementia or mild cognitive impairment. It can occur in an older adult who, prior to his acute illness, was independent and cognitively unimpaired. But patients with Alzheimer's are at heightened risk to fall and suffer a hip fracture (President Reagan, five years after his diagnosis of Alzheimer's disease, fell at home and fractured his right hip).[1] They're also at heightened risk for delirium.

For patients with Alzheimer's disease and other diseases of the aging brain such as Parkinson's or Lewy body disease, delirium and hip fracture are the common culprits in a sad story of how, in an instant, someone who was doing reasonably well despite these diseases became terribly ill. In a sense, hip fracture and delirium are to Alzheimer's disease what a heart attack is to heart disease and pain is to cancer.

The end is often either profound disability requiring moving to a long-term care facility such as a nursing home or death. In any given year in the United States, these two events kill or maim millions of older adults and cost billions of dollars.[2] When Robert Katzman called Alzheimer's a serious and life-threatening disease in his 1976 call-to-action essay, these were among the events he was referring to.

Ironically, at death, Alzheimer's disease—and also delirium—is often forgotten as the cause of death. Death certificates notoriously undercount the role of Alzheimer's in this lethal cascade. On my grandfather's death certificate, I made sure the leading cause of his death was listed as "Alzheimer's disease." But what I really wanted the doctor to write was "the American health care system."

For much of human history, physicians thought about delirium in an older adult like they did of dementia in an older adult. It was either ignored or dismissed as an inevitable and uncontrollable natural disaster. In contrast, physicians cared about an older adult with a hip fracture. They had a broken bone in need of repair, but the repair job was an iconic display of the best and the worst of the American health care system. By the end of the twentieth century, however, revolutions in care began to break out.

In the weeks following Dr. Sharon Inouye's first month as an attending physician she experienced a career-changing revelation. The health care system had a big problem, and she was part of it.

An attending physician leads a team of doctors in training, a mix of medical students and residents and interns training to become internists. The work is busy and emotionally intense. The twenty-five-year-old geriatrician was responsible for overseeing the care of as many as forty-five acutely ill patients on the medical service at the United States Department of Veterans Affairs' West Haven VA Hospital in New Haven, Connecticut. Her dominant emotion throughout the month was anxiety. In an interview thirty-four years later, the events that created those emotions were as vivid as the April when she lived them.[3]

"The buck stops with you," she reflected. And at the end of her month she realized that she'd dropped the buck not just once but at least six times. Some things had really gone wrong.

In that extremely busy month, there were six patients she didn't know how to care for because the problem that made them so ill was unlike any of the other common problems her team cared for. "Every other patient I felt confident. Heart failure, diabetic ketoacidosis, lung disease, stroke, anything like that, throw it at me. I can totally deal with that. . . . But I had these six patients who were cognitively intact on admission and they became acutely confused on my watch." They came in with the common problems she was quite skilled in caring for, problems like pneumonia and heart failure. Each one of them, however suffered in ways that were vast and disproportionate to those problems.

Two went to the intensive care unit, two died, and two left not to go home but to nursing homes. "It was like, oh my goodness. They were wildly confused and did really poorly."

She needed to figure out what happened. What caused these patients who, though bothered by long-standing memory problems, started out alert and conversant but then became wildly confused and disoriented to time and place?

She conducted her own morbidity and mortality conference. These conferences are medicine's centuries-old method to sort out why a patient suffered a bad outcome. They follow a ritual of discernment that begins with the clinician's detailed case presentation leading up to the admission that the diagnosis was wrong and so the treatment unsuccessful. Next, the pathologist presents the slides depicting the results of a careful anatomic dissection that explains the correct diagnosis. Implicit in this discernment is that if the diagnosis had been correct, the patient might still be alive.

I recall one such case I was involved in as a resident. We thought the man died of alcoholic liver failure. The pathology showed an obstructing cancer of the gallbladder. To this day, I wish I could apologize to him for the shame he felt over our misdiagnosis and for the fact that if we'd been correct in our diagnosis, he might have lived.

Except Inouye didn't go to the basement pathology morgue. Instead, she went to medical records. She dissected each patient's chart. Page by page—this was in the age of paper medical records—she reviewed what she and her colleagues had done, and the thick charts began to tell a story. She wrote it out on a gigantic sheet of graph paper, each day organizing the events of care plotted against the summary of the patient's cognitive well-being. She started to see a pattern. The morning of the day when acute lethargy and confusion struck, a patient was prescribed a dose of an antihistamine to accompany a blood transfusion. A catheter to ease the drainage of urine predated a fever and urine infection and ensuing agitation. And so on.

She figured out what happened. "We, through our care, we contributed to the problem."

Armed with her spreadsheets, she presented her findings to her colleagues, but they were essentially indifferent, explaining: "That just happens to older people when they come to the hospital." One of the department's clinical leaders suggested she deliver a lecture on appropriate prescribing to the elderly. That lecture she knew was premature. To be sure, medications were part of the problem, but Inouye's spreadsheets showed that medicines weren't the only cause of what went wrong. The problem was a lack of knowledge: which of the countless things that happened to the patients caused the delirium? Once known, could we intervene on them and so prevent the delirium? She and her colleagues were ignorant, and her more senior colleagues were doubly ignorant. They didn't know what they didn't know and therefore what they needed to discover. A nonjudgmental process of reflection and self-discovery was needed, a kind of discernment to arrive at not just knowledge but also the willingness to change.

She decided to learn the scientific methods used to discover the causes of a disease. The disease she wanted to figure out was just a few years old, having been first named and defined in 1980 to replace a variety of terms such as "hospital-induced psychologic decompensation." She set out to discover what caused a person to develop delirium.

She began to audit epidemiology classes at Yale University.

The more she read about delirium, the more she learned, and the more she began to change. Instead of returning home to Los Angeles, California, where her family expected she would join her father's busy solo primary care practice, she decided to remain at Yale and become a researcher. She had a vision: to prevent delirium as one might prevent polio. The available research literature suggested this would be a notable challenge. Polio is a disease caused by a virus and prevented with a single vaccine. Delirium was more complex. There were likely a multiplicity of factors at work, including a sudden disease or trauma like a hip fracture, changes in living situation, such as spending hours in a loud emergency room, and things that made the person vulnerable, such as their impaired cognition. Her goal was to figure out which ones were the culprits.

Problems, though, soon multiplied. Her training director, the eminent physician and epidemiologist Alvin Feinstein, dismissed her research proposal, explaining that he couldn't think of a topic less interesting to anyone than older people becoming confused in the hospital, and also there was nothing to be done about it.

Feinstein was a titan. His approval launched careers, and his dismissal often ended them. She moved on to other topics, each time preparing a research proposal, and each time he sent her away. Five rejected proposals later, she made a decision to defy a powerful man. She returned to her first idea and simply told the director: "Alvin, this is what I want to do." What she ended up doing transformed how medicine and society understand hospital care for older adults, especially older adults with dementia or MCI.

She was thinking like an epidemiologist. What factors explained why an older adult who came into the hospital without delirium ended up developing this acute confusion? The research to answer this question was rough going, requiring daily assessments to meticulously record the details of over one hundred inpatients at Yale's busy hospital: their diagnoses, medications, labs, and outcomes.

Complications ensued. At the last minute, a collaborator withdrew permission to use his instrument to measure delirium. She scrambled and devised her own—the Confusion Assessment Method, or CAM. She traveled to Canada to meet a potential mentor, but he no-showed. Researchers in Sweden never replied to her letters. Nevertheless she persisted, and in September 1993 published a foundational paper: "A Predictive Model for Delirium in Hospitalized Elderly Medical Patients Based on Admission Characteristics."[4]

An older adult free of delirium at admission developed it because of four things present on the day of admission: impaired vision, dementia, dehydration, and severe illness. Each of these added to an older adult's risk of transforming from being alert and attentive when she came into the hospital to deteriorating into a state of frightened inattention and confusion. These were exciting results because they suggested potential points of intervention such as rehydration. But she needed to do one more study. After admission, when doctors like her were in charge of the patient's care, what did *they do* to the patient that caused the patient to develop delirium?

Three years later, she had her answer. "Precipitating Factors for Delirium in Hospitalized Elderly Persons" reported how five noxious insults and events following hospital admission independently conspired to cause delirium.[5] Physical restraints that kept the patient from moving about, a urinary catheter that also restrained the patient (and also increased the risk of a bladder infection), adding three or more medications (among the most common were psychoactive medications, especially sedatives for sleep), low blood proteins suggestive of malnutrition, and, finally, harms from the things doctors did, their diagnostic procedures or treatments.

Ten years of meticulous research had transformed what had been dismissed as just another downside of being old into a diagnosis. Clinicians had the Confusion Assessment Method, a tool to easily detect delirium, and also now knew the matrix of events that explained why delirium happened. And Inouye still wasn't done. It's all very well for a researcher to describe the world. The goal of a doctor is to improve it.

One more study was needed. She ended "Precipitating Factors for Delirium in Hospitalized Elderly Persons" with the idea that all five of the noxious insults and hospital events were modifiable. These were the targets of an intervention.

Three years later, the lead article of the *New England Journal of Medicine* reported how a multicomponent intervention reduced the risk of developing delirium from 15 to 10 percent and, among those who developed it, reduced its duration.[6] An accompanying editorial praised the study as "myth busting."[7] The devastating confusion older adults experience in the hospital was not like the winter, something that just happens, but the consequence of a cascade of events and, like polio, it was preventable. The Hospital Elder Life Program, or HELP, was born.

The intervention is a set of sensible things. To read them is to wonder: *Why wasn't this routine?* During the day, someone helps the person get up and walk about and assists with eating and drinking. There are conversations about current events and a sign board with the day, date, and the names of the treating nurses and doctors. At night, silence and calm reign—the pill crushers are noiseless and phones are set to vibrate—and instead of a sedative, a glass of warm milk or herbal tea and a back massage are provided. Restraints are strictly prohibited and bladder catheters are used with great caution if at all.

In college, Inouye trained to play the harpsichord, and the concert performer's confidence and command of both her score and her audience endure. Her direct and inviting gaze, the emotions of her story, and a compelling command of the facts compel the listener to genuinely care about delirium and to believe in the possibility that we can do something about this bleak, dark, and seemingly intractable problem.

The press paid attention. For two weeks, reporters called. The Associated

Press headline read: STUDY SUGGESTS COMMON SENSE STEPS ALLEVIATED CONFUSION CONDITION.[8] Among the results reported was the cost per patient: $327. HELP was not only effective, it was also cheap. But in the years to follow, HELP struggled through a rough translation from idea into standard practice.

The reason was the health care system. HELP wasn't a prescribed medication treatment for a defined disease, and Medicare wasn't designed to rigorously support prevention interventions, especially an intervention as both complex and simple as HELP. Complex because to learn it requires studying a set of six binders and six training videos and inculcating it throughout a hospital. Simple because each of the interventions is just that: simple. A glass of warm milk instead of a tablet of Ambien.

HELP wasn't a pill with a business model to propel it into practice. It was a way of thinking and behaving. It was culture. It's hard to change culture, even when that culture is causing people to suffer and die at the hands of the health care system.

Unless that health care system is losing money.

After twelve years of practicing geriatric medicine, Dr. Bob McCann knew a number of valuable maxims. One of them is, a hospitalized older adult is a kind of canary in the coal mine. "If you can make a hospital safer and more user-friendly for them, it'll be better for everyone," young and old, he reflected.[9] And if the hospital isn't safe, these are the patients who sound the alarm.

He told me this as he was recounting his early years as chief of medicine at Highland Hospital in Rochester, New York. In 1999, when he started the job, the older adults being cared for there were sounding the alarm. Highland, founded in the late nineteenth century by homeopathic physicians, was a "community hospital," and McCann was among its new leaders, brought in by the new owner, the University of Rochester Medical Center.

The affiliation was part of the large academic medical center's strategy to survive in the changing twentieth-century medical marketplace. Insurers were threatening their business model. Their practitioners were subspecialists caring for complicated patients in need of expensive specialty care (sometimes called tertiary care). Insurers—both Medicare and the private companies—were cutting reimbursement. Rochester sought to diversify the number of patients it cared for—meaning, billed for—so as to stabilize sources of revenue. An affiliation with Highland Hospital, a 250-bed community hospital located a few miles from the academic medical center, was an opportunity to gather thousands of patients cared for by the practitioners in the community. These primary care practices would "feed" the more expensive tertiary care subspecialists. Many of these patients were older adults with dementia, particularly the residents of nursing homes.

McCann recalled repeated calls from the director of the emergency room. Something was terribly wrong. Older adults were coming in with fractured hips, but no one wanted to take care of them.

"The doctor in the emergency room would call medicine and say, 'We've got a person with dementia from the nursing home who's on twenty medicines and is delirious.' And medicine would say, 'We don't accept fractures. Call orthopedic surgery.' And so they'd call orthopedics, and they'd say, 'Oh my God, admit them to medicine!'"

Each patient instigated a constant back-and-forth over who would have charge of an acutely ill older adult with dementia and a broken hip. The longer the patient waited in the emergency room, the sicker she became, and the clinicians' approach to caring for her became more and more risk averse. The anesthesiologists insisted on a cardiology consult and the cardiologist then ordered tests, and so surgery was further delayed. Fluids were limited so as to avoid heart failure. The now-dehydrated patient developed worsening kidney function. As a result, once-safe doses of medications became toxic. Not surprisingly, delirium often ensued and as it did, antipsychotic or sedative medications were prescribed, and so they became even sicker.

Mistakes were building on mistakes were building on mistakes.

The story of how they changed this is an unusual confluence of circumstances, of people willing to take risks in a place that was willing to let them. And why not? There was nothing to lose. Highland Hospital was falling apart.

A modern American hospital is chock-full of technologies, some of which are capable of generating breathtaking tallies of revenue, and yet its financial viability can be summed up by the use of one simple and prosaic item of furniture: the bed.

The metric of a successful hospital is that *every* bed is *always* "filled." An empty bed means no patient is being billed, no technology is being used. When McCann took over as chief of medicine, Highland had 261 beds. On any given day, only about sixty of them were filled. The institution was at least $10 million in debt. He recalled how it felt like the hospital was going to be "mothballed at any minute."

This was an opportunity to try anything, something, to save a failing institution, and the people in charge were the right people to try. McCann recalled the turning point. It was after a conversation between one of the orthopedic surgeons, Steve Kates, and a young geriatrician, Daniel Mendelson. They had a unique approach to care for patients with a hip fracture. They worked together.

One day, Mendelson recalled, Kates opened up to his young colleague. "Daniel, what's it like when you have to work with an orthopedic surgeon that's different than me?" What followed was a mutual confession.[10]

"I said to Steve, 'Well, you know, to be honest, sometimes it's like pulling teeth. We don't talk the same language. The other surgeons don't seem to have the same interest as you, and the patient outcomes aren't really as good as they could be.' And Steve said to me, 'Well, would it surprise you if I said that the same thing happens when I have to work with a different medicine doctor?'"

"No," Mendelson admitted. "It wouldn't surprise me at all."

They agreed that it made no sense that there were two different standards of care at Highland Hospital: the "Steve and Daniel standard" and the "everybody else standard." There should just be one, and it should be better than what was happening. Worse, they knew that what was happening was the standard of care across the country.

They went to Bob McCann and explained their plan. Kates had been studying management theories and processes to improve industrial production. McCann said simply, "Let's do this." After all, he recalled, they had nowhere to go but up.

So they set about to change the way they delivered care to older adults admitted with a hip fracture (most, but not all, persons with dementia). Among all their goals, the one Mendelson recalls as their "eye on the prize" was preventing the harms they committed in their acts of care, and the number one harm they sought to eliminate was delirium.

They started not by doing but by listening.

They reviewed the medical literature, searching for the best evidence on how to care for an older adult with a hip fracture. Inouye's HELP program was an obvious intervention. More important than listening to the medical literature was listening to each other. They went to the emergency room and listened to everyone who cared for older adults presenting with a hip fracture. What do you do? What don't you do? What do you wish you could do?

They did the same with the pre- and postoperative care suites, the operating room, and the wards. They defined all the steps in a patient's care. No detail was too trivial. McCann recalled, "We looked at each step with a critical eye to see what was missing or what was there that was unnecessary."

And then they set to doing things differently.

Implementation was an act of politics. They needed to gently rebut the accusation that they were implementing a one-size-fits-all approach or otherwise imposing on physician autonomy.

Patience was an essential virtue. McCann recalled constant and repetitious messaging. "We probably said the same things thousands of times. I mean the amount of time we talked to people in the ER, saying, 'No, you need to hose these patients with as much fluid as they can take until they start making urine, that's when we know their tank is full.' And they'd say, 'Yeah, but then we might put them into heart failure.' And we'd say, 'Well, we can treat heart failure, but we can't treat acute kidney failure.'"

Among their most revolutionary changes was a new answer to the decision that vexed the emergency room physicians, the decision of who "owned the patient." Admit to orthopedic surgery? Admit to medicine?

An older adult with a hip fracture was no longer admitted to either orthopedics or to medicine. They were admitted to the Geriatric Fracture Program. Both professions comanaged the patient, each bringing their expertise, each charged with writing their own orders, and when a nurse called a physician about a problem that should be addressed by the other team, the answer to the nurse was no longer: "Why are you calling me?" Instead, the doctors contacted the other team member. The buck stopped with the Geriatric Fracture Program.

Slowly, this revolution in care took hold.

Eight years later, with the assistance of a researcher trained in epidemiology, they set out to study their program. The once-upon-a-time failing community hospital compared the outcomes of their hip fracture care to the hip fracture patients cared for at the flagship academic medical center. Patients at Highland were older, sicker, and more likely to have dementia compared to those who received "usual care" at the flagship hospital. The outcomes of their care, however, were uniformly better. The Highland patients stayed fewer days in the hospital. There were fewer patients with infections or blood clots. There were fewer cases of delirium.[11]

And Highland turned around. Mendelson facilely recited how these numbers add up to everyone's benefit. "You've improved the patient's outcome and experience. You've improved the staff's experience. You've improved the surgeon's experience. And you've improved your bed utilization. When you shorten length of stay from seven to five days, you're getting about one thousand bed days back. One thousand bed days are also worth a lot of money." Remember, in a successful hospital *every* bed is *always* "filled."

But Bob knew the program was working before the researchers and accountants ran their numbers. The alarms stopped sounding. "I stopped getting calls from the head of the emergency room saying, 'We've got someone here no one will take.'"

A common theme unites the work of Sharon Inouye, Bob McCann, Daniel Mendelson, and Steve Kates. They set out not simply to discover things but rather to use their discoveries to change the ways their colleagues thought, interacted, and communicated with each other and their patients. They set out to change culture.

This theme of revolution resonates across the history of Alzheimer's disease. Robert Katzman's 1976 essay was a call to change the way medicine and society thought about senility, to see it not as an extreme stage of aging but as a disease worthy of medical attention. The next—and tragically delayed—step in this revolution has been the recognition that to care for these millions of patients and their families, we need to change. There are still more revolutions to come, revolutions in how we decide to use technologies that could upend the very practice of a memory center.

19

SOME THINGS TO
WATCH OVER US

When the day is done the only thing that matters is function. If you had a terrible disease, but it didn't affect your function it's not a terrible disease. You're not demented, technically, till you have a problem with your function. That goes for everything in medicine.

—Jeff Kaye, MD

LEAN, BEARDED, AND modest, with a preference for blue blazers, Dr. Jeff Kaye is the stereotype of the usual male neurologist studying Alzheimer's disease. His ideas and approaches, however, are most unusual and quite revolutionary.

In 2001, thirteen years into his career as an Alzheimer's disease researcher, Kaye experienced a career-changing aha moment. It came to him during a lunch break at "Alzheimer's and Technology," a conference hosted by Intel. Jeff said to his tablemates: "Why don't we use technology to get a better understanding of what's really happening, instead of this artificial layer that's been going on for decades or even centuries."[1]

The "artificial layer" was the well-trod routine of studies done at Alzheimer's disease research centers throughout the world, the large, yearslong cohort studies that follow a group of older adults, such as ADNI or the ADPR at Mayo. As he explained in an interview eighteen years later, the approaches researchers use in these studies in order to understand Alzheimer's disease and the other diseases of the aging brain have a fundamental limitation.

"You see somebody, you interview them, you get all their self-report that you can, and you have to believe in it because what else are you going to do. You do some cognitive testing. You see them for a brief period of time, and then you send them home and you wait. And then you do the same thing. You do this year after year after year. Then you try to connect the dots."

This approach, he decided, was too removed from the day-to-day lives of older adults. He and his colleagues weren't really studying the disease. They were studying their representation of the disease. His tablemates nodded. The young neurologist had a good idea.

Kaye returned from the Intel meeting to his office at the Oregon Health and Science University, OHSU, with a plan. He was going to disrupt OHSU's Alzheimer's center's cohort study, using new technology made possible by funds appropriated by Senator Hatfield.

No more requiring older adults to come to his research center. He would go to them, gathering data in a manner that was as passive and unobtrusive as possible. Instead of asking a subject, for example, to fill out a form to report how often they went out of their house in a typical week, a door sensor would record each time the subject opened her door. And so, too, for moving around her home, traveling outside her home, even sleeping. He launched what he came to call the platform.[2]

I toured one of his research subjects' homes. From a twenty-first-floor apartment, Anne and Ed have a spectacular view of the Willamette River and tree-filled Ross Island. The snowcapped Mount Hood is in the distant east.

Glorious nature surrounds them, but they reside amid technology. It is everywhere, even under their mattress. Their main hall has sensors in the ceiling to record gait speed, and in the corners of every room to record passage in and out of the room. Beneath their mattress, a sensor records when they're lying in bed. The bathroom scale records their weight and heart rate. Their car is continuously tracked. A sensor knows when their computer is turned on and when it is turned off.

Even Ed is monitored. He shows me his thin black wristwatch. It's also an activity monitor that tracks his daily step count. Each time he opens the lid of his medication box a signal is sent to the router and so yet another piece of data goes to Jeff Kaye's monstrous database.

Sensors everywhere, continuously capturing their day-to-day activities. This suite of technologies is the "platform." As the technology changes, the platform changes, but the logic of the platform never varies.

Kaye explained the logic. "Better ways to capture data that is objective, real time, and as unobtrusively as possible." Like all Alzheimer's disease centers, the team gathers data on each subject's cognition and a physical exam (these, too, at an in-home visit), blood samples, and MRI and other imaging, but unique to OHSU, they add in the data from the platform.

Within a few years, month after month of daily recordings from the sensors in the homes of hundreds of older adults in Portland began to accumulate vast quantities of data. The test was whether any of these data fit together. Was there any signal in all that noise? Meaning, would measures of the use of technologies like the computer or the car or of moving about one's home have any relation to changes in cognition or to the other important clinical events, like slow decline from being cognitively unimpaired to having mild cognitive impairment?

The challenge was formidable. The platform generates so much data that traditional summary statistics and the common bar charts and pie graphs simply fail to show the results. Novel methods were needed to tease out the patterns. They stumbled on an idea. Let the data make a picture of each day.

Imagine a day like a circle, akin to the face of a clock but instead of numbers and hands, imagine dots along the circle. Each dot signals, say, when the person moved about the house. Around noon, there are lots of dots. Not so at midnight, save perhaps a trip to the toilet.

Now draw another circle, this one just outside the first. Again, fill in the dots. And so on with another circle. Day after day, circle after circle.

The result is a series of concentric circles, a wheel with hundreds, thousands of dots. It is out of the pattern of dots arrayed along the concentric circles that the truth emerges. The image is a kind of mandala, a Buddhist term for a circular geometric pattern that a person gazes upon.

The platform's mandalas were notably vivid and provocative expressions of truth. Walking speed,[3] medication usage,[4] the time spent on a computer,[5] even the use of the mouse[6] all correlated with changes in cognitive function or detected cognitive impairment.

The mandalas were also disruptive.

The researchers compared cognitively unimpaired adults' mandalas to their responses to an email asking them to look back and self-report what they were doing, when they were doing it, and where. One-quarter of the subjects' self-reports of what they were doing didn't match the mandala that displayed what in fact they *had* been doing.

Kaye reflected on the implications of the result for traditional cohort studies that rely on self-report data. "The moment I saw the results, I thought, 'We really don't know what we're doing because we're suffering from a data desert.'"

In time, he had results that put it all together. A colleague mapped the results of brain atrophy measured using MRI with the mandala patterns of declining computer use.

The images were arresting. "When Lisa Silbert showed me how the MRI templates of volume loss had the highest correlations with less computer use, I said to her: 'You must have painted those on.'"

Dr. Silbert, a neurologist whose research uses MRI and PET scans to discover the nascent signs of disease in the aging brain, was confused. These were the results, she insisted. The greater the decline in computer use, the more atrophy in the brain's medial temporal lobes.

What amazed Kaye was that the medial temporal lobes are the regions of the brain where Alzheimer's pathology starts. They had demonstrated that a measure of computer use was associated with atrophy in brain structures affected by Alzheimer's disease. This was a "digital-biomarker correlation."

These are the kinds of results that could settle the interminable fights over what the best way is to measure whether a drug effectively treats Alzheimer's disease. Never mind the scores on pencil-and-paper tests of memory and concentration. Set aside the frustrations of asking people to recall what they or someone else did weeks ago. Measure what the person actually does, such as how long she is on her computer.

Listening to Kaye explain his research and its implications is refreshingly free of technical jargon. He's not interested in what's inside the gadgets and how they work. He himself lives relatively unadorned of the latest devices, preferring a PC over the more fashionable Mac. What enthralls him is how technology opens up a new way of thinking about the Alzheimer's crisis.

"It's not the platform. It's the approach," he insisted. The approach yields results that are objective, real time, and gathered as unobtrusively as possible. They are ecologically valid, meaning not a person's biased self-report or an intrusive observer's recollection of another person, but a report of a person's real life.

Kaye explained, "When the day is done, the only thing that matters is function. If you had a terrible disease, but it didn't affect your function, it's not a terrible disease. You're not demented, technically, till you have a problem with your function. And that goes for everything in medicine."

In the closing lines of Katzman's 1976 essay "The Prevalence and Malignancy of Alzheimer Disease: A Major Killer," he declared that Alzheimer's was "a single disease, a disease whose etiology must be determined, whose course must be aborted, and ultimately a disease to be prevented."[7] His call cast aside social and psychological models of dementia. In their place was a full-on biomedical assault. Go after the amyloid plaques and this problem will be solved.

Jeff Kaye, Sharon Inouye, Bob McCann, Daniel Mendelson, and Steve Kates don't reject the biomedical, but each recognizes our approach to Alzheimer's disease ought to be more all encompassing. Clinicians are part of a social ecosystem that we can manipulate to achieve the same kinds of outcomes of care we desire from a biological treatment. This will address the overcorrection of the late twentieth century when the biomedical crowded out more psychological and social interventions. A rebalancing among the biomedical, psychological, and social models will allow us to achieve a more complete understanding of what the problem is and how best to treat patients and their caregivers.

Continuous, unobtrusive monitoring of our day-to-day lives offers unique opportunities to improve care, but these technologies come with challenges. Technology in medicine has long been judged as a barrier to intimate doctor-patient communication. The computer screen intrudes on the doctor's gaze on her patient. Arguably, though, mandalas of function will have a different effect. They'll bring doctor and patient even closer together but in a very different way than before.

Patients will be able to come alone to a memory center. The requirement to bring someone else to the visit, to serve as an informant and caregiver, will transform from an expectation that starts a visit to a prescription at the end of a visit.

This transformation will happen because doctors will not have to start a visit by interviewing a knowledgeable informant. Instead, they will start with the patient and begin not by asking the centuries-old question: "*What's the problem? How can I help you?*" They will start by looking at images that display a vivid, graphic narrative of a person's function in their real world. It will replace our most powerful technology, the four-word question: "*What's a typical day?*" In this new and deeply intimate practice, Alzheimer's doctors will need sophisticated conversational skills. They will need to be able to ask, without threat or condescension: "*Do you see what I see?*" And then they will need to learn how to manage a back-and-forth conversation to arrive at a common understanding of what the problem is, how significant it is, and what needs to be done to address it.

The diagnosis and care of older adults with cognitive problems is a talk-intensive practice, and mandalas such as Kaye's will require even more talking. But these conversations will need to be very different. We need to shed fixed and settled habits that disrespect the very same autonomy we're trying to preserve.

20

NOT (LEGALLY) DEAD YET

I am the master of my fate,
I am the captain of my soul.
—William Ernest Henley, "Invictus"

I HAVE TOO many plaintive stories of people struggling to live with Alzheimer's disease, whether as patients or caregivers. Among the most arresting are the stories of men and women who were treated like they were there but not there, alive but also sort of dead. One was told to me by a caregiver, the wife of one of my patients. In addition to dementia caused by Alzheimer's disease, her husband had disabling heart disease. A leaky heart valve that backed fluid up into his lungs rendered him breathless after just crossing a room. Alzheimer's and heart disease together were racing to carry my patient to his death.

They were at a visit with his cardiologist when the doctor lifted his stethoscope from the man's chest, eased one of the ear buds out of his ear, and said to her, "It won't be long now." Just like that, right in front of his patient, like he was there but not there.

In the care of persons with Alzheimer's disease, this experience of people talking about or over the person even as she is in the presence of the talker is common. It is as if the person is dead. The behavior is inexcusable, but it is understandable. It's hard to talk to a person with Alzheimer's disease, even a person who has mild cognitive impairment, but it's especially difficult talking with a person who has dementia.

In his 1971 text, *Dementia*, the physician Charles Wells wrote how "poor judgment usually results from the individual's inability to attend to details and to assimilate the multiple factors that are usually weighed in decision-making, so that choice is directed on the basis of one particular bit of information with disregard for multiple other factors."[1] Wells elegantly calls attention to perhaps the most vexing problem of living with Alzheimer's or caring for that person. Sometimes patients make choices that are inattentive to essential facts, even after the best efforts to teach them those facts.

Early in my studies of the ability of patients to make decisions about whether to enroll in research, Wells's insight became evident. Patients with severe-stage dementia would hold on to one bit of information, such as "this is a study to test a drug for Alzheimer's disease," and with this and only this bit, they'd decide to enroll in the study. Some would insist on enrolling. Notably, these patients didn't grasp the other important facts, such as the risks and burdens of the research.

Simply put, patients with Alzheimer's disease can make bad decisions, such as refusing to see the doctor or to take a medication, or they purchase an unsuitable investment. But not always. And that's the problem.

A busy, time-pressured clinician soon finds caring for such patients can be frustrating and time consuming. Talking to the family member is easier, and this ease elides into a habit of only talking to the family member. The patient fades away into an object of care. And when the health care practitioner does talk with the person, this degradation amplifies.

The problem is evident even with the most basic communication. Mrs. Johnson witnessed this at her husband's hospitalizations.

"Hi, sweetieeee! How are *we* today?"

"Do . . . we . . . want . . . to . . . get . . . *up*!?"

"Darren, you look so *cute* in that gown!"

And on and on. Simple sentences spoken at a slow, high pitch. "We" instead of "you." "Darren" instead of "Mr. Johnson." Or just "sweetie." The Johnsons found the experience surreal. It was like he was an infant.

The phenomenon of speech they experienced is well described and documented. Linguists call it patronizing speech or, more vividly, elder speak.[2] It is a common form of communication care providers use when talking with an older adult, particularly one they think has cognitive impairment. One researcher assigned college students recordings of teachers talking to nursery school students and nurses' aides talking to older adults. For each, the students rated whether the speaker was a nurse or a teacher (the recordings were de-identified of clues to the ages or roles of the speakers). Three-quarters of the nurses' aides' conversations were mistakenly rated as conversations between a teacher and a nursery school child.

Simplifying complex sentences and the information they convey makes sense when, for example, the information is novel and complex. That's just good teaching. A gentle tone in address to a person in a panic and a term of endearment to an intimate are each acts of sensible social cognition. The problem with elder speak is that it spreads like a weed into all acts of communication between the older adult and the professionals who care for them. Older adults find that the speech insults their dignity and is disrespectful.

Ending the Alzheimer's crisis is going to take a lot of work. We need more memory centers and competent clinicians to run them. Patients and their caregivers need treatment for the whole person that includes caregiver training and day-to-day care in the community such as adult day activity programs. They need better care for the common complications of the disease and technology that will obtain truly personal data about daily function. All these corrections share a common desideratum: to preserve and protect the person's autonomy.

One more correction is needed. Physicians and other professionals and family members need to transform the ways they communicate with people with Alzheimer's disease. People don't know what to say or how to listen. This leads to experiences like my patient at his visit to his cardiologist and to opposite and equally flawed encounters with clinicians who entirely ignore the caregiver and insist on speaking only to the patient. They defend this practice as an effort to respect the autonomy of the patient. Both practices reflect how people don't know how to decide whether they ought to respect the person's choice or instead attempt to intervene, to persuade, or even to take over the decision. They don't respect how the patient and caregiver are a kind of monad of interconnected minds.

At the office visit when I prescribed an adult day program for Mr. Johnson, Mrs. Johnson cut me off. "He won't agree," she insisted. She was right. When I presented the idea to him, he refused it. I could have stopped there. Decades of twentieth-century litigation and legislation have finally secured that a fundamental right of all adults is the right to refuse care, even care that most adults accept routinely. It was his right to say no and my duty to obey. I knew, however, that I must obey an ethical obligation to balance his right to be the captain of his self with my duty to protect him from harm. The fulcrum upon which I determined this balance between respecting his will versus advancing his good was to assess his capacity to decide whether to attend an adult day activity program.

I knew that a person with his disease and his kinds of cognitive impairments can have problems making a decision about how to care for the disease that is causing his impairments. I wasn't going to make a categorical judgment about him, meaning that his diagnosis—dementia caused by Alzheimer's disease—meant that he couldn't make this decision, and I wasn't going to use his performance on my cognitive tests to make that decision. Instead, I assessed his ability to make this particular decision. This was going to take some time (unreimbursed time at that), but this was my duty as his doctor. A disease of autonomy requires the clinician to make every effort to preserve, protect, and respect what remains of autonomy even in the face of disabling cognitive impairments.

It wasn't always that way.

In 1987, the Associated Press published *Guardians of the Elderly: An Ailing System*. This special report was the biggest investigative effort in the history of the near century-old newswire service. Fifty-seven AP reporters, spread out over all fifty states and the District of Columbia, "traveled thousands of miles to nursing homes, shacks, condos, cow pastures and courtrooms; they interviewed hundreds of judges, lawyers, social workers, doctors, court clerks and academics."[3] The lead story's disturbing headline of the twenty-six-page summary report read: DECLARED "LEGALLY DEAD" BY A TROUBLED SYSTEM. The AP had uncovered a national scandal.

Guardianship describes a legitimate legal procedure to protect an adult who can no longer manage his day-to-day life, such as after a devastating brain injury that causes a persistent unconscious state. A judge decides a person needs a guardian and then appoints someone to serve in that role.

A guardian possesses a powerful role. An adult under guardianship has none of the rights of an adult: to own property, manage finances, sign herself into or out of a long-term care facility, refuse or accept treatment, even to vote. The court-appointed guardian makes all these decisions (except for voting). The lead article quoted Dennis Koson, an expert in law and psychiatry: "Guardianship is a process that uproots people, literally 'unpersons' them, declares them legally dead. Done badly, it does more hurting than protecting."[4]

The AP had uncovered a graphic, systemic, and nationwide scandal. The array of harms and indignities included failing to even tell the person a guardianship was being pursued, short and perfunctory court hearings, and abusive guardians who, for example, raided the property of their ward for their own personal gain. The findings were so compelling that Congress held hearings and formed a Select Committee on Abuses in Guardianship of the Elderly and Infirm, efforts that led to reforms to state guardianship laws and a model guardianship law.

Among the potential hurts, one stood out. The core of guardianship is a judge's decision that a person is not competent to manage her day-to-day life. To make this important decision, judges often rely on the testimony of medical professionals. The AP story showed that physicians possessed little if any skill in determining that a person can make day-to-day decisions. In other words, a judge might just as well have decided whether a person was competent or incompetent using the outcome of the flip of a coin.

In 1987, the same year the AP ran its blockbuster report, Paul Appelbaum, a young psychiatrist and assistant professor at the University of Massachusetts, received a telephone call that would transform his career and the lives of patients with Alzheimer's disease and other diseases that impair the ability to make decisions. The call was from a representative of the influential John D. and Catherine T. MacArthur Foundation. Would he be interested in serving on a MacArthur-funded research network to develop a research agenda on issues at the intersections of law and mental health? In an interview thirty years later, Appelbaum described the call like an episode of *The Millionaire*, a TV program from his childhood whose plots centered on the aftermath in the life of a random person who'd received an unconditional gift of $1 million.[5]

Appelbaum was among a small cadre of scholars wrestling with the problem of decision-making capacity. Following his psychiatry residency at Harvard, he moved to the University of Pittsburgh to train at an innovative program in law and psychiatry set up by the psychiatrist Loren Roth. Roth had assembled a multidisciplinary group of scholars in law, social sciences, psychiatry, and ethics to tackle important issues at the intersections of these disciplines. Among the most important was, how should a clinician assess whether the patient had the capacity to make a decision? In other words, how to decide whether a patient was competent?

The AP report showed this was an urgent problem. I recall early in my geriatrics training, informing the senior physician that his long-standing patient whom I was caring for at a rehabilitation unit had dementia. His response was reflexive. "We need to pursue guardianship." Most clinicians thought just like this physician. They conflated diagnosis with incompetency. If you were psychotic, "senile," or "demented," you were not competent. Others used their own idiosyncratic approaches. Incompetency, for example, was defined by the refusal of a clearly indicated medical procedure or performance below a cutoff on a short test of cognition. Charlie Sabatino, the head of the American Bar Association's influential Commission on Law and Aging since 1984, summed up the state of affairs: "The power that the clinicians have in these cases was just remarkably unlimited with these perfunctory analyses and opinions being taken with very little challenge."[6]

The scholars at Pittsburgh were patiently working through the legal and ethical literature to both explain the problem and propose solutions. In 1987, the same year as the astonishing AP report, Loren Roth, Alan Meisel, and Charles Lidz—a psychiatrist, lawyer, and sociologist, respectively—published a foundational paper in the *American Journal of Psychiatry*. "Tests of Competency to Consent to Treatment" summarized the cacophony of terms and then made the case for a set of five possible tests to assess whether a person was competent.[7]

The MacArthur network set out to refine these tests and translate them into clinical practice. In the ensuing decade, Appelbaum was among a team of researchers who created a conceptual foundation to a disordered, idiosyncratic field. They developed a model to assess capacity. Diagnostic labels and cognitive test scores were cast aside. Instead, the clinician needed to assess at least one of a person's four decisional abilities: the ability to understand facts, to recognize how risks and benefits applied to daily life, to infer outcomes, and to express a choice. In other words, the abilities to understand, appreciate, reason, and choose.

Each ability was defined in ways that gave clinicians a common language to talk about a person's capacity. Of particular value, they created short interview guides and instructions for a clinician to assess a patient's capacity to make a particular decision. These interviews came to be known as the Mac-CAT tools, short for MacArthur Competence Assessment Tools.[8] To assess a person's understanding of, for example, a drug's risks, the clinician asks: "Can you tell me in your own words what are the risks of this drug?" And to assess his appreciation, the clinician asks him to explain if he thinks it's possible the drug could harm him.

This work was groundbreaking. Like PiB, the imaging agent for amyloid, it transformed the ways physicians thought about and communicated with people with Alzheimer's. What had once been mysterious and seemingly impossible to measure now had a common and coherent language and tools to measure it. Instruments soon multiplied to assess the ability of a person to make all kinds of decisions: voting, appointing a proxy, writing a will, executing an advanced directive, and solving a day-to-day functional problem.

Research took off. The results of studies of persons with dementia caused by Alzheimer's disease disrupted old norms. A diagnosis of dementia does not map to incapacity, especially among patients with mild- to moderate-stage dementia. Notable fractions of these patients in fact retain the ability to decide whether to take a treatment for Alzheimer's disease,[9] enroll in a clinical trial,[10] or appoint another person to make decisions for them.[11] Some even retain the ability to solve a functional problem, such as finding help to manage their medications or prepare a meal.[12] Decision-making capacity varied within a person; that is, a person may lack the capacity to consent to enroll in a risky research study, but she still may have the capacity to appoint someone else to make the decision for her. The overall message of the research was clear and consistent. The physician needed to talk, adult to adult, to her patient.

In some clinical settings, this model of capacity assessment has taken hold, but like memory centers, HELP, and hip fracture programs, it hasn't spread far and wide into the day-to-day lives of persons with Alzheimer's. Old ways of thinking (diagnosis equals incompetence, for example) and acting (talking only to the patient or only to the caregiver) need to change.

One setting where it is especially needed is in the care of patients who are not embedded in trusting networks of care like Mr. Johnson is. These are patients without a spouse or who have children at odds with one another over what is the right thing to do for their parent. For these patients, help comes from social service agencies. At these agencies, busy caseworkers are charged with an ethically fraught decision. Is this older adult living the life he wishes to live, or is he in need of help? Alone and refusing help, is he a proud captain of his self, or is he a victim of himself or others, the people who claim to help but are abusing him, most commonly by stealing his money? The skills of capacity assessment apply here, too.

Sadly, they're rarely used. Caseworkers typically decide whether the person has the capacity to choose by relying on the results of short cognitive tests. Colleagues who teach these caseworkers how to correctly assess capacity describe a profound, eye-opening light bulb moment, when the caseworker realizes that her focus should not be the person's score on a short test of cognition or the diagnosis or even a judgment about the rightness or wrongness of the decision the person made—their choice—but to judge the person's ability to make the decision.

In the lives of adults with Alzheimer's disease, guardianship is the exception, not the rule. Families work things out. Property is shared with spouses. Someone has a power of attorney limited to finances. Advance directives and informal conversations guide decisions. Laws and ethical codes recognize that close family can make a decision for a patient who cannot. Though these day-to-day and clinical settings are far from a courtroom, capacity still matters.

I used the questions from the MacCAT-T (the MacArthur Competence Assessment Tool—Treatment) to guide my conversation with Mr. Johnson about my prescription of an adult day activity program. I uncovered impairments in his capacity. This was revealed in his answer to the question: "Do you think it's possible that attending the activity program could benefit you?"

He couldn't. In the language of capacity, he couldn't appreciate the possible benefit of the treatment. In the care of persons with Alzheimer's disease, this is a common problem. Patients will often recognize they have some degree of impairment but simply fail to connect the benefits of a treatment to their impairment. When such patients refuse an intervention, as Mr. Johnson refused the adult day activity program, what to do next depends on the problem the intervention will treat and the benefits and risks of the intervention. This step is of course an ethical judgment. It requires weighing risks and benefits—and the harm of setting aside a person's self-determination.

Arguing that Mrs. Johnson should force her husband to attend would be coercive—even abusive—and likely unsuccessful. Still, displaying to her that he lacked the capacity to refuse was revealing. She shouldn't simply rest on his refusal. Instead, she ought to work to persuade, cajole, and reframe their options. "Do this for me. I need some time to shop for us." In this way, she would not so much be making decisions for him but asking him to support each other.

The list of corrections is long and complex, but the point of part 3 is simple. It is possible to reintegrate the biological, psychological, and social so that patients and families can live well and with dignity with Alzheimer's disease.

In the early twentieth century, an equally elegant argument could have been made about what do about the polio epidemic. As cases of the crippling and sometimes deadly neurological disease multiplied, we'd train more pediatricians and physiatrists and build better and more convenient iron lungs and rehabilitation centers and develop the necessary social and financial supports to provide patients access to them.

We could do that for Alzheimer's, colleagues chide me. Build more memory centers, nursing homes, and adult day activity centers. Noodle our way to better team-based care. Set our hospital cell phones to vibrate at night.

Or, they insist, we could just cure this damn disease.

21

TARGETING AMYLOID

The only drug that is best used after symptoms is Viagra.
—Reisa Sperling, MD

THE SEPTEMBER 1, 2016, issue of *Nature,* the prestigious 147-year-old "international journal of science," displayed big news: the discovery of a breakthrough treatment for Alzheimer's disease. The all-capital-letter headline of the magazine-style cover read: TARGETING AMYLOID.[1] Above it were two identical images of brain Amyvid scans.

On the right was a cool blue brain without amyloid. To its left was a hot red brain with a yellow rim, a cross section of a brain on fire with amyloid. The story was a report on the effects of the drug aducanumab ("a-doo-can-noo-mab") on 165 persons with Alzheimer's disease. The two pictures told the message of the study report's thousands of words. The drug turned a red brain blue. It cleared toxic amyloid from a patient's brain.

After fifty-four weeks of monthly intravenous infusions, the subjects—persons with either MCI or mild-stage dementia who had positive amyloid scans—showed the striking contrasts displayed on the cover. The patients who received the drug had less amyloid than patients who received a placebo. Beneath TARGETING AMYLOID was the study's take-home message: "Antibody aducanumab reduces Alzheimer's disease–associated amyloid in human brains."

Alone, these results were a provocative science experiment. What put the study on the cover of *Nature*—as well as made it headline news—were the results of the "clinical measures," the regularly scheduled assessments of the patient's memory and function. These measures were labeled as "exploratory" (the study's main focus was measuring amyloid), but the responses seen in persons on the drug suggested that the researchers were on to a breakthrough treatment.

Some but not all of the measures suggested lowering brain amyloid slowed the usual rates of decline in cognition and function experienced by persons living with MCI or dementia caused by Alzheimer's disease. In an accompanying commentary on the study, Eric Reiman, a prominent Alzheimer's disease researcher at the Banner Alzheimer's Institute, wrote: "If that hint of a clinical benefit is confirmed, it would be a game changer in the fight against Alzheimer's disease."[2]

A SUCCESSFUL FAILURE

For Dale Schenk, the 2016 *Nature* cover story was the apotheosis of a career as a groundbreaking neuroscientist dedicated to discovering a disease-slowing treatment for Alzheimer's disease. Seventeen years earlier, he'd led a team of San Francisco–based researchers working with him at the Irish pharmaceutical company Elan. Like TARGETING AMYLOID, their study made the cover of *Nature*. The July 8, 1999, issue announced: "PURGING THE BRAIN OF PLAQUES."[3]

The research report remains among the cleverest and most creative approaches to treating neurodegenerative diseases. Schenk entirely cast aside the well-trod approaches, particularly boosting neurotransmitters with drugs like the cholinesterase inhibitors. His inspiration was to go after amyloid as if it were a kind of bacteria or virus, a foreign invader of the brain that could be removed by the body's immune system.

The idea of an "immunotherapy approach to Alzheimer's disease" was at first so unusual that Elan resisted devoting resources to support the studies, but Schenk—ever amiable, well liked, and deeply respected as a scientist— persisted. The executives who controlled the budgets finally relented and authorized funding his experiments.

"Immunization with amyloid-β attenuated Alzheimer disease–like pathology in the PDAPP mouse" reported the effect of injecting mice with the fragment of amyloid known to lead to the toxic plaques. Would this stimulate the mouse immune system to attack these fragments and so prevent the development of plaques?

The answer was unequivocal. The mice who received the injections were cleared of amyloid plaques, whereas those who received a placebo showed the characteristic buildup. The results in young mice who were destined to develop the plaques were even more provocative. They did not develop plaques. The report concluded: "Collectively, these results suggest that amyloid beta immunization may prove beneficial for both the treatment and prevention of Alzheimer's disease."

The study of an experiment in mice genetically engineered to produce toxic amyloid was so revolutionary it was a headline story. *PBS NewsHour*'s headline was: A NEW POTENTIAL FOR AN ALZHEIMER'S VACCINE. And Dr. Steve DeKosky, an Alzheimer's Disease Research Center director at the University of Pittsburgh and spokesman for the Alzheimer's Association, described the result as "striking, even to the scientists who did the study. I don't think they thought it was as effective as it turned out to be."[4] Lary Walker, an Alzheimer's disease researcher at Emory University, recalled that in the days following the 1999 publication he considered shifting his research to a new disease because "it looked like the Alzheimer's problem had been solved."[5]

Elan and other pharmaceutical companies quickly mobilized their resources. Within three years, immunotherapy for Alzheimer's disease was being tested in humans. The first of these studies, with a drug called AN-1792, stumbled. It caused dangerous brain inflammation that necessitated halting the study. Detailed subanalyses of the results offered hope. Some persons who had received AN-1792 had amyloid cleared from their brains and, in some of these cases, this correlated with clinical stabilization. The study was ironically dubbed a "successful failure."

The field retooled the immunization strategy, switching from an "active approach" that injected amyloid in order to stimulate antibody production to a "passive approach" that infused a manufactured antibody targeting amyloid. It was this retooled attack on amyloid that led right up to the study of aducanumab in humans. The immunotherapy approach to Alzheimer's disease had crossed the chasm from mice to men.

On September 30, 2016, just twenty-nine days after *Nature*'s "game-changing" report that aducanumab cleared a human brain of amyloid, Dale Schenk, fifty-six years old, died of pancreatic cancer. Eulogies and memorials uniformly and unconditionally described him as an industry scientist who was uniquely collaborative and open in his approach to research. A brilliant career was prematurely ended.

By 2016, his breakthrough had spawned multiple potentially game-changing drugs that were under study. Joining aducanumab were bapineuzumab ("bapi-nez-ooo-mab"), crenezumab ("creh-nez-oo-mab"), gantenerumab ("gantan-eer-oo-mab"), and solanezumab ("sola-nez-oo-mab")—all bearing the signature *ab* ending to indicate the passive antibody approach to clearing amyloid from the brain (moreover, early-phase safety studies of revised active immunization strategies were promising).

Large studies using these *ab* drugs were underway or in planning, and several of these have taken a bold step forward. Unlike the study published in *Nature*, whose subjects were persons either with MCI or mild-stage dementia, these studies were testing drugs in persons without *any* cognitive impairment. A race was on to discover a treatment to prevent people from developing Alzheimer's disease dementia or even MCI. In 2016, the first of these "Alzheimer's prevention studies" was already three years underway.

PRECISION MEDICINE FOR THE BRAIN

The vast ballroom at the Westin San Diego Gaslamp Quarter was filled to capacity as Dr. Reisa Sperling stepped up to the podium on the morning of November 17, 2013. The latecomers stood in the back beside the coffee service tables. Sperling needed a stepping stool to reach the microphone (she's four feet, eleven inches tall), but her stage presence was commanding and confident. Before embarking on a career in academic neurology, she performed musical theater. It was her grandfather's and father's suffering with Alzheimer's disease that compelled and sustained her switch to medicine and a dedication to Alzheimer's disease research.

I first met her years before at a conference for promising young researchers in aging research. "You've got to see this," she enthused as she flipped open her laptop. "Look at this!" They were images of amyloid PET scans from participants in the Harvard Aging Brain Study, or HABS, a study that serially assesses the cognitive function of several hundred older adults in the Boston area, many, like her, Harvard faculty.

As she balanced the computer on her palm, with her free hand she gestured to the screen. "We've been amyloid imaging people in HABS. These are squeaky-clean normals, all over sixty-five" ("normal" means that their cognitive function was unimpaired; they had neither MCI nor dementia).

As expected for a normal, the images were the cool blue ones of a brain without amyloid, but several weren't. They were the red-hot images of PiB binding to brain amyloid.

The scans of about one-quarter of the "normal" HABS participants were these "abnormal" results. What excited her—and me—were her graphs of the annual results of the two groups' measures of their cognition. Both started

out the same, but over time they diverged. The curve of those without amyloid wasn't a curve. It was flat. Those with amyloid, however, displayed a
steady downward decline. In time, some were diagnosed with MCI and later,
dementia.

"This is Alzheimer's," she explained, "unfolding in a normal person."

Now, less than a decade later, she was putting a bold idea to the test.

This meeting was the kickoff of the Anti-Amyloid Treatment in Asymptomatic Alzheimer's study or the A4 Study, for short, a multimillion-dollar
clinical trial designed to test solanezumab, an experimental drug manufactured by the pharmaceutical company Lilly, in one thousand adults, ages
sixty-five to eighty-five, whose cognitive test scores fell within a range of normal but whose amyloid PET scans showed elevated amyloid. Half of these
subjects would receive a monthly infusion of solanezumab, a drug like aducanumab that binds to brain amyloid, and half would receive a placebo.

After four and a half years, the study would end and investigators would
compare the two groups. If the people who received the drug showed less
cognitive decline compared to the people who received a placebo, doctors
like Sperling and me would radically change our clinical practice. We'd diagnose the disease at a stage even before MCI, when an Amyvid scan shows
elevated amyloid, and prescribe solanezumab to delay the time before a person develops MCI or dementia.

Sperling summarized the strategy. "Cancer, stroke, HIV, diabetes—they're
all better treated earlier—before a patient is symptomatic. The only drug that
is best used after symptoms is Viagra."

The Alzheimer's field was energized about an idea: drugs like aducanumab
and solanezumab that targeted amyloid will extend the time before a person
transitions from being normal and healthy to having a diagnosis of MCI or
dementia. Our goal was to discover "disease-modifying therapies" to prevent the onset of symptomatic Alzheimer's disease. These same drugs were
also being tested in persons with MCI and dementia. The "test-drug" logic
of these studies was to give the drug to a person who has a test result signifying a heightened risk of cognitive impairment or, if they were impaired, risk
of suffering more cognitive decline.

Researchers were using one of two strategies to identify persons at risk.
The A4 Study was among several studies that used an "Alzheimer's disease
biomarker enrollment strategy." To enroll in these studies, a person must have
elevated amyloid. Dr. Reiman led a research team whose strategy focused on

testing drugs in persons with a genetic risk of developing Alzheimer's disease dementia.

His team created GeneMatch, a massive online registry that enrolled people who'd undergone testing for the APOE gene. First described in 1993, persons with a particular form of this gene, called the APOE ε4 allele, have an increased but not definite risk of developing dementia caused by Alzheimer's disease. In GeneMatch there were tens of thousands of volunteers willing to be contacted to learn their APOE result, and, if it was the APOE ε4 allele, they would enroll in a trial.

Researchers at Washington University in Saint Louis led a research team that used a similar but even more targeted genetic risk approach. They were testing drugs in persons with rare genes that inevitably cause a person to develop Alzheimer's disease by their fifties (less than 1 percent of all cases of Alzheimer's disease are caused by these genes).

Immunotherapy was just one promising drug being tested. By 2016, when aducanumab made headlines, potentially disease-modifying drugs were being tested in humans that targeted the enzymes that precipitated the cascade of events that broke amyloid into toxic fragments that then accumulated into plaques. These "secretase inhibitors," so named for the enzymes they blocked, were like the immunotherapy approaches. They promised to slow or even shut down the production of toxic amyloid fragments.

With drugs targeting amyloid pathology, given to persons with an Alzheimer's biomarker or gene along the continuum of cognitive abilities, the Alzheimer's field seemed poised to take a great leap forward into the twenty-first-century world of "precision medicine for the brain."

Dr. Paul Aisen, the lead presenter at the disastrous 2013 MEDCAC hearing that led to Medicare's decision to deny coverage for amyloid scanning, enthused of a day when an amyloid scan would be akin to a "colonoscopy for the brain." His idea was that just as this test for colon cancer is universal for all who turn fifty, so, too, there would be an age when an amyloid test would be part and parcel of routine care. Colleagues speculated over strategies: an APOE test at, say, age sixty, and if you are an APOE ε4 carrier, get an amyloid test; and if the test shows elevated amyloid, start treatment. Otherwise, wait perhaps five years and then receive an amyloid test.

Looking back, it's amazing these large and costly studies were happening. In the years that followed Schenk's 1999 paper, America experienced a series of staggering and demoralizing economic and international challenges, beginning with the terrorist attacks of 2001 and the subsequent wars in Iraq and Afghanistan costing trillions of dollars per year. And then in 2008, the world's economy nearly collapsed. The country and its leaders were deeply divided along partisan lines, arguing over just about everything and especially over federal spending. It was a horrible set of political conditions under which to advocate for the massive and sustained increases needed for funding for Alzheimer's research.

Moreover, enduring and seemingly intractable congressional customs stifled any dramatic increase in spending federal dollars specific to Alzheimer's disease research. Divided as Congress was, they remained unified in obeying an unwritten rule. Congress doesn't do "disease-specific" research funding. Instead, Congress allocates funds to the NIH. The NIH directors decide how best to spend the dollars.

From its inception, the Alzheimer's Association obeyed this rule. The December 4, 1979, minutes of the nascent board of directors recorded an enthusiastic rollout of multiple committees eager to get to work. The Public Policy Committee, however, was launched but then instructed to be cautious in advocating in Congress for research funding. Its leaders could contact a few members of the congressional appropriations committees but again "care must be taken because Congress is not receptive to the 'Disease of the Month' concept."[6]

Since 1980, all increases to Alzheimer's disease research at the NIH were from incremental increases to the *overall* NIH budget. The National Institute on Aging then took from this the portion for Alzheimer's disease.

And then something happened that was as revolutionary as Schenk's 1999 *Nature* study. In 2011, America had a national plan to tackle Alzheimer's disease. In language reminiscent of President Kennedy's 1963 deadline-driven call to land a man on the moon and safely return him to earth before the decade's end, goal number one of this plan was that America would "prevent and effectively treat Alzheimer's disease by 2025."

America had launched the Alzheimer's moonshot.

Millions of dollars were now available to Drs. Sperling and Reiman and other researchers for their massive, yearslong studies. And more funding was on the way. America was beginning to tackle at least part of the problem of Alzheimer's.

The story of how this came to pass in a deeply divided Washington is a fascinating tale of power and persuasion, or in a word: politics.

22

HOPE IN A PLAN

The Alzheimer's crisis, like the disease itself, will unfold gradually, making
it all too easy to ignore until we have little opportunity to alter its impact.
—Alzheimer's Study Group, *A National Alzheimer's Strategic Plan:
The Report of the Alzheimer's Study Group*, 2009

ON THE MORNING of Wednesday, March 25, 2009, room 106 in the Dirksen Senate Office Building was packed. The audience for this hearing of the Senate Special Committee on Aging was loud and lively. The occasion was *The Way Forward: An Update from the Alzheimer's Study Group*. Alzheimer's disease had come a long way since its first Senate hearing in July 1980 when Jerry Stone and Bobbie Glaze testified to a single senator in an empty hearing room.

The personal remarks from the eight senators showed this, too. Senator Susan Collins, Republican of Maine, explained how Alzheimer's is so common in her family that they call it the family illness. Her and her colleagues' candid and forthcoming sharing of their personal experiences demonstrated the social and cultural transformations since the 1990 hearing when Senator Hatfield's disclosure of his father's Alzheimer's disease silenced the hearing room. The stigma of Alzheimer's was, perhaps, abating.

In a deeply divided, often hyperpartisan Washington, DC, this hearing was an unusually bipartisan event. Testifying to the committee were two former congressional opponents, former Speaker of the House Newt Gingrich, a Republican, and Bob Kerrey, a former Nebraska senator and a Democrat. Together, they chaired the Alzheimer's Study Group whose nationally prominent members included former directors of the NIH and Centers for

Disease Control. At this hearing, together with another group member, the retired Supreme Court justice Sandra Day O'Connor, they were presenting the results of a two-year project to examine the federal response to Alzheimer's disease.

Justice O'Connor's opening remarks summed up their conclusion. "Our nation has no real plan for a Federal effort to find a solution or to help manage costs, and we need to do both."[1]

The study group's forty-nine-page report framed the urgency of the problem with dire, even apocalyptic rhetoric. The opening paragraph evoked recent environmental and economic crises—the multibillion-dollar damage and thousands of lives lost in 2005 to Hurricane Katrina in America's Gulf Coast and the 2008 economic collapse—to set up an argument. "If we fail to address the Alzheimer's crisis now, we face the prospect of losing lives and dollars on a much larger scale."[2] The word "crisis" appears twenty-four times.

The crux of their argument was money, specifically the cost of the disease to the United States economy and the federal budget. "Over the next 40 years, Alzheimer's disease–related costs to Medicare and Medicaid alone are projected to total $20 trillion in constant dollars, rising to over $1 trillion per year by 2050." Dr. Katzman's 1976 essay that framed the disease as a "major killer" was being recast. Alzheimer's disease was like the budget deficit, unemployment, or inflation. It was a national economic problem in need of a national solution.

This framing of the disease as a threat both to the nation's economy and to two of the largest federal expenditures (Medicare and Medicaid) was a politically unifying strategy designed to capture bipartisan congressional attention. Among the plethora of figures in the report, one gained traction. "For every dollar the Federal government spends on the costs of Alzheimer's care, it invests less than a penny in research to find a cure."

After Susan Collins spoke these same words at the hearing and then proclaimed, "It is time for us to put our foot on the accelerator and redouble our research efforts," the audience in room 106 broke out in applause.

This line about the disparity between the dollars spent on care versus on a cure was the pivot from dire warnings of economic disaster to a plan of action. The Alzheimer's Study Group called for the Alzheimer's Solutions Project—a bold national plan to discover a cure. "In 1961, the Apollo program was the right mission to spearhead our exploration of the great frontier of outer space. . . . Today, overcoming Alzheimer's disease is the ideal mission to spearhead a new era of exploration of the human mind, with great potential benefits across the entire spectrum of human health and activity."

By 2020, the United States will discover a cure. Congress was being asked to unleash a momentous, truly breathtaking commitment of resources.

The report included a table of five prior "Great American Projects," their "champion," and their start and completion dates, beginning with the transcontinental railroad championed by President Lincoln and ending with the Human Genome Project championed by President Clinton. For the sixth project—the Alzheimer's Solutions Project—the spaces for its champion and dates were blank.

The group's call for a deadline-driven, all-out assault on Alzheimer's disease modeled after ambitious national projects such as the invention of the atomic bomb and construction of the transcontinental railroad and the Panama Canal was the inspiration of one man, Zaven Khachaturian, a childhood refugee from Syria who had emigrated to the United States to study neurobiology.

He'd led the NIA's Alzheimer's disease research program since its inception in 1978. After he retired in 1995, in cooperation with the Alzheimer's Association, he organized a series of symposia devoted to socializing the Alzheimer's disease research community to a plan. The United States should fund a national mission: prevent Alzheimer's disease by 2020. He formed the advocacy group PAD2020, for Prevent Alzheimer's Disease by 2020, and became an adviser to the Alzheimer's Study Group.

Khachaturian was therefore ready when selected members of the group, notably two former NIH leaders, objected to a deadline-driven national plan for Alzheimer's disease. Drs. Harold Varmus, a Nobel laureate, and Steve Hyman cautioned against the harms of an analogy to successful engineering projects, warning that it would encourage unrealistic expectations of progress and distort research priorities set without a foundation of knowledge needed to guide decisions.

Khachaturian responded with a petition. Appendix F of the report lists 139 Alzheimer's researchers, Khachaturian among them, who endorsed the goal of preventing Alzheimer's disease by 2020, provided that the effort was backed by sufficient funding and "pursued an appropriate, disciplined strategy."

A commission led by former colleagues whose members were undisputed leaders in science, business, and medicine had presented Congress with a fact-packed assessment and plan to take bold action to address the Alzheimer's crisis. Three months later, in July 2009, a bipartisan group of senators and representatives followed their lead. They introduced the Alzheimer's Breakthrough Act. The act called for a doubling of funds to the NIH for Alzheimer's research and the convening of a National Summit on Alzheimer's to bring together scientists, policy makers, and public health professionals to work out the strategies and tactics needed to spend these funds in the race to a cure by 2020. The Alzheimer's Association called the Breakthrough Act "a tremendous step in the fight against Alzheimer's" that would "change the paradigm" of research.[3] It was Congress's opportunity to join the 139 scientists who endorsed the 2020 moonshot.

The act never became law. It never even came up for a vote. And this wasn't the first failure to massively increase funds for Alzheimer's research. It was the fourth since 2000.

Before we examine why it failed and the political theater that followed, we need to look deeper into the events that made the Alzheimer's Study Group happen. In just a few years before 2009, Alzheimer's disease advocacy had transformed. The polite and collegial world of not-for-profit advocacy that steered clear of elections, donations, and lobbying was now melded into the hurly-burly partisan world of national politics. This transformation can be traced to the efforts of two men: George Vradenburg and Harry Johns.

Together, they were the founding fathers of Alzheimer's disease as a political movement.

George Vradenburg stands tall and confident. Following college at Oberlin, where he studied economics, and his service in the navy, the Harvard-educated lawyer—he was a partner at the centuries-old prestigious firm Cravath, Swaine and Moore and in-house counsel at CBS—capped his career as one of the founders of America Online, or AOL (in its time, one of the largest internet service providers). That work made him wealthy. In 2001, after a near-fatal heart attack, charitable work became his full-time occupation. He raised funds for the victims of the 9/11 attack and also to prepare the DC region against another terrorist attack. But then he began to perceive how America faced an even greater threat than terrorism. And it was right at home: Alzheimer's disease.

His wife, the writer Trish Vradenburg, instigated this. She was becoming increasingly concerned about her risk of Alzheimer's disease. Her mother had died of it.

The couple soon embraced the customary activities expected of charitable, wealthy, and well-connected Americans. They held parties that raised lots of money.

Their annual National Alzheimer's Galas raised over $10 million for the Alzheimer's Association. After their April 2011 gala, Trish Vradenburg blogged that the attendees included senators and representatives. "These are, after all, the ones who vote on funding so we want them to see the problem and be part of the solution."[4] The evening at the National Building Museum ended with all raising lit candles to sing "The Times They Are A-Changin'" to persuade those congresspersons to increase funding for Alzheimer's research. The creator of ADNI, Dr. Mike Weiner (piano), and the director of the NIH, Dr. Francis Collins (guitar), led the performance.

But then the parties ended.

The Vradenburgs were frustrated. The pace of incremental progress was too slow. They disagreed with the association's strategy that respected the unwritten congressional prohibition against "disease-of-the-month funding." Cancer and AIDS both received targeted, sustained, and massive increases in their research funding. Why not Alzheimer's disease?

They changed their strategy and tactics. No more raising money for other groups' efforts. They announced they'd transformed from philanthropists to "philactivists." They were going to persuade those senators and congressmen to make Alzheimer's disease a priority in need of a response commensurate with the nation's response to terrorism.

Theirs was an aggressive, multipronged strategy.

They created UsAgainstAlzheimer's, a not-for-profit advocacy organization, to lead a network of "[group]AgainstAlzheimer's" brigades, including WomenAgainstAlzheimer's, ClergyAgainstAlzheimer's, and ActivistsAgainstAlzheimer's, and coalitions of willing partners, including the Latinos Against Alzheimer's Coalition, Youth Against Alzheimer's Coalition, and the Global CEO Initiative on Alzheimer's Disease.

They added politically powerful weapons to their arsenal: a 501(c)(4) organization, or "(c)(4)," and a political action committee, or PAC. With these, they could take on activities prohibited to a 501(c)(3), a not-for-profit to whom donations are tax deductible. From offices on K Street in Washington, DC, they commanded forces that could engage in partisan and political activities such as advertisements during an election year, fundraising for candidates' campaigns, and donations to politicians.

The Alzheimer's Study Group was their brainchild. The inspiration was the Iraq Study Group, a bipartisan group of ten prominent Americans formed to advise the government on a way out of the escalating quagmire in Iraq. To lead this, they needed a very particular person, a nationally prominent public official who, though out of office, still commanded media attention and cared passionately about Alzheimer's disease. After attending a speech at the FDA by former Speaker of the House of Representatives Newt Gingrich, Vradenburg knew he'd found his national champion. Gingrich had argued that Alzheimer's disease was the greatest health crisis of the twenty-first century.

"I said to Newt: 'Let's do an Alzheimer's Study Group.' And Newt said, 'That's a great idea.'"[5]

At the same time that UsAgainstAlzheimer's was advocating to Congress in ways never before seen in the history of Alzheimer's disease, the Alzheimer's Association also was preparing to enter the political battlefield. In 2006, the board of directors hired a new president and CEO, the master's in business administration–trained Harry Johns. In his prior work as executive vice president for strategic initiatives at the American Cancer Society, Johns worked on laws to protect employees with cancer from being fired and to facilitate access to mammography and colonoscopy.

If Vradenburg is rock and roll, then Johns is mellow country music. Bearded and self-effacing, he started his education at a community college in his native southern Illinois, worked on Capitol Hill for his district's representative, and earned an MBA at Northwestern University's weekend executive training program. He was intent on figuring out how to instill in not-for-profits the mission-driven approach of a for-profit business and a master in deploying an armamentarium of political tools such as a (c)(4) or a PAC to achieve mission-driven strategies and tactics.

Johns was taking command at a low point in the association's history. Five years earlier, the association embarked on a radical plan to change how Americans think about Alzheimer's disease and the association. Market research found that 80 percent of Americans weren't aware of any Alzheimer's support organization. A general sense of hopelessness surrounded the disease. They launched the trademarked "Maintain Your Brain" campaign designed to both raise the association's profile and inspire hope in America that *right now* something could be done about this most feared disease.

The messages delivered in print and video advertisements promoted brain-healthy activities. They included "Think Round" to promote eating fruits and "Eat Blue" to focus that choice on blueberries, a fruit that is rich in brain-protective nutrients. To promote a physically and socially active lifestyle, there was a video of an elderly woman dressed in parachute gear, the wind whipping her gray hair, grinning as she exited the plane's hatch and leapt into thin air.

The campaign was an undisputed flop.

Researchers and clinicians conceded that decent evidence did support that these behaviors reduced the risk of dementia, but little if any evidence supported the claim that they prevented Alzheimer's disease. Moreover, it was a message that seemed to distract from the research mission. None of the anti-amyloid drugs—or any other drug for that matter—had been proven to be effective. America needed to invest its hope in research, not eating blueberries. It was the wrong message at the wrong time.

The public was also confused. "Maintain Your Brain" suggested people who developed Alzheimer's disease did so because they didn't live a healthy lifestyle. The association seemed to be blaming the victims for their misfortune and suffering.

The campaign was quickly scrapped, the president resigned, and a period of retreat and reflection ensued. Out of that came a renewed conviction and sense of urgency that immediate and bold action was needed to promote research to discover a cure. Under Johns's leadership, the association embraced a vigorous commitment to promoting research. They were going to dramatically increase, from millions to billions, sustained funding to the NIH. They assembled their arsenal.

In 2007, the association published the first edition of its annual *Alzheimer's Disease Facts and Figures Report*, described on its cover as "a statistical abstract of U.S. data on Alzheimer's disease published by the Alzheimer's Association." The text is dry and the rhetoric cool (terms such as "epidemic" and "crisis" don't appear). The terms "America" and "Americans" are used frequently. Data are presented both nationally and, most notably, state by state. The messaging is to politicians. The facts and figures that tiny Rhode Island has 37,000 caregivers who provide 32 million hours of care worth $310.7 million was likely of not much interest to a caregiver living there, but it was of great concern to her federal and state senators and representatives.

To ensure that those officials were concerned, the association created the Alzheimer's Impact Movement, a (c)(4), and a PAC. Now they could, like UsAgainstAlzheimer's, dive into the thick of Washington politics.

In a 2012 interview, George Vradenburg explained the difference between the two organizations. "The Alzheimer's Association is the battleship; we're the destroyer."[6] The failure to pass the 2009 Alzheimer's Breakthrough Act was the armada's first battle and its first defeat. They were truly caught in a dilemma. Each member of Congress seemed like Hamlet. They cared a lot about the disease (it was Senator Collins's family disease), but they were incapable of doing anything about it.

The times were not changing.

NO MORE BREAKTHROUGHS
WITH BREAKTHROUGH ACTS

The failure of the Alzheimer's Breakthrough Act was a tremendous disappointment to the Alzheimer's movement. It was the political equivalent of the failure of AN-1792, the first of the amyloid immunotherapy drugs in humans that caused the dangerous brain inflammation in persons with Alzheimer's disease dementia.

Things got worse. The association and Alzheimer's Impact Movement made a strategic decision to retreat. There would be no more breakthrough acts, no more frontal assaults on Congress with grandiloquently titled bills.

In an interview nine years later, Robert Egge, the association's chief public policy officer and executive director of the Alzheimer's Impact Movement (and former executive director of the Alzheimer's Study Group), remembered vividly the intense emotions this decision provoked. "We were so desperate to get things done and the idea that we would have to step back in order to step forward to set up for success was a lot to ask of this community. But our sense was we haven't done our homework yet. We're not going to break through with another breakthrough act."[7]

UsAgainstAlzheimer's disagreed. Behind George Vradenburg's desk is a tremendous reproduction of the actor George C. Scott outfitted in his role as General Patton in the 1970 movie *Patton*. Asked if he agreed with the general's dictum "a good plan executed right now is far better than a perfect plan executed next week," he replied decisively: "Absolutely."

He redoubled efforts for another act and advocated for changes to laws and regulations to create public-private partnerships and extend a drug's patent life to incentivize the pharmaceutical industry to study Alzheimer's disease. He used the (c)(4) and PAC to make Alzheimer's the issue in the 2012 presidential race. Gingrich tried the same in his 2012 bid for the Republican nomination. Both campaigns failed to capture the voters' imaginations.

Meanwhile, the association took stock of the political landscape. The country and the capital were deeply divided along partisan lines. If President Obama emulated President Kennedy's grandiloquent political act of a national address to a joint session of Congress to call for America to discover a cure for Alzheimer's disease by 2020, he'd most likely receive a chilly reception. Fierce and partisan bickering—not national unity—was the norm in Washington.

Moreover, the endless wars in Afghanistan and Iraq and the 2008 economic collapse were continuing to sap the will of legislators to spend federal funds. When congresspersons were asked in private to increase funding, they'd often respond incredulously: "Why do you need more money? In the five years between 1998 and 2003, we doubled NIH funding from thirteen to twenty-seven billion dollars."

The work that followed is perhaps best understood not with military metaphors but as an intellectually demanding game of chess. Johns and Egge were deliberate, quiet, and very decisive. They launched a series of targeted and incremental steps, a steady movement of the pieces up to a checkmate. They started not by asking for money but instead for yet another Alzheimer's plan.

On January 4, 2011, on the eve of his Christmas holiday vacation at Hawaii's Kailua Bay Paradise Point resort, President Obama signed the National Alzheimer's Project Act into law. There was no speech, signing ceremony, or address to Congress or the American people. Just a short press release. These low-key optics were the complete opposite of the Great American Project Vradenburg, Khachaturian, and Gingrich desired.

It was precisely as the association planned.

The law came to be known by its abbreviation, NAPA. It was a short set of instructions to the secretary of the Department of Health and Human Services to create and maintain an integrated national plan to overcome Alzheimer's disease. All federal agencies whose work touched Alzheimer's disease were authorized to participate in an advisory council to create a plan to accelerate the development of treatment, halt or reverse the disease, improve diagnosis, and coordinate care and treatment. Joining the council were twelve members from outside the federal government, including caregivers, patient representatives, researchers, and "voluntary health association representatives, including a national Alzheimer's disease organization that has demonstrated experience in research, care, and patient services."

Notably, it called for absolutely no money.

"It was," Egge reflected, "an underwhelming bill. I imagine some people were thinking, 'We just did the Alzheimer's Study Group. This is another variation on the theme of 'Let's do another plan.'"

It was exactly the move they intended. Another plan.

The report the advisory council produced was a detailed, dispassionate presentation of the problem of Alzheimer's disease in America. It proposed five goals, each with detailed strategies, and those strategies were tagged with action items. Three of them—to enhance the quality and efficiency of care, support patients and their families, and promote public awareness and engagement—reiterated the decades-old goals of advocates like Hilda Pridgeon, Bobbie Glaze, and the other founders of the Alzheimer's Association. Goal number one was the most provocative: "Prevent and effectively treat Alzheimer's disease by 2025."

The moonshot was on but with a deadline pushed five years later—and most notably without a dollar to support it or for that matter any of the plan's other ambitious goals. Remember, all the law authorized was a committee to create yet another report.

The chess pieces were moving closer to victory.

The report was part of a strategy to open up Congress to increase funding specifically targeted to Alzheimer's disease. Egge summarized this strategy in an imaginary conversation with Congress. "We would go back to Congress and say, 'What part of this do you take issue with? You asked for this, Congress. You asked for this report to be done by government. It's come back to you. Are you going to ignore what they say?'"

In fact, they didn't take the report back to all of Congress. There were no packed hearings or press conferences. Persuading all of Congress to massively increase funding for Alzheimer's disease research and care was a Sisyphean task. Instead, the association used the full power of its (c)(4) and PAC to persuade the powerful chairs of the House and Senate committees that allocate funding to the NIH.

This targeted exercise of power and persuasion worked. In 2013, Congress added $100 million in funding to the NIA for research on Alzheimer's disease. In the history of the Alzheimer's crisis this disease-specific appropriation was probably the single most important moment, both for the dollars and the revolution in how the dollars were allocated. The fundamental objection that Congress could not increase disease-specific funding was dropped.

The final move in this quiet game of political chess was to sustain the massive increase in funding. One more short, targeted piece of legislation was needed. In December 2014, Congress passed its massive annual spending bill. Tucked into the 702-page document was a hundred-word paragraph, section 230, the Alzheimer's Accountability Act.[8] It authorized the director of the NIH to prepare an annual budget to meet the benchmarks and goals of the National Alzheimer's Plan.

This budget was unique. It would bypass the usual process that begins with congressional review and revisions. Instead, the NIH request would go directly to the president for approval. The NIH had been granted the power to ask for exactly how much it needed to address the Alzheimer's crisis.

Alzheimer's disease had joined a privileged group. Only cancer and HIV/AIDS research were the focus of the same budget-making authority.

It was the breakthrough! Four decades after the seven families banded together to form their voluntary self-help organization, the United States was finally taking on the disease of the century.

And yet, frustrating ironies endured. President Obama did embrace the call for a national investment in a "moonshot cure," but not for Alzheimer's disease. In his January 12, 2016, State of the Union address, he rallied America: "For the loved ones we've all lost, for the families that we can still save, let's make America the country that cures cancer once and for all."

WHERE WERE YOU ON MARCH 21?

The mood at the November 2017 Clinical Trials on Alzheimer's Disease, or CTAD, meeting was congruent with its gilded setting, the Grand Ballroom in the elegant Boston Park Plaza. Researchers were upbeat over the progress to discover Alzheimer's disease–slowing therapies. Several anti-amyloid immunotherapy drugs were in "late-stage" phase 3 trials (phase 3 is the final step of study before the FDA decides whether a drug is safe and effective and so can be prescribed for the care of patients). These studies—with enticing names like Expedition, SCarlet RoAD, Engage, and Emerge—were being conducted worldwide at hundreds of clinical trial centers. They typically enrolled from one to two thousand persons with either MCI or dementia. After a PET scan confirmed elevated amyloid, the subject was randomly assigned to either drug or placebo and then assessed at regular intervals for as long as one and a half to two years.

Privately, however, many researchers were beginning to worry. Two of these promising studies had failed. Would the nearly two-decades-old idea of immunotherapy approach work? Some were even questioning not just this particular approach but whether amyloid was the right target.

The first failure was Pfizer's bapineuzumab, among the earliest of the passive immunotherapies. Its promising 2007 start ended in July 2012, when Pfizer issued disappointing news. The clinical trial studying patients with mild- to moderate-stage Alzheimer's disease dementia showed that one and one-half years of drug treatment did reduce amyloid, but this reduction didn't translate into a benefit to the patients' cognition and day-to-day function. In the months to follow, three other similar trials of "bapi," as it was commonly referred to, failed.

Bapi's failure taught the field lessons. Immunotherapy approaches weren't a simple exercise in vacuuming up so-called mature amyloid plaques. The studies needed to test even more targeted approaches, such as removing the fragments of amyloid that would coalesce into plaques. Moreover, bapi caused the small blood vessels in the brain to leak tiny amounts of blood and fluid into the brain. This risk came to be called ARIA, for amyloid-related imaging abnormalities. It was a side effect that while easily detected with MRI, required either lowering, interrupting, or even stopping the drug altogether.

ARIA introduced a number of complexities into these studies. Of greatest importance, the drug might in fact harm the very same organ it was intended to treat. Early detection seemed to limit that harm to an individual, but detection effectively "unblinded" the person and their caregiver, meaning it revealed they were receiving the risky active drug and not placebo. Such unblinding biased patient and caregiver reports of how the patient was doing. Hope and its attendant expectations of benefit are powerful medicines in and of themselves.

The finding that the risk was more common in persons with the APOE ε4 gene led some studies to test patients for the gene in order to dose the drug with greater care in APOE ε4 carriers. Knowledge of this genetic risk for Alzheimer's disease gave a patient and caregiver information to understand and consent to the risk of ARIA, but it also introduced bad news to their family. Blood relatives may have this gene and therefore are at heightened risk of developing Alzheimer's disease.

Even more frustrating than the bapi results were the results of studies of solanezumab, or "sola."

The lessons from two failed studies of the drug instilled great hopes in Lilly's third try, the Expedition 3 study in 2,129 persons with mild-stage Alzheimer's disease dementia. A single word in AlzForum's November 23, 2016, report on Expedition 3's results described the frustration. "Lilliputian."[9]

Persons on the drug benefited, but the difference between their scores and persons on placebo was quite small and just on the wrong side of statistical significance. This result divided experts. Some concluded it was experimental proof that the immunotherapy approach worked, but others concluded differently. Immunotherapy approaches were not the way forward.

Dr. Sperling articulated the consensus position. Giving drugs like sola to persons with mild-stage dementia was likely "too late" in the course of the disease. Amyloid accumulation started early in the natural history of Alzheimer's disease. It was bittersweet support for the A4 Study's strategy of testing the drug in persons without cognitive impairment. The A4 Study would continue, using a higher dose of solanezumab in the expectation that this higher dosage would transform a Lilliputian blip into a gargantuan benefit.

The data from bapi, sola, and other studies clarified the promise of immunotherapy approaches. It was far more nuanced than their initial 1999 success in mice. Monitoring for ARIA added complexity. And yet, hope endured. Not only aducanumab but also crenezumab and gantenerumab were in large late-phase studies.

Two years later everything seemed to come crashing down.

In January 2019, Roche halted its studies of crenezumab in persons with mild-stage dementia and two months later did the same with its studies of gantenerumab. Like bapi and sola, the drugs affected amyloid levels and caused ARIA. Unfortunately, the effects on amyloid didn't translate into a clear slowing of the disease. By July of that year, at the annual international gathering of Alzheimer's disease researchers in Los Angeles, the mood was grim and desperate.

"Where were you on March 21?" was asked with the same dark meaning as catastrophic dates like September 11 or November 23 (the dates, respectively, of the terrorist attacks on the United States and President Kennedy's assassination).

I was at my university office reading email when a colleague sent me Biogen's press release. Engage and Emerge, their two phase 3 studies of aducanumab in persons with MCI and mild-stage dementia caused by Alzheimer's disease, were being terminated. The company was shutting down further development of aducanumab.

The problem was the results of a planned interim review by an independent safety monitoring board. The drug wasn't working. Further study and so exposing persons to the risk of ARIA was judged futile. The studies were discontinued.

More bad news piled up. Several studies of the secretase inhibitor drugs, the drugs that targeted an enzyme that cut amyloid into its toxic fragments, had failed across the continuum of persons living with Alzheimer's disease. Persons with dementia, MCI, and cognitively normal persons with elevated amyloid experienced *declines*, not improvement in cognition, while taking these drugs.

The field was gathering failed trials like a stamp collection.

And then came October 22, 2019. "Check out the news from Biogen" was the simple message of an early morning email from a colleague. I clicked on the link: "Biogen plans regulatory filing for aducanumab in Alzheimer's disease based on a new analysis of a larger dataset from phase 3 studies." Biogen was going to ask the FDA to approve their drug. "If approved," the press release read, "aducanumab would become the first therapy to reduce the clinical decline of Alzheimer's disease and would also be the first therapy to demonstrate that removing amyloid beta results in better clinical outcomes."[10]

Biogen's stock rebounded from its March plummet.

Two months later, at 8:00 a.m. on December 5, 2019, I was among the crowd packed into the Hilton San Diego Bayfront's Indigo Ballroom. The occasion was the opening scientific presentation for CTAD 2019. The buzz and feel in the room was of a celebration. There were hugs, smiles, laughter, and friendly backslaps. In the ensuing forty minutes, Samantha Budd Haeberlein, Biogen's vice president for clinical development, delivered the company's reanalyses of Engage and Emerge.

It turned out that at the same time as the independent data and safety board was reviewing the data that caused them to conclude the drug was futile and that the two studies should stop, more data were coming in. Analyses that included these additional data reached a different, though still nuanced, conclusion.

The Emerge study was a success. Patients taking the drug had slower decline in their cognitive scores than the patients taking placebo. Engage, however, wasn't successful.

Haeberlein explained that a deeper dive into Engage suggested a subset of persons on the highest dose of the drug, like the subjects in Emerge, had slower decline in cognition. Biogen was so confident with these results that they planned to ask the FDA to review them and, they expected, approve the drug for sale.

The chatter in the coffee lounge wasn't as bullish and confident. Midstudy changes to the design of the studies—one study positive but the other negative, unblinding because of ARIA, teasing out results using subanalyses and, also, results not presented—all added up to disquiet. *Something* might be happening to the patients who received the drug, but the results could also be random events. Another study was needed to sort out the disturbing uncertainties.

Twenty years after Dale Schenk's revolutionary study, an immunotherapy approach targeting amyloid had crossed the finish line—or maybe not— but the initial promise at the dawn of the twenty-first century of a cure for Alzheimer's disease, a result so provocative it made headlines and some researchers pondered switching to another disease, was exhausted. At best, this drug slowed the disease. The benefit to patients was modest, perhaps a few months' delay before a person cascaded downward from being inefficient in her daily activities to being disabled and needing a caregiver to monitor and help her.

For the millions of people with MCI or dementia caused by Alzheimer's disease and the millions more at risk of these conditions, aducanumab presented a complicated and nuanced message of a very qualified hope. Drugs targeting amyloid might alter the natural history of disabling cognitive impairments, but if they were like this drug, they only made a dent.

These ambiguous results added to an escalating criticism that the Alzheimer's field was captured in service to a decades-long error. Beta-amyloid—the protein at the core of the senile plaque that Robert Katzman described in his April 1976 editorial and that Glenner and Wong sequenced eight years later, that PiB imaged and that Schenk cleared with his immunotherapy approach—wasn't the cause of Alzheimer's disease. It was therefore the wrong target for treatment.[11] Critics pointed to the results of nearly two decades of research. The mice get better but the humans don't.

The mice in question were "transgenic animal models" of what was claimed to be Alzheimer's disease. These "transgenics," as they came to be called, were created using elegant engineering to insert rare human genes that caused the disease at the unusually young age of fifty years old. They were the mice Schenk used in his 1999 *Nature* study.

Anti-amyloid drugs given to these transgenics produced spectacular successes. As the mice were cleared of amyloid, they performed better on tests of mouse memory, such as remembering to quickly paddle to the dry spot in a tankful of water. But in humans with the common late-onset form of the disease, the same drugs were either consistent failures or, if aducanumab in fact worked, not a cure but instead modestly beneficial. This gargantuan mismatch between the disease engineered in mice versus the disease in humans suggested that the field was in a sense captured in the costly service of raising and caring for thousands and thousands of mice rather than spending those dollars on studies of humans with the actual disease.

The goal was care of the patient with the disease. But which disease?

The story that older adults with dementia typically had Alzheimer's disease caused by amyloid plaques and tau tangles was too simple. A single word summarized the results of decades of research: heterogeneity.

This term described how persons with Alzheimer's disease pathology had other pathologies as well. A colleague quipped to me, "The least common form of Alzheimer's disease is Alzheimer's disease." Meaning, patients with only Alzheimer's pathology were the exception, not the norm.

A convergence of findings supported this. They included how among older adults, vascular lesions—not strokes but rather patches of fuzzy white dots seen on MRI thought to be micro infarcts—were quite common and had a notable role in causing the disease to become symptomatic.

Further support for heterogeneity was that persons with dementia caused by Alzheimer's disease who were over eighty had an additional, distinct pathology not seen in persons who were under eighty. These patients not only had the classic amyloid and tau pathologies of Alzheimer's but they also exhibited a third, not-well-understood pathology called pathologic TDP-43 (TDP-43 is the abbreviated name of a protein that normally controls how cells read their DNA). The younger patients didn't have pathologic TDP-43.

The discovery of TDP-43 presented potentially devastating consequences to patients, their families, and society. Persons over eighty, sometimes called the oldest old, are the largest proportion of persons with dementia. The aging of the baby boom population ensures they're the fastest growing proportion. Experts worried whether this common pathology might confound the ability to measure the success of a drug targeting amyloid or tau. Some even argued that drug studies to discover a treatment for Alzheimer's disease might have to *exclude* persons over eighty. The discovery of an effective drug treatment for Alzheimer's disease might, therefore, not be a breakthrough for these millions of persons and their families.

Fortunately, innovation has been at work. By 2020, the field was responding to heterogeneity. The drawing board listing other possible targets for Alzheimer's disease was quite full. They included, to name just a few: drugs targeting tau protein, inflammation, the brain's metabolism of its essential fuel, glucose, and even drugs for viral infections. These multiple candidate pathways to treatments kindled hope, but together with the heterogeneity in the common late-onset forms of the disease they led to an unsettling consensus.

Alzheimer's disease is like cancer. It isn't one disease but many (some spoke of "Alzheimer's *diseases*"). And like cancer, we should expect we're going to discover better treatments, but we're not going to drug our way out of this complicated enormity of a problem. George Vradenburg summed up this assessment in a 2017 interview. "I think we're going to be in a world in which we have some successful drugs, but the drugs are only going to be partially effective and where we're going to need high-quality care institutions for a very, very long time."[12] Addressing the Alzheimer's crisis with a strategy that relies on discovering "the cure" is like planning for retirement with lottery tickets.

The other goals of the national plan—to improve the system of care—demand work equal to our search for better treatments.

The challenge is to finally end the bitter fight that broke out on the Monday afternoon in October 1979 when the founding families of what would become the Alzheimer's Association debated what their mission was: a world without Alzheimer's disease or a world that cared for all persons with dementia, regardless of the cause.

Our mission has to be both, because the problem of Alzheimer's disease isn't simply a scientific puzzle to be solved, a menace of "druggable" pathologies to be conquered. It's the vortex of the scientific, political, cultural, and social problems of aging and disability.

It is a humanitarian problem.

PART 4

. . . .

A HUMANITARIAN PROBLEM

Reports of a decline in age specific incidence and prevalence of dementia in some regions, concurrent with improvements in living conditions,
education and health care, suggest that dementia is indeed preventable.
—Graeme J. Hankey, "Public Health Interventions
for Decreasing Dementia Risk," *JAMA Neurology*, 2018

There is no such thing as a self-made man or woman. Never was, never
will be. We are all, as were those in whose footsteps we follow, shaped
by the influence and examples of countless others—parents, grandparents, friends and rivals.

—David McCullough, commencement address
to the University of Oklahoma, 2009

23

SOMETHING *MUST* BE WORKING

What if I had grown up in Boston? If I believe my research, I think I would
be in much poorer health.

—Lisa Barnes, PhD

LOOKING BACK ON my years of medical training in the closing decade
of the twentieth century, I now recognize that I was witness to events that
were distinct, sometimes quite sudden, and entirely without precedent in the
history of medicine. Dramatic expansions in the numbers of patients and
transformations in what it means to be a patient were occurring. Disease in
general was becoming chronic. The exemplar was heart disease.

At least two forces were at work: longevity and technology. Courtesy of advances in public health, such as vaccines and infection control, people were
living longer lives, but as they did, they were more likely to suffer a heart attack or heart failure. Fortunately, advances in technology began to transform
lives once crippled or even ended by heart disease. By 1991, the year I interviewed for residency in internal medicine, cardiology was the king of all specialties. Cardiologists used "clot buster" drugs to dissolve away the blockage in
a coronary artery and lower cholesterol and blood pressure, and they installed
devices to pace a lethargic heart, arrest a deadly rhythm, and channel blood
flow through narrowed arteries or leaky valves. Surgeons had their dexterous
hands in some of this, too, of course. The point is that what were once crippling, even deadly events often became manageable chronic diseases.

At the same time, advances in diagnostic technologies relentlessly pushed heart disease into the land of the healthy. During my medical internship, the meaning of an elevated blood pressure in an older adult changed. At the start of internship, I explained to my elderly patients how their elevated pressure was their aging body's "natural response" in order to push blood through their hardened arteries. By the end of internship, I told my patients something quite different. What was once considered normal cardiac aging was now a disease called systolic hypertension of the elderly. I prescribed medication to lower their elevated blood pressure. Fast-forward three years to my fellowship in geriatric medicine. Nearly all my patients were on antihypertensive medications.

In the years to follow, the cutoffs for "normal levels" of blood pressure, as well as cholesterol, kept changing. Each time they did, more and more "asymptomatic patients" were added to the tally of the millions of patients who survived events such as a heart attack or stroke. The sum of all these events was a staggering increase into hundreds of millions of patients with what we loosely called heart disease.

Oncology has a similar history. Cancer still kills, often quite mercilessly and dreadfully, but for many patients, treatments have turned cancer into a chronic or even a curable disease.

Now, as the twenty-first century unfolds, Alzheimer's disease is experiencing a similar revolution. As people survive their heart attack, as heart failure and some cancers become chronic diseases, people are living into their eighties and beyond. This is the age of dementia.

Cancer and heart disease are of course diseases of the body. There is something different—truly peculiar—about the experience of a disease that disables the mind. The husband and adult children of one of my patients revealed this to me. Midway through his detailed account of her illness, her husband paused the recitation of his day-to-day tasks and decisions and expenses and gripped his chest like a man signaling a heart attack. But his gesture was the sign of the experience of a very different illness.

He insisted, "*I* have Alzheimer's disease!"

He's right. For every patient with dementia, there's a caregiver—or should be—to manage time, task, and truth and who must cope with experiences of ambiguous loss and worries about the future. The number of patients doubles.

Their son and daughter, out of earshot of their suffering parents, taught me other ways the numbers and disease experience are changing. The son implored me with a question and the daughter with wide-eyed worry. "Doctor, is there anything *we* can do about this?"

"This" was their worry of becoming like their parents.

Their worry was legitimate. Katzman's 1976 call to redefine senility as Alzheimer's disease transformed it into a prevalent disease affecting millions of families and thus entire communities. The biomarker redefinition will multiply these numbers. As my colleagues discover how to diagnose and treat the disease before a person has dementia or even MCI, the diagnosis of Alzheimer's disease will spread to include a stage defined not by cognitive decline but instead by biomarkers and only biomarkers. A 2018 study estimated that as many as 46.7 million persons have this "preclinical Alzheimer's disease," a term that describes a diagnosis before cognitive impairment.[1] The net effect of biomarker discoveries is that each of us is more and more likely to learn we are at risk of dementia—or at risk of becoming a caregiver. Or both.

The complexity of Alzheimer's disease (really diseases), the lack of a simple and single "druggable target" so that we might tame it like influenza, measles or polio, the threat of chronic escalating disabilities, the staggering costs of time and task, the stigmas that corrupt dignity and identity together converge on a call to action. Nations must tackle the Alzheimer's problem as a humanitarian problem. They must muster the full range of medical, scientific, social, civic, and cultural resources. Good data from well-done studies are showing us the way.

We just have to listen to their results.

The 2017 Alzheimer's Association International Conference unfolded over four days at London's inspiring hundred-acre ExCel center. The London Docklands is somewhat out of the way from central London, but the visit is worth the journey. Following the collapse of London as the world's largest port, the Docklands became synonymous with decay. Now, it displays a city transformed. There are architecturally provocative meeting spaces, stylish hotels, and restaurants.

In the evenings, my colleagues and I rode the cable car across the River Thames to take in the spectacular view from 295 feet over the river and then wandered through the entertainments at the O_2, a venue for cultural events. We needed these distractions and entertainments. The proceedings of our conference left us despondent. As we lamented the myriad of failed clinical trials and the complexity of the disease's biology—"heterogeneity" was *the word* at the conference—the prestigious British medical journal *Lancet* tried to lift our spirits.

As much as 35 percent of the lifetime risk of developing dementia was caused by things people could do something about.[2] To reinforce the promise that taking action could reduce the risk of developing dementia—and therefore reduce the burden of dementia on a society—the report summarized multiple studies showing that in the past thirty years, the risk of developing dementia has been declining. There still are millions of people with dementia. There just aren't as many as we expected and, if we take action, there may be fewer than the 13 million projected in 2050.

The implications for policy makers, for society, are immense. The crisis may not bankrupt us—may not be as bad as we fear—provided we act on the answers to the questions: What have we been doing? And what more do we need to do?

The residents of a town some thirty miles to the west of Boston, Massachusetts, are showing us the answers. On September 29, 1948, the first of Framingham's twenty-eight thousand residents enrolled in the Framingham Heart Study.[3] In the decades to follow, thousands of residents participated in hourslong study visits that included physical exams, blood tests, cardiograms, and questionnaires about their habits, such as smoking and exercise. Every two years, they came back to the research center and repeated this work.

The study they were in, commonly called Framingham, became a treasure chest of data to explain the natural history of heart disease, one of the twentieth century's greatest killers. Framingham was among the key studies to demonstrate that the rise in blood pressure seen commonly in aging was not "normal" but rather the sign of disabling, deadly events to come, namely a stroke or heart attack.

Framingham even created a new lexicon of health: the "risk factor." The term describes a measurable and defined quality such as elevated blood pressure or cigarette smoking that if present, increases a person's likelihood of suffering a heart attack or stroke and, most importantly, if addressed, reduces her risk. These risk factors have been assembled into the Framingham Risk Score, widely used by doctors to calculate a patient's overall risk and thus to prescribe interventions to reduce that risk.

In the 1970s, the researchers broadened their interests to include diseases of the brain. They added tests of cognition, brain scans, and neurological exams to take on the new problem of dementia. Forty years later, their results made headlines.

From 1970 to 2008, the risk of getting dementia has been steadily declining. A 20 percent drop per decade.[4] This seemed ironic. In that same time period, the only treatments for dementia caused by Alzheimer's disease were the minimally effective cholinesterase inhibitors. Researchers hadn't discovered disease-slowing treatments for Alzheimer's. But something must be working to keep aging brains healthy despite Alzheimer's pathology. A dive into the data showed what they were.

Over thirty years, the residents with access to health care took more and more treatments to prevent heart disease, such as antihypertensive medications, and if they developed heart disease, particularly a heart attack or stroke, they received care. The more care they got, the healthier their brains were. Their risk of dementia was lower. Drugs to lower blood pressure and cholesterol were one intervention. The residents of Framingham also benefited from reductions in rates of tobacco smoking and other heart-healthy lifestyles.

Framingham wasn't unique. Similar large studies from Sweden and the United Kingdom showed the same results.[5] The *Lancet* report summarized their results into a compendium of early- to late-life interventions that can reduce the risk of dementia. The message to individuals, communities, and policy makers was loud and clear. Access to health care, such as in America through the Affordable Care Act, and communities that promote exercise by, for example, building sidewalks and recreation centers, and those that incentivize healthy habits with nudges like a soda tax and bans on smoking, are steps that will address the Alzheimer's crisis.

Framingham reported another finding with tremendous policy implications. EDUCATION MAY CUT DEMENTIA RISK, STUDY FINDS was the headline of the *New York Times* story reporting the decades-long decline in the risk of developing dementia.[6] Only residents with at least a high school education experienced the reduced risk.

Multiple studies have shown that education—the years of our youth spent in a classroom—protects us from the ravages of a disease of our aged selves. How is this possible? Among the clues to explain what might be at work were the men and women who ferried my colleagues and me to and from our hotels and the ExCel center—the cabdrivers of London.

Gaze at a map of the streets of London. The image is quite distinct from Manhattan's neat and ordered quadrille of streets and avenues. It seems the work of an expressionist painter, a collage of lines going in all directions. Imagine that you had to memorize this map well enough to negotiate a car trip without the aid of either a map or GPS. That's the daunting requirement you need to fulfill to become a licensed taxicab driver in London. It will take you about two years to do this. If you succeed, if you pass the test, you're now among those "being on the Knowledge."

The Knowledge is among the purest natural experiments of how education affects our brain. Our capacity to learn a place—where things are and how to get about—resides in a very specific part of our brain, the posterior portion of the hippocampus. Researchers at University College London took advantage of learning the Knowledge as a natural experiment in the effects of education on the brain.[7] Does a London cabdriver who has passed the exams have a particularly large posterior hippocampus?

The answer is they do. The posterior hippocampus of taxicab drivers on the Knowledge is larger than that seen in people who do not have the Knowledge. To increase confidence that this difference is the result of rigorous learning of a complicated geography and not regularly driving about the busy streets of London, the researchers compared the hippocampi of London's cabdrivers to its bus drivers.[8] Their work is similar to a cabdriver but simpler. They need to learn not the map of London but just one route.

The comparison firmed up the result. Cabdrivers have larger hippocampi than bus drivers. Learning and practicing the Knowledge was the thing.

Findings such as these support a decades-old theory called cognitive reserve. Among its earliest proponents was Robert Katzman, who picked up on a puzzling finding from his neuropathology colleagues. The brains of some older adults Katzman pronounced as *without dementia* had Alzheimer's disease pathology like a person *with dementia*, but their brains were often larger than a person's with dementia. They had the disease—the pathologist could see it—but something seemed to be protecting them from showing the signs of it. The theory is that a larger brain has more neurons with multiple connections to other neurons, a kind of matrix of neural protection against the slow ravages of pathology. This is cognitive reserve.

The finding that mastering a cognitively demanding activity—navigating the streets of London, playing the piano, learning a second language—causes a strengthening of the regions of the brain where we execute that activity is immensely appealing. It confers a biological story to the consistent results of multiple studies. The more years of education a person has, the lower her risk is of developing dementia. Her brain is better able to withstand the vicissitudes exacted by pathologies such as amyloid, tau, and TDP-43.

Cognitive reserve is a biological argument for a public policy. To prevent dementia, we ought to make a robust investment in public education and other cognitively stimulating venues such as museums and cultural centers. This argument offers the opportunity for consilience between generations. Money spent on the young will doubly aid the elderly. The young shall have better jobs so as to help pay for care (through taxes or meeting direct expenses), and they'll be less likely to develop dementia.

But there was more than just schools and other educational programs at work in Framingham. Something else was keeping their brains healthy.

The psychologist Lisa Barnes discovered this firsthand.

Barnes is a professor at Rush University in Chicago and an expert on how social and behavioral factors affect the aging brain. She didn't start out with this interest. As she studied psychology, the Chicago native was planning to pursue laboratory studies of memory. In college, she studied patient HM, the renowned research subject whose capacity to form memories was irrevocably lost following a neurosurgery that destroyed the hippocampi in his otherwise healthy brain. As a consequence of this brain damage, he became a living laboratory to study how memory works.

"I was of the view that the brain is the brain is the brain," she recalled in an interview some thirty years after her studies on HM.[9] But then she took a ride on the Boston T.

The year was 1985. She was a student at Wellesley College, a prestigious college on the shore of Lake Waban some fifteen miles west of the city of Boston, surrounded by well-off suburban towns like Brookline and halfway to Framingham.

"I'm from Chicago. Chicago city girl, South Side. Even though I wasn't physically in Boston, because I'm a city girl, I did like to go to the city occasionally, and I had some bad experiences there and I never really felt welcome." She remembers fellow riders on the metro (known as the Boston T) got up from their seats and moved away from her.

She loved her Wellesley education, but right from the start something didn't feel right. College is an opportunity to explore and try new things, but at her new-student orientation she and her fellow African American students were instructed on where they should not explore and what they should not do. They should avoid certain Boston neighborhoods. They were told the residents there did not like Black people. Some of her friends ignored the advice, made a visit, and suffered insults and even assault.

This was quite different from where she grew up. The University of Chicago's Lab School was, like her Hyde Park neighborhood in Chicago, integrated. In a city segregated by race and social and economic status, her school and neighborhood were a kind of oasis. Boston and Wellesley were quite different.

"I always felt like an outsider," she recalled. "I didn't have a lot of money growing up, and most of the women at Wellesley were very wealthy, people who were driving Porsches, and I was on work study."

A semester away at the historically Black Spelman College in Atlanta, Georgia, was transformative. She felt welcomed and nurtured. She belonged to a community. She never returned to Wellesley. In time, she dropped her plans to study the precise mechanisms that explain how brain regions produce cognition. Instead, she returned home to Chicago and joined the faculty at Rush University to begin a career studying big questions: Why do African Americans perform lower on tests of cognition? Do they have a greater risk of developing dementia? And, if they do, why?

Finding answers to these questions requires more than the application of the biological sciences. The brain is the brain is the brain, and yet, all brains live in and interact with the world around them. Race in America is about how you are treated because of the color of your skin. What Lisa and her fellow students of color experienced were the effects of people perceiving them as different and thus treating them differently. Researchers therefore have to use a diversity of sciences including psychology, epidemiology, anthropology, and sociology in order to measure complex constructs like stress and discrimination.

This research remains a work in progress but among the results, one is particularly compelling.[10] Answers to questions about how you were treated beginning at a very young age—questions such as "Where were you born and where were you living when you were twelve years old?"—explain some of African Americans' performance on measures of cognition.

If you are Black and answer with regions of the American South, particularly those in what was once the Confederacy, that explains the lower scores. Schools in the South were segregated and the schools for persons of color were notoriously underresourced. They were given fewer teachers, shorter class time, and fewer textbooks. Remember, the count of the number of years of education is only a proxy for cognitive reserve. These data show the obvious: the quality of those years of education matters.

Lisa's experiences were, however, not in the South but rather in the North, in Chicago and then Boston, the city that calls itself "the cradle of liberty." She found salvation in the South, in an Atlanta-based college community that cared for her, much like the community where she grew up. Which shows another important finding.

When others repeatedly mistreat a person, they cause chronic stress. This stress is toxic to neurons, especially neurons in the hippocampus, the region of the brain that is often first affected by Alzheimer's pathology.[11]

Lisa suffered two years of acute stress. Imagine a lifetime of repeated discrimination, people hurling insults and objects at you, moving away from you on the metro. Imagine going to a school that is a school only in name. These microaggressions and deprivations accumulate. Over time your brain is at greater risk of dementia.

As the Framingham study was getting started, Framingham was changing. Like much of America, the sleepy town of farmers and small businesses was experiencing America's post–Second World War boom of growth and opportunity. These included the Servicemen's Readjustment Act of 1944, known more commonly as the GI Bill. By the late 1950s, millions of veterans were benefiting from assistance to obtain loans for a mortgage or to start a business. They were paid tuition to attend college or a vocational school. Some of these veterans settled in Framingham and so the town grew and prospered.

But not every veteran and town benefited. Persons of color were routinely denied mortgages and loans. Admission to schools would require an act of the Supreme Court in *Brown v. Board of Education* and other rulings that slowly chipped away at entrenched discrimination. Culture was slower to change. Lisa experienced that.

I asked her if she'd grown up in Boston, what would that have done to her? "What if I had grown up in Boston?" she reflected. "If I believe my research, I think I would be in much poorer health."

HM, the man she studied early in her career, suffered brain damage at the hand of a neurosurgeon treating his disabling seizure disorder. His seizures vanished but so, too, did his ability to make new memories. The message from the studies done by researchers like Lisa Barnes is that poor-quality schools, discrimination, and the social and economic deprivations that ensue are like HM's neurosurgeon's knife. The disease that impairs our ability to live as individuals is in part the consequence of our failure to live well together and the damage we inflict on each other's brains.

Out of this sad fact emerges an inspiring idea. Ending the ways we mistreat and fail to care for each other are tools to address the Alzheimer's crisis.

And yet, even in the "brain-healthy" world that we can create, we should expect people who, despite the best of our collective efforts, despite a quality education and good health care, will be at risk. I have many patients who enjoyed well-nurtured childhoods and prospered in well-paid professions, who, but for Alzheimer's disease, are quite healthy. Clearly, we need treatments that target the pathologies.

We haven't yet discovered these treatments. We also haven't discovered the right combination of tests to accurately measure an individual's risk of developing dementia. Imagine a sort of Framingham Risk Score for the brain that combines measures such as age, biomarker tests, and perhaps a genetic test. Above a certain score, a drug is prescribed.

This is a promising future, but it is also challenging. Once these discoveries are part of standard clinical practice, we'll live in a world with our "brains at risk." This will threaten the very selves we're trying to protect. This isn't speculation. The following chapter explains how the subjects and their families in the A4 Study and other biomarker-based Alzheimer's disease studies are living in existential dread.

24

EXISTENTIAL DREAD

I feel very sensitive about the PET scan result. It speaks to who I am. My brain is a very critical part of me. I also, in some sense, define myself by what my brain is like. If my brain goes, I'll feel really, really bad.

—A person who learned his amyloid PET scan result
showed "elevated amyloid"

I'LL ALWAYS REMEMBER Paris in July.

It was there and then that I experienced one of life's events that opened me up to new worlds. I was at the Paris Expo at the 2011 annual meeting of Alzheimer's disease researchers. Dr. Reisa Sperling and I struck up a conversation during one of the breaks. She was describing her plans for what would become the A4 Study.

After she summarized the idea—test an anti-amyloid drug in several hundred cognitively unimpaired people ages sixty-four to eighty-five whose Amyvid scan shows amyloid—I asked her the question.

"What do we tell a person who enrolls?"

"About the scan result?" she replied.

"Right."

"That's what I wanted to ask you."

It was the beginning of our yearslong collaboration.

Three years later, one hot and humid August morning at the Penn Memory Center, I met the first person who was seeking to enroll in the A4 Study at the center. I'd known Mr. Hooten for several years. After a career as an engineer, he was now a vibrant, active cyclist, a painter, and an enthusiastic participant in the center's research studies. This visit was what the A4 Study called the amyloid imaging disclosure visit.

"Your scan," I told the seventy-six-year-old man, "shows elevated amyloid."

He exhaled slowly through his nose. "That's not good news."

Perhaps it wasn't but I was confident it was news he could deal with. I was confident because my colleagues and I had worked for months to create what we called the amyloid imaging disclosure process.[1] As we worked, I was haunted by a name: Rita Philip, the woman with MCI and a positive amyloid scan who, after I told her she had Alzheimer's disease, suffered crippling anxiety, wished she'd never met me, and whose daughter said she feared how her mother would become a zombie.

I was determined not to repeat that disaster.

We used as our guide the practice of disclosing the results of tests for genes associated with a disease, such as a BRCA gene that if present, means a woman is at heightened, though not certain, risk to develop breast and ovarian cancers. In many respects, the practice for disclosing the results of a genetic test is analogous to delivering an Alzheimer's disease biomarker result to a person who is cognitively unimpaired. The biomarker test result explains the likelihood of a future health event—developing MCI and later, dementia.

This rationale is different from my rationale for ordering Mrs. Philip's test. For her, the test was diagnostic. It, together with her MRI, explained her year or two of mild memory problems. We were mindful, however, of two important differences between an Alzheimer's disease biomarker test and a gene test: (1) biomarkers are not hereditary and (2) biomarkers are dynamic, meaning, the test result is a snapshot in time of the beginnings of a disease unfolding in a person's brain. Put another way, we are born with our genes; we develop our biomarkers.

The process had two components—education and an assessment of psychological well-being and motivations. The assessment of well-being used measures of mood and took a careful psychiatric history of suicidality. To undergo the amyloid scan, a person's scores on the measures must be within ranges deemed healthy and the person must not endorse a plan for self-harm or have a history of such behaviors in the face of bad news. At my study site, I excluded a man who explained to me that if he had elevated amyloid and, in time, developed more problems with word finding and recall, he would asphyxiate himself in his garage. His life as an actor, he explained, depended on his memory.

The education was our qualified, first-step effort to turn the language of amyloid-imaging research into a clinical lexicon that made sense to people like Mr. Hooten. We settled on two terms to describe a scan result: "elevated amyloid" and "not elevated amyloid."

One of our key messages was delivered using an analogy to heart disease. The relationship between elevated amyloid and Alzheimer's disease is like the relationship between elevated cholesterol and heart disease. Decades of research in hundreds of thousands of people show that an elevated cholesterol is associated with an increased risk of a heart attack. Amyloid, we explained, is similar but in these early days of research we didn't have the robust results needed to tell someone like Mr. Hooten what his personal risk of developing MCI or dementia was. The best we understood at that time was that a person with elevated amyloid was more likely than a person with not elevated amyloid to later develop disabling cognitive problems.

This was exciting work. My colleagues and I were carving out of normal aging a new illness experience. Our hunch was that if solanezumab worked, if the drug slowed cognitive decline, then amyloid testing—and for that matter other biomarker measures such as tau or TDP-34—would join a list of tests that is quite familiar to aging Americans, a list that includes blood pressure, bone mineral density, cholesterol, mammogram, and colonoscopy. Each of these tests, if positive, initiates a prescription. A positive test means you are at risk of a hip fracture, for example, and the prescription—a medication to strengthen bone density—is given to reduce this risk. The unifying strategy is risk reduction.

The analogy made sense logically but emotionally it didn't. An amyloid test was quite unique. We soon discovered that the aftermath of learning an amyloid test result was worlds apart from learning the results of a cholesterol test.

Our assessment of psychological well-being and education kept matters safe. Mr. Hooten didn't develop disabling depression or worry. In general, people like him who learned they had elevated amyloid and so enrolled in the A4 Study to try out whether a drug would reduce their risk of Alzheimer's disease dementia handled the news without catastrophe. They weren't depressed or traumatized. They were, however, transformed.

"It's less about medical than about my personality. A colonoscopy isn't going to change who I am. This is my brain involved," was one woman's answer to the question how the amyloid test compared to other medical procedures.[2] Her answer expressed a common theme among people with elevated amyloid. The result was different from other medical tests because the disease this test foretold was not an attack on the body but on the mind and her self-determination and identity.

The existential significance of the test translated into action. One woman explained to me how she shared the result with her husband, but they decided not to tell their daughter. "I don't want to worry her, and plus, I think she may start building that into the ways she interacts with me. I don't want that." She didn't tell her friends with whom she played bridge out of concern that an error at the game, such as forgetting the suit designated trump, would cause them to ease her out of the game. Another woman noted that when a person in her retirement community develops Alzheimer's disease, fellow residents begin to separate from them. These personal and particular experiences share a common theme. People who learned they have elevated amyloid were concerned about stigma, concerned that they would be treated as "less of a person" and suffer as Lisa Barnes did when her fellow passengers on the Boston T got up from their seats and moved away from her.

People also described how knowledge that they had elevated amyloid caused them to think differently about their future and the plans they were making. I recall one woman explaining how she was caught up in a dilemma created by a feeling that "the clock is ticking." Before she learned she had elevated amyloid she expected to live into her eighties. The prospect of Alzheimer's disease prompted her to think about those last years and how to pass her remaining time.

"Part of me says, 'OK. I want to enjoy myself more. I'm going to cut back on working even though that would mean less income of course.' But working is stimulating for me, and it keeps me going. I don't know. I'm conflicted. Yes. I'm a little more conflicted about how I want to spend my time based on the fact that I may have limited time left."

She was, she explained, "more 'planful.'"

A scan result affected other people, too, especially adult children and spouses. An elevated result fostered sometimes difficult conversations about the future, of being a "pre-caregiver" and of becoming a caregiver. Couples pondered moving closer to family. One man reflected how his dog would likely be his last pet.

Persons who learned they had a not elevated test result by contrast recounted joyful conversations with family members, celebrating that they would not have to become their caregiver. One simple word, repeated over and over in conversations, summarized their reaction to "not elevated." Relief.

These experiences and concerns were of course not uniform. Some A4 Study participants were quite matter-of-fact and open about their "elevated amyloid" result, explaining how they shared it widely. Some reported no changes in their life or plans save for the monthly visit to receive the infusion at the research center. Still, the message was clear: telling a cognitively unimpaired older adult a positive Alzheimer's disease biomarker test result creates an existentially fraught experience.

The drugs being tested in studies like the A4 Study are of course the key to shaping this illness experience. If one worked, if it slowed down the time before a person developed MCI or dementia, how would it change how these people reacted to learning they had elevated amyloid? Other existentially fraught diseases provide guidance.

In the early years after HIV became prevalent—when it was untreatable and so a serious and life-threatening illness—persons with the infection were shunned and despised. The test for the virus required in-person, pre- and post-test counseling, akin to the model of genetic testing. In time, as treatments were discovered, attitudes and behaviors changed. It is possible now to test oneself in the privacy of your home.

An effective treatment for Alzheimer's disease could cause a similar transformation of the illness experience, especially stigma, but short of a cure, people like Mr. Hooten are going to have to cope with an existential dilemma. The interests of him in the here and now are pitted against the interests of him in a future state of cognitive impairment. He is living a competition between his "now self" and his "future self."

The way to address this dilemma and so to live in a world of biomarker-labeled and drug-treated brains is to live with a paradox: we dread Alzheimer's disease because of its assault of our hard-won autonomy. Yet, to maintain independence in spite of the disease, we're going to have to accept some changes to the ways we exercise our autonomy. The remainder of the book examines how we can do this and still live well.

We need to create a society we can trust to monitor our lives outside the usual medical spaces, especially at home and work when we perform the cognitively demanding tasks that first reveal incipient cognitive decline. Monitoring will then lead to interventions to allow us to live well and flourish, to maintain an identity we cherish. To do this, we will need to think deeply about what is home and how to pass a typical day that is safe, social, and engaged.

The chapters to follow will show how we might achieve this. We must engage diverse people we don't typically include in the solutions to the Alzheimer's crisis, including bankers, lawyers, artists and performers, engineers, and architects.

The problem each of them will work on is the answer to the overwhelming question: How to live a good life when you're slowly losing your ability to live life?

25

CARING FOR EACH OTHER

There are only four kinds of people in the world: those who have been care-givers, those who are currently caregivers, those who will be caregivers, and those who will need caregivers.

—Rosalynn Carter

We must ask whether a technology expands our capacities and possibilities or exploits our vulnerabilities?

—Sherry Turkle, *Alone Together: Why We Expect More from Technology and Less from Each Other*

SUPPOSE YOU HAD a disease that caused a slow, relentless loss in your ability to use your hands. The first signs would be subtle, say, for example, trouble writing with a pen. A tablet device with a keypad would solve that. In time, however, typing would become too clumsy. Voice recognition software would solve that. Still later, you might struggle to hold the tablet and tap the icons. More voice recognition software. As troubles opening a door developed, doorknobs would be replaced with sliding doors. And so on.

The possibilities of reasonable accommodations are manifold. All we need is to imagine how to integrate the skills of engineers, clinicians, software designers, lawyers, and policy makers to ensure patients like you enjoy equal access to these "user-friendly," life-affirming interventions.

It could be like that with Alzheimer's disease. Imagine a world reconfigured to support our failing minds. Some of these innovations will be technological fixes to the environment, sort of sliding doors and voice recognition devices for the mind; others will be changes in the ways we interact with, look out for, and support each other. Imagine a revolution in technology, society, and our culture.

It begins right at home.

BEING AT HOME

Each time I saw Dr. Deacon at the Memory Center, he caused me to reflect about the future, cognitively impaired me. He was a retired physician, former researcher, and he loved opera. His family had moved him to a retirement community close to where they lived.

"My memory's lousy!" he'd tell me. "But I'm OK as long as I have this."

"This" was his smartphone. He kept it in a sort of holster attached to his belt (I keep mine in my pants pocket). He showed me how he used it to remember the day's plans, alert him to take his medications, and show him where he was in his walks about the still-unfamiliar (and probably forever so) neighborhood where he'd moved to. It also kept him entertained. Like me, he played operas on it.

"Without this, I'd be lost. Literally!"

In part 3, we met Dr. Jeff Kaye and his "mandalas of function," a vivid example of how technology can transform physicians in their efforts to diagnose and track a patient's illness. Dr. Deacon and his smartphone is an example of how technology assists a patient's day-to-day function and thus enhances his quality of life. The phone's ability to guide him through his neighborhood is a kind of wheelchair for his mind.

And that wheelchair is used not just by him but also by his son. He explained in private to me how with his smartphone he monitors his father's whereabouts. One hot summer afternoon, he saw his father walking far away from the community.

"I drove out to where he was, pulled over, and said, 'Dad, what a surprise to run into you!'" He drove his father home, where they sat and talked as they drank several glasses of ice water.

Two smartphones and an app saved my patient from one of the most common hazards of living with dementia, getting lost on a hot day and suffering dehydration and the ensuing devastating cascade of life-threatening complications such as delirium. I admire how his son, rather than call out to his father that he'd wandered, instead artfully "ran into" him and so spared him the stigma of calling out his disability.

Smartphones with apps to monitor and remind a patient are just one example of the possibilities for technologies to track, remind, alert, help, and connect us as we live with cognitive impairments: medication-dispensing devices, motion-activated cameras, wearable trackers that can detect a fall and sound the alarm to 911, devices that answer common questions such as what the date is or that play a song, a service that provides a car with driver and, someday, a driverless car.

With technologies like these, we may still have an only partly treatable disease, but at least, for a while, we won't be disabled. They're a kind of cognitive prosthetic, devices to fill in the gaps in our ability to remember, orient ourselves to time and place, or negotiate a space. They are in a sense parts of our extended mind.

Technology offers patients the opportunity to preserve and even enhance a sense of control, independence, and comfort, that sense we feel when we are at home.

Home is of course one place where we pass our days. The other is work.

BEING AT WORK

Professor Martin Miller's wife noted her sixty-two-year-old husband was "showing his age," but she wasn't worried. He had always performed the stereotype of the absentminded professor—forgetting to close doors and forgetting his students' names, misplacing pens—but in the classroom, he was a rock star. His Twentieth-Century American Novel Since Hemingway course was routinely filled.

She became worried, though, when she read his students' reviews on "RateMyProfessors": "I gave up sleeping in for this ramble?" "Not the star show it was billed to be. Should have taken Brit Lit." "Skip the lectures; befriend the teaching assistant." "Hello, but how weird was it that he gave the same lecture twice in one week???"

Something was wrong and, after his new patient visit to the Memory Center, I agreed. His troubles in the classroom (the teaching assistants entirely took over the grading) were the earliest signs of Alzheimer's disease.

His story makes tragic sense. Work is among life's more cognitively demanding activities. Many of my patients' histories begin with the sometimes embarrassing and too often sad end of their working days because of errors, missteps, and lapses in performance leading to awkward confrontations or even firing. For some professions, such as law, finance, teaching, and medicine, the consequences of failing to detect a problem can be harmful to others.

Dr. Kirk Daffner, a neurologist and director of the Center for Brain/Mind Medicine at Brigham and Women's Hospital in Boston, like me, had accumulated enough of these kinds of cases that he became afraid, so he decided to take action. In 2018, he confessed in an essay in the *Washington Post*: "I want to stop working before I embarrass myself."[1]

He described the all-too-frequent stories of not only patients but also colleagues working past their abilities. What bothered him was how some, when confronted with their problems, became resistant to all suggestions for help.

He wanted to avoid two unappealing options: on the one hand retiring early before there is a problem or, on the other hand, working past his abilities and having others finally force him out. The former cut off the opportunity to enjoy at least some of his work, while the latter risked harm to his patients—and to his reputation. Like china, it's easily cracked and once damaged, hard to repair.

His solution was to chart a middle ground. He created an "occupational living will."

His effort is ambitious. It includes sharing with colleagues a document that articulates his personal commitment to how, in the future, he would want to behave if faced with cognitive impairment. He has confided in these colleagues to make a fair and reasonable assessment of his work performance and to share their observations with him. If these observations trigger a concern, a plan is in place for a formal assessment with a physician.

A most provocative component is a video. He recorded himself communicating his wishes to his future self, telling that very different future Dr. Daffner what the past Dr. Daffner wanted.

Advance directives for health care are common. These documents designate others to make decisions if the person cannot make a decision. They instruct them on what to decide, for example, whether to undergo dialysis in the event of kidney failure. Advance directives for work are not common.

The experience of the subjects in the A4 Study—their existential dread over their knowledge that they were at risk of losing their cognitive abilities—shows how the age of living with a brain at risk will encourage society to address Alzheimer's disease in the workplace, which is, in some sense, a daily cognitive test.

In my and Dr. Daffner's practices, for example, the computerized medical record periodically confronts us with an upgrade we need to master. Moreover, our performance is monitored—how long before we complete and close our clinic notes, review labs, respond to patient calls. All these are data points that over time may show incipient cognitive decline. So, too, the ratings from our patients. A similar kind of real-time, on-the-job monitoring is possible in other professions that rely on computers.

There are challenges in implementing this kind of workplace monitoring. A disclosure to an employer of a diagnosis of Alzheimer's disease (or "elevated amyloid" or some other marker of a brain at risk) puts a worker at risk of being ostracized, placed under excessive scrutiny, and ultimately being fired. But we can also put in place workplace protections modeled after those in place for persons with a physical disability or for those who learn they have a gene that puts them at risk for a disease. These, together with occupational advance directives and an unbiased monitoring of performance, offer a way to continue working in some capacity that is productive and rewarding while at the same time avoiding what Dr. Daffner dreaded. The embarrassment of the now self by a future self and harms to patients or colleagues.

Patients like Professor Miller are relatively uncommon. The typical person has retired before the beginnings of memory problems. There is, however, one activity common to nearly all of us, and, like work, errors made doing it are a kind of canary in the coal mine, an alarm that a brain is at risk of failing.

Managing money.

WHEALTHCARE

One year before Mr. Yang came in with his grandson for his new patient visit, he was comfortably well-off. When we met, he was on the edge of poverty. What happened in between was a woeful story of the failure of the banking and financial services industry to protect a client from modern-day bank robbers.

It all started with a telephone call. The woman who called was polite. My patient said it was hard to hang up on her. Several weeks later, he confessed to his grandson: "I think I've been had." Nine-tenths of his wealth was lost to a lottery scam.

At first, the criminals took just a little money. The woman explained that he needed to pay fees to transfer his winnings. She got to know him. "What will you do with your winnings?" she asked. He told her about his grandson and his plans to support his college education. Later, she called him to explain that he needed to pay taxes on his winnings. And then they cleaned him out.

He'd been financially destroyed.

The size and scope of this problem is hard to pin down. Unlike central reporting of motor vehicle accidents, the United States does not have a central
reporting system into which banks and investment firms relay these crimes.
Still, the common knowledge among banks and firms is that this is a big
problem. Bankers admit that it takes off in their clients who are seventy-
five years and older, precisely the ages when the risk of cognitive impairment rises.

The kinds of scams are multiple and ever changing and admittedly clever
efforts to trick a mind that is a little less vigilant, a bit more susceptible to
misjudging social cues. They include elaborate stories of a lottery winning
that requires paying taxes, calls from the IRS for back taxes, calls from a
"grandchild" in jail and now desperate for money wired to pay bail: "But
please, Grandma, don't tell Mom and Dad."

In addition to these scams, there are self-inflicted errors such as the purchase of unsuitable investments or unpaid bills. Sometimes these errors,
too, cause irretrievable losses of life savings. All these events are among
the earliest signals that a brain is having a hard time managing one of life's
cognitively demanding activities.

This is largely preventable. Financial transactions are electronically recorded. When, where, and how much was purchased, given away, or transferred are all recorded in data warehouses. These transactions are like cognitive
tests or biomarkers—signals of a brain interacting with its environment.

We can build a better collaboration with banks and financial services
providers. Mr. Yang's transfers of money from his accounts to other banks
were not suspicious in and of themselves (unlike, say, an effort to wire
money abroad). They were, however, utterly out of character for him, in
both their dollar amount and frequency. They were unusual. What if this
change in behavior sounded an alarm to the bank, a family member, or a
social worker?

"Client Yang may be experiencing cognitive problems. We recommend a
visit to his doctor."

A better collaboration would not only help to detect cognitive changes
but it would also help care for persons who have MCI or dementia. After
Mr. Yang lost his wealth, the funds he needed for his care were gone, and he
lacked the time and the cognitive skills to go back to work. Someone else, his
family or the state, needed to step in and pay for his care. This ramifies across
the generations. Mr. Yang's grandson will either forgo an expensive college or
will incur tens, even hundreds of thousands of dollars of loans.

This kind of fusion of monitoring wealth and health, or what I have come to call whealthcare, could ensure that the earliest signs of cognitive decline are detected and wealth is preserved.[2] Banks and financial firms are beginning to transform their business practices to achieve this. The U.K. Coventry Building Society is just one example of how technology, law, and communication can be integrated to identify cognitive problems and intervene before a disaster.[3] The bank has in place a monitoring system that flags transactions out of a person's usual habits or that suggest fraud. The transaction is put on hold within the time limits allowed by law. Meanwhile, an employee trained in tactful communication with an older adult calls the person and inquires about the transaction. Coventry reports many of these transactions are often canceled.

Dr. Deacon's and his son's smartphones, Professor Miller's RateMyProfessors ratings, Dr. Daffner's video to his future self, and whealthcare alerts to signal unusual financial transactions are all examples of the potential for technology to be an essential part of caring for each other so that we can live well with a disease that we dread because it chips away at our ability to live as we choose, to be free to shape our identity as we desire.

The challenge to achieving this isn't a technological or engineering problem. We have the tools in hand. They include the internet, data integration, artificial intelligence, and machine learning. The challenge is us: we have to figure out how we should allow these tools to monitor us and create boundaries on our behavior.

LIVING WITH MONITORED, EXTENDED, AND INTERCONNECTED MINDS

All technologies have risks and downsides. The electric light bulb may cause fires. The car emits carbon that contributes to pollution. The technologies we use to monitor, extend, and interconnect our minds present us with risks and downsides, too.

Dr. Deacon's son wasn't the only one who discovered his father had wandered. The makers of the app he used to track his father also knew. Such is living with an extended and monitored mind hooked up to the internet of things. To live it, we have to surrender some privacy.

We trade off some privacy to achieve things we value, such as security from attack or in the case of a person like Dr. Deacon, gains in function, independence, and safety, or in the cases of Dr. Daffner and Professor Miller, assurance that their function and independence are monitored and reasonable accommodations are put in place.

This trade-off, this loss of privacy, may cause stigma. People—strangers—now know something deeply personal about you. You're a person living with dementia or MCI, or you are at risk of becoming such a person. Or you're a caregiver with a "family history" of dementia.

Ironically, this stigma threatens the very identity and privacy we're using the technology to preserve. So do the technologies that gain independence and function to preserve or enhance Dr. Deacon's, Dr. Daffner's, and Professor Miller's identity. Each surrenders some identity and privacy to these technologies that talk to each other. The often-annoying experience following an internet purchase paid for with a credit card illustrates this. Subsequent web browsing displays ads curiously tailored to our recent purchases.

In the world of monitored, extended, and interconnected minds, we'll experience "tailored" or "curated" ads, news items, and other information. Dr. Deacon and his son will receive stories about and promotions for "brain-health" products. The world around them is nudged, shaped, and reshaped according to someone else's motives. The experiences of being a patient and a caregiver are in a sense shaped by others. These unknown others' intentions are sometimes to care but also to sell, market, or otherwise persuade us to choose one thing over another.

Felix the cat is an even more insidious capture of our mind.

I learned about Felix from the daughter of a woman with advanced-stage dementia complicated by horrible and unremitting anger and agitation. Nothing seemed to calm Mrs. Gatteaux. Until the family gave her Felix the cat.

She always had a pet cat (her prior cat was also named Felix), but as her dementia worsened, caring for a cat became yet another formerly pleasant task she had to shed. She could, however, care for and enjoy being with her new Felix.

Her affectionate touch would cause him to purr, gaze at her, and blink. He didn't flee her efforts to feed him yogurt. The only care he required was to wipe the yogurt from his fur and a periodic battery charge. Felix was a robot.

We now manufacture robotic pets to behave in the ways we desire the living creature they represent to behave. Felix could be dismissed as merely a toy, but what about an FDA-approved robot as a treatment for persons with dementia? At Alzheimer's meetings, between the booths sponsored by pharmaceutical companies and journals, I always make a point to visit Paro the baby seal.

As I gently stroke his soft head and even softer belly, he looks at me, blinks, and sort of chirps. The more I do this, the more he responds with affection. Sold by AIST, Paro is marketed as an "advanced interactive robot" (AIST, National Institute of Advanced Industrial Science and Technology, is based in Japan and "paro" is Japanese for robot). In FDA regulatory language, Paro is approved as a "class 2 device" (a motorized wheelchair is an example of a device in this category).

Paro's sensors for touch, light, sound, temperature, and position allow it to interact with me as if it were my very own pet baby seal. Over time, it would learn the name I grant it and respond to my greetings and praise. It's the gift of love. The more I give, the more I will receive.

In time, I suppose, it will take on the gender of the name with which I baptize it.

Multiple studies report the robotic baby seal's ability to reduce agitation and to promote socialization and interaction between persons with dementia and their caregivers. The representatives at the information booth explain that FDA class 2 device status allows me to prescribe Paro and for insurance to pay for it. Paro is like donepezil. It is part of the model of care for persons with dementia.

But it's not just a pill. AIST explains on its website: "By interacting with people, Paro responds as if it is alive."[4]

I have no fundamental objection to using a robot pet to care for persons with dementia, just as I have no fundamental objection to cars to transport them to adult day programs. Felix the cat wasn't a panacea for Mrs. Gatteaux's sometimes explosive anger and irritability, but he was far safer and more effective than the blunt armamentarium of sedative drugs that would typically be prescribed to calm her. And talking about Felix gave her family an activity to engage with her.

The FDA categorizes Paro as a "biofeedback device." Such a device gives you a signal about yourself so that you can in turn control something about yourself. A classic biofeedback device is a measure that reports your heart rate. With that information, you can then run faster so as to increase your heart rate.

With Paro, the feedback isn't your heart rate but your emotions. You show Paro affection and it feeds affection back to you. Robot cats or baby seals (there are also otters and dogs) are designed to stimulate good feelings and to change behaviors.

We ought to have concerns about this.

My patient didn't ask for a robot cat. Other people decided to prescribe it to her. Her family in a sense deceived their disabled relative in order to change her behavior.

What becomes even more morally problematic is when we put together machines that can feel and think to make a human robot that becomes a caregiver.

This isn't science fiction.

In 2016, the *China Daily* news reported that Korean robotics researchers were launching a company to develop and market Silbot the dementia-care robot. Silbot will be equipped with sensors capable of reading the person's emotions, actions, and vital signs "so as to master their status." The detection of negative emotions will cause Silbot to play calming music or dispense a medication. If emotions worsen, an alarm is sent to a human or even 911. "All records will be stored in big data."[5]

For some caregivers this is likely a valuable tool, especially for staff in the time- and task-intense world of care homes. Japan, for example, has championed robots as a means to address the shortage of humans to care for the multitude of persons with dementia.

The robot can also take on the emotional aspects of caregiving. The designers of the carebot Mario, an acronym for the somewhat clunky "*Man*aging *A*ctive and healthy aging with use of ca*R*ing serv*I*ce r*O*bots," explained: "People with dementia enjoy their interaction with Mario and they often refer to Mario as he or she, and some referred to Mario as 'a friend.'"[6]

This new friend learns about a person and her typical day and uses that story to improve that day. Mario's designers explain how the machine can learn the person's past and use this data to feed back images and stories and, like Paro, engage the person as he responds in order to kindle positive responses and avoid unpleasant ones. Think of the robot like a music app on a smartphone. As it learns the kinds of music you favor, it presents performers "you might like."

Imagine a robot programmed to execute this on a grand scale—taking up data about your typical day, together with other bits from your past to curate not just songs but also images, stories, and conversations that engage you.

A thought experiment limns out how this might work.

❂

As president, Ronald Reagan met all kinds of people, learned their secrets, and participated in world-changing events. He also had a reputation, a sense of being presidential. The office gave him meaning and dignity. Suppose that in the years after his diagnosis of Alzheimer's disease, Ronald Reagan was prescribed a carebot.

There is a story of Reagan meeting visitors at his Bel Air, California, home. He asked one of his nurse caregivers: "Who is that man sitting with Nancy on the couch? I know him. He is a very famous man."[7] The man was George Shultz, his former secretary of state.

How would Reagan's caregiver robot answer this question? What would the robot tell the former president about George Shultz? More generally, what memories of his eight years as president would the robot recount? As Reagan's cognitive impairment grew, he, like some patients, might begin to mix up memories or dwell on past events as though they were in the present. Should the machine follow the former leader of the United States' imaginary direction? Or should the robot attempt to reorient Reagan to the truth?

This thought experiment reveals the profound ironies created by prescribing a robot caregiver to care for persons with Alzheimer's disease. For all of human history, in the face of numerous recastings of what we called the problem (first insanity, then senility, and then dementia, perhaps someday amyloidosis with tauopathy, etc.), we've relied on moral beings to understand the problem and take care of it. Humans, people like Nancy Reagan, answer the question: "What's a typical day?" And she, together with hired nurses and secret service agents, had charge of her husband's typical day. They helped him get dressed and out of the house, kept him happy, and answered his questions. We call these people caregivers.

Prescribing a robot to perform this care surrenders at least some of the person with dementia's identity and self-determination to a mindless and therefore amoral machine. Of course, humans will design and program these machines to care for humans who are losing their ability to care for themselves. How should we responsibly do this? What should the robots do and not do?

To answer these questions, we need to scrutinize quite closely the culture that programs, prescribes, and promotes these technologies to persons with dementia or who are at risk for dementia and the people who care for and about them and will decide when to turn them on and when to turn them off. The next chapter examines how we must examine the worlds we create.

26

THE WORLDS WE CREATE

I have been a stranger in a strange land.
                                        —Exodus 2:22
Your house will be my home for as long as I live.
                                        —Psalm 23

YOU RISE JUST after five thirty in the morning, when the sky begins to glow and so the stars fade away. You step out to your porch just in time to see the streetlamps go out. The air is warm and has the faint scent of peppermint. Across the lane, a neighbor is on a rocking chair on her porch. Like you, she's a poor sleeper. And like you, she lives alone.

A woman greets you. She holds out a bottle of water but, as usual, you decline and ask for coffee.

She says it's time for breakfast. "Follow me."

You're hungry. You follow her along a road, passing other houses. Some are red, others green. You pause before your favorite. The one with the brick façade. You tell the woman your friend lives there. His father is a lawyer. They have money. The lines of white classical columns frame his front door, capped by a pitched roof that points to the sky.

Cumulus clouds. A fountain gurgles. The grass is emerald green. It is spring.

It's always spring in Chagrin Falls, Ohio. And the sun always rises at five thirty and sets at seven thirty in the evening. It never rains, and yet the fountain has never run dry.

You're not actually outdoors. You're inside the Lantern.

The Lantern is the inspiration of Jean Makesh, an occupational therapist and businessman.[1] His idea was to create a space in Chagrin Falls, Ohio, that responded to where he thought persons with dementia said they wanted to live. He reproduced 1930s Chagrin Falls.

The entry to each room has a miniaturized facade of a house of that era. The wooden front doors are framed by brick or wood-clabbered walls, windows with shutters and a front porch whose pitched roof is supported by columns. The porch has space enough for a small bench or rocking chair.

The rooms face a hallway whose floor is decorated to appear as a grass lawn. Along "Main Street" there is a post office, the Moosejaw Trading Post, and the offices of the Standard Oil Company. The streetlamps are black, straight, vertical, torchère-style lanterns. "A Rockwell painting condensed," "your own little town," "home" are visitors' descriptions from a promotional video.[2]

Everything is by design.

The aroma of peppermint in the morning stimulates appetite. Eucalyptus throughout the day supports the immune system, and, in the evening, lavender calms. So, too, the setting sun at half past seven and starlight that follows. A "smart ceiling" adjusts the light according to the time of day.

The Lantern is just one example of design and decoration that adheres to a philosophy of dementia care. "The future of caring for those with dementia begins in the past," explains the narrator at the opening of a video of the Glenner Town Square day program in San Diego, California.[3] As a spunky, saxophone-heavy big band tune plays, the viewer beholds a space organized according to the same principles as the Lantern.

It is an interior made to look like a circa 1950s Southern California town. Patrons at Rosie's Diner sit on bright robin's-egg blue chairs before Formica tables. A jukebox sits along the wall. The library has a card catalog and 1950s issues of *National Geographic*. A portrait of General Eisenhower hangs on the wall.[4]

There are many other places like the Lantern and Glenner Town Square. In New Canaan, Connecticut, the Village reproduces the Main Street of circa 1960 New Canaan. This New Canaan is in fact old New Canaan.

Ordered and modest middle America, sun-soaked Southern California, quaint New England. As distinct and specific as these spaces are, they share a theme. They are facades not just in structure but also in the use of an outward appearance to create a new reality: a kind of perpetual high school reunion.

This approach to care is quite different from the still all-too-common spaces where persons with dementia live or pass their days. Nursing homes and adult day centers have typically been designed according to a perverse principle. We are born and die in a hospital, so the spaces where persons with dementia live should look like a hospital.

The nursing home where I trained was one long, alternating green-and-brown-tiled fluorescent-lit hallway bisected by a "nursing station." Floor-to-ceiling curtains strung up on slick, ball-bearing runners were set between the beds to create the "private" part of its ironic "semiprivate rooms." We were so obsessed with safety that the beds had rails to keep the person from exiting and falling. Few could manage the call button to summon help to get out of bed and so some injured themselves in attempts to climb over the rails. A large black mat before the elevator doors kept the residents from rushing into the elevator. We reasoned they would (mis)perceive it as a hole they could fall into.

No one wanted to live there. Or work there. Sometimes, in the course of the bitter end of a long day, in a candid reflection on the state of care for our patients, a colleague would ruefully describe the place as "a death house."

Nursing homes, adult day activity programs, memory care units, robots like Paro and Silbot, all have a common and essential theme. They're efforts by well-meaning people to create a world for a person living with dementia. How should we design these worlds? What principles ought to guide us?

HOMELOOSENESS

In the lives of persons with dementia, one of the most emotionally arresting moments occurs when they ask us a question. Typically, this happens at a stage of disability that requires someone to assist the person with dressing, bathing, and grooming. She may struggle with the toilet. She cannot be left alone for fear she will wander.

In this stage, he may stand in the living room of his house of some fifty years and ask his spouse: "Whose house is this? I want to go home." He may also ask her if she is married or when Mother (or some other long-ago-deceased relative) will be coming home.

I have come to understand these questions as an extreme stage of one of the most common symptoms of the disease. The person is losing her sense of feeling at home. She's experiencing what I call homelooseness. Like much of the working of the human mind, in both health and disease, homelooseness occupies a continuum. It spans from the contented feeling of being at home to the unsettling feeling of homelessness, of being a stranger in a strange land, of suffering the distress and impairments of a separation from home, or, in a word, homesickness.[5]

For caregivers, these questions are utterly devastating, even frightening. They dread them. The person seems a different person, obedient to a different mind.

Caregivers tell me this is among their worst experiences. Bill Walters, caregiver for his wife, described how the experience created a vast and sad loneliness. "When she did talk, it was always, 'I want my mother.' 'I want my father.' She never asked about the kids, never asked about me. It was always backward. 'I want my mother.'" These experiences heightened his depression and a welling but ambiguous loss. His wife, the mother of their children, was there but not there beside him in bed.

This extreme expression of homelooseness explains a paradox observed in mourning among caregivers of persons with dementia.[6] In the months and years *prior* to their relative's death, their depression and grief are greater than in the months *after* death. In a sense, mourning precedes death. This pattern of bereavement among caregivers of those with dementia is precisely the opposite of the experience of caregivers of people dying from cancer and other diseases that typically ravage the body but spare the mind.

A person who asks these questions often wanders, may have bowel or bladder accidents and episodes of agitation. This assembly of disturbing events is the genesis of the zombie metaphor. A daughter once told me that this word that I argue is stigmatizing and entirely inappropriate was, for her, in fact comforting. It allowed her to make sense of her mother as no longer her mother but instead as some sort of monster created by the disease.

Treating these extreme symptoms of homelooseness is morally challenging. Professionals at a memory center counsel family to tell the truth: "This is your home." "I'm your wife." "Mother died, years and years ago." But we also counsel that the truth may cause distress. The person may become angry over not being told that Mother died, then grieve, only to repeat again, and yet again, the question. Or they may feel embarrassment that they forgot such an essential aspect of their identity.

Another response is to lie. Tell your spouse: "We'll be leaving soon for home." Tell her that you'd like to get married or that Mother will be home soon. These words are intentional and sometimes highly creative acts of "loving deception."

The Lantern, the Town Square at Glenner, and the Village are also our answers to these extreme symptoms of homelooseness. They are acts of loving deception committed with architecture and design.

Makesh recounted how his inspiration for the Lantern came from his work as an occupational therapist. He was born and raised in Puducherry, India, and educated in Bombay. Then, after he immigrated to America in 1995, his first job was as an occupational therapist at an assisted-living facility. In India, he'd never been among older adults save for his grandparents, and so a stranger in a strange land, like an amateur anthropologist, he assumed nothing and took in everything.

There was Norma, a woman who would ask to go to the bus stop. She wanted to return home to her children. His efforts to reason with her—you're in your home and your children are all grown up—failed.

Within an hour after dinner, Walter would pace the fluorescent-lit corridors and repeatedly ask for breakfast. Efforts to reason with him were futile. He'd forgotten he'd just eaten dinner. Frustration would soon give way to anger. These were among repeated experiences that taught Makesh something. Manipulating the environment might have a great effect on changing behavior.

At the Lantern, Norma would live in the home she wanted to return to, more or less, and so might not ask to go home. The faux night sky would cue Walter, who'd forgotten he ate dinner, that it is night and so not yet time for breakfast. The absence of peppermint and the scent of lavender might also help to redirect his appetites from hunger to sleep.

Loving deceptions can be committed not only in words and decoration but also in the activities we have people participate in.

At Glenner Town Square, attendees comfort baby dolls they lift from cribs in the health clinic. At city hall, a woman is given printed invoices to manage. At the Country House Residence in Davenport, Iowa, the staff perform faux weddings complete with a bride in a gown and a groom in a suit, a pastor to officiate, a kiss, and then cake.[7] The organizers explain they don't consider the events lying. These are "special moments" for people with short-term memory loss.

Faux weddings, communities made to look like another time, saying Mother will be home in an hour, robot pets, the treatments for homelooseness lay plain the moral challenge that living with Alzheimer's presents us. Persons with the disease experience what might be a decade or more when they struggle to self-determine their lives. We—other people—have to decide with and, in time, for them. From person to person, family to family, these choices are typically private and highly personal, akin to how we allow parents tremendous discretion and latitude in how they raise their children.

Matters become more morally complex when we have to decide what worlds we'll create for persons living with dementia, spaces like the Lantern and the activities at Glenner Town Square and the Country House Residence.

No doubt these interventions help some people with homelooseness. The daughter of the woman who manages fake invoices at Glenner Town Square town hall recounts how the activity gives her mother a sense of purpose. Residents at the Country House are visibly moved by the weddings. Felix the cat was the only treatment that calmed Mrs. Gatteaux.

But do these treatments affect us, the perpetrators of the deception? How do they affect how we feel about the persons we deceive? Arguably, deception kindles feelings of separation. It creates a distance between persons living with dementia and the rest of us. They are an audience and we are actors. Between us and them is the invisible fourth wall at the edge of the stage. Despite the best of intentions, deception risks reinforcing a sense that we're different from them and also that they feel different from us. Deception risks reinforcing the stigmas of Alzheimer's disease.

And yet, we have to do something. There is no "neutral position" in the worlds we create for persons living with dementia. All the world's a stage. We have to make choices about how to perform.

I first realized this when I was in the day room of an assisted-living facility. On the wall was a poster of Alfred Hitchcock's 1954 film *Rear Window*. "That's nice," I thought. For now. I wonder when they'll swap it out for *Star Wars*. Or should it be *Rocky*?

We have to make choices. We have to put on some sort of show.

Makesh recounted how, in the first year of running the Lantern, the sky ceiling was sensibly programmed to follow the cycle of Ohio's four seasons. As the year progressed from summer into fall, the sky ceiling's days grew shorter and shorter, leading up to the shortest day of the year.

"It was a big mistake," he admitted.

The residents became confused and eager to retire to bed hours before the proper bedtime. He decided to keep the hours of day and night constant throughout the year. The days in the town that looks like circa 1930s Ohio have the daylight of an equatorial town and the climate of a perpetual American spring.

Proponents for deception often draw on theories of neuroscience, asserting, for example, how old memories are the most well networked and so most resistant to the loss of neurons. Other possible explanations are well-described neurological syndromes in which lesions to particular regions of the brain cause a person to fail to recognize faces or insist that the person they see has been occupied by some other person. The most common of these is Capgras syndrome, named after Jean Marie Joseph Capgras, the French psychiatrist who described the delusion in the early twentieth century.

We need to learn from the neuroscience research that explains what we observe and use this knowledge to guide how we treat homelooseness, but science will not tell us what show we should put on.

From the earliest stages of dementia, when the disabilities are quite subtle, such as troubles preparing a holiday meal, to the very end stages, care blends some of what the person wants and also what we want for them. In other words, care admixes the person's choices and decisions and also our choices and decisions.

There is a way out of the dilemma between whether to tell the harsh, perhaps embarrassing truth ("Mother died fifty years ago" or "I am your wife") or to dare to deceive. We can find it by creating worlds for all of us—persons with and without dementia—to live in together and feel loved, protected, and secure.

TIMESLIPS

Anne Basting knew that what she was doing at the Morgantown Care and Rehabilitation Center in Morgantown, Kentucky, was working when the policeman came asking if he could help. No crime needed his investigation but, in his mind, a crime had been committed. Years ago, his grandfather had died there. In the decades to follow, the boy, now in his fifties, promised never to return to the center. The Morgantown Care and Rehabilitation Center was a death house.

He'd now finally broken his decades-old promise. He was back and he wanted to help. Basting was grateful. The staff and the residents really needed a lot of help. They were putting on a play.

"We were rehearsing this scene, kind of the final scene. We called it the wheelchair ballet. We really needed a lot of help," she recalled in an interview in 2019.[8]

The police chief explained that his office was right next door to the center. "I cannot believe what is happening here and I want to help in any way I can. How can I do that?"

This wasn't the first time people opened up to Basting. The more they did, the more she knew that *Wendy's Neverland* was going to be a success.

What was happening was a performance intended not simply to amuse the frail residents of this long-term care facility and to provide a few hours of respite for the staff who cared for them. The stage wasn't this Kentucky town set forty years ago. This performance was the culmination of two years of work. The residents, the staff, and the residents' families had been writing, designing, and rehearsing a play about Wendy, a resident at the center. For years, Wendy told stories of Neverland.

Basting's inspiration was an insight she had when she was a doctoral student in theater studies at the University of Minnesota. As part of her research for her dissertation, "The Stages of Age," she'd been observing a troupe of performers in a senior theater, actors in their eighties and nineties. She discovered something.

Contrary to the stereotype that, compared to younger adults, older adults are more rigid and distilled in their ways of being, she witnessed actors not only learning new roles but also being changed by them. A ninety-year-old woman voicing Shakespeare's King Lear rage against the storms was also showing her rage against her impairments in hearing and vision—and her uncomfortable dentures.

Could theater have the same effect on older adults with dementia? she wondered. Could they benefit from the transformative power of theater? Or were their fragile minds simply too impaired to learn lines and follow a plot? Theater is after all quite memory based, and memory is among the first skills to fade from a failing brain.

She tried anyway.

Her inspiration came out of her own failure to connect with the residents living in their locked dementia unit (often these are called memory care units) of the Marian Franciscan Center in Milwaukee, Wisconsin. The space was the usual cold, hospital-like arrangement. The residents were people who needed help with life's most basic activities, like dressing and grooming, who spoke very little and when they did, might ask to go home or inquire about long-ago-deceased relatives.

She'd been using the standard approaches of the time for activities for persons with advanced dementia. The key was remembrance, tapping into those well-learned memories of the past. "Memory mapping" involved prompting people to tell the story of when they were younger. She would be a kind of director coaxing and prompting people to tell their life stories and so, like the woman who played King Lear, they might be transformed by this performance of their past lives.

"None of it worked very well," she recalled.

Asking people to fill out the details of their past lives only seemed to heighten their anxiety. They were afraid to say something wrong. So they fell silent, fearful of the self-inflicted pain caused by what Basting came to describe as "story extraction."

For six weeks, she tried other approaches at reminiscence. Each time, she failed.

"It was pretty bleak," she said.

And then she made a decision. Never mind memory.

She brought in a large image of a man, placed it on the wall, and then stood before a plain white, two-by-three-feet writing pad set on a writing easel. She had in hand a large marker.

"We're going to make up a story about this image," she announced. "Anything you say, I'll write it down."

The image was the iconic picture of the Marlboro Man.

They named him Fred.

"Fred who?" she asked. "Do you want to give him a last name?"

"Fred Astaire," someone said.

She wrote that down. She wrote down anything they said. Any words.

"And where does Fred Astaire live?"

He lived in Oklahoma.

He was married to Gina Autry. They lived among skinny rivers and skinny trees, eating fish. Two for lunch and two for dinner.

And then someone said, "They're so sick of fish they wouldn't eat another fish if you fried it in gold."

They carried on like this for nearly an hour, laughing, repeating the story, embellishing points, even singing. Lost in the story they were creating.

And then Basting looked up from her lively circle.

"The staff were gathered around us and they were laughing and singing alongside of us."

She'd discovered something. This wasn't just a special moment of entertainment. This was a powerful intervention for people with dementia. It wasn't a drug, but it seemed to have the same kinds of effects as drugs popularized by the neurologist and author Oliver Sacks that caused an awakening in people once comatose.

She decided to test her idea. Can I awaken creativity and communication between persons with dementia and also between them and the people who cared for them? The key was her method. She was using the theory of improvisation.

"In improvisation, you're listening intently, you're observing intently what's happening around you in the moment, and you're adding to it in a positive way."

The essence of improv is "Yes, and . . ." When the resident said Fred Astaire ate fish, she wrote that down and then asked: "Yes, and fish for which meals?" The message to the person with dementia was: "I've heard what you said, whatever you said, and I'm writing it down, and so let's build on that."

"How many fish at breakfast?"

In time, she realized people with dementia were, with assistance, capable of creating something, and their work ought to be performed where they live. These plays were different from the usual linear flow of a drama, of one scene leading to the next. There could be a character with four names in three places at once. She decided to call her idea Timeslips.

The premiere was a play prepared by the residents, staff, and residents' families at Luther Manor in Wauwatosa, Wisconsin. They called it the Penelope Project. Basting chose the title based on her fascination with the ancient character from Homer's epic, *The Odyssey*. Penelope is the wife of Odysseus, a warrior and king who's been off at war for years.

Much like a caregiver of a person with dementia, she at times feels neither wife nor widow. Suitors seek to persuade her that her husband must be dead. They seek her hand. She struggles to maintain a home for her and her teenage son.

For residents at Luther Manor, Penelope is an affecting character. Strangers are about them. They wait for family to visit. They struggle to feel at home, strangers in a strange land.

Students studying theater and the residents and staff of Luther Manor set to work. They wrote dialogue and songs, made sets, wove decorations, and constructed origami birds to represent the birds who carried letters to and from Odysseus and Penelope. Professional actors and the residents themselves performed in the production. Those who could not learn a line participated in a chorus, where all as one, on cue, would recite a line or perform a movement.

As they did this, something happened. The walls between people began to come down. The residents in the independent living areas began to commingle with the residents in the skilled area. The families began to participate in the workshops.

The ninety-minute performance of *Finding Penelope* unfolded as a mobile play that began in Luther Manor's entrance. The actors explained to the audience how they would proceed from the Health Center ("where people receive the most nursing care") to the Courtyards ("the assisted-living area"). They were going to find Penelope Papadapolas, a resident of Luther Manor.

The final scene is in the chapel. Penelope is found and reunited with her husband and daughter. Odysseus recites how Penelope has made a home for all of them. Each line begins: "You are the one . . ." and then adds bits of the residents', families', and staff's lives.

"You are the one who passed away last Tuesday."

"You are the one who visits her husband in the nursing home every day."

"You are the one who answers the phone, 'Luther Manor, how may I direct your call?'"

This recitation concludes: "You, you are the ones who make this place home."

"A pretend wedding, a fake place, is not authentic," Basting reflected when I asked her to compare Timeslips to approaches like the weddings at the Country House Residence, the Lantern, and Glenner Town Square. "A place like that might be meaningful to the person with dementia, but you're ultimately not changing anything about the toxicity of the environment or people's attitudes toward dementia or changing the way we embrace vulnerability at the end of our lives."

Wendy's Neverland, the performance at the Morgantown Care and Rehabilitation Center that the police chief wanted to help with, is, like *Finding Penelope*, scripted to the place it is performed. The premise is that Wendy, who had been living at the center for about ten years, is in hospice and the residents, staff, and families have come together to honor her in her final days. What follows are eight stations, or scenes (the first three are "Music," "Welcome to Neverland!" and "Positive Thoughts") that end in "Belief," in which the residents, staff, and their family members are invited to create an "I am" poem.

The key to Timeslips, Basting explained, is how both persons with dementia and the people who care for them work together for months to create and perform the play whose script draws on their stories. The production transforms how people feel about the facility and the residents who live there. The fears and stigmas that turn persons with dementia into untouchables dissipate. An environment that is made toxic from bitter memories like the one the policeman harbored for decades, changes. The death house became a home he wanted to visit.

In a sense, the fourth wall came down.

In the opening of this book, I revealed that my most powerful diagnostic and treatment tool is a simple four-word question: "What's a typical day?" It elicits from a person, typically a caregiver, a vivid account of a brain interacting with its world, a kind of biography of the disease talking through a particular person and interpreted by another. The story has unique and identifiable characters living in a distinct time and place. I use this biography/autobiography not only to diagnose but also to treat the patient and the caregiver.

We all should use this tool to create days that are safe, social, and engaged. As we use it, we need to recognize that these days cannot be replete with activities that are fully safe, completely social, and totally engaging. Each of these has to give a bit. There has to be a balance. Safe, social, and engaged are three axes in a kind of triangle that describes a world where a person with dementia can exercise her tastes and creativity.

Persons with dementia struggle with this. The person providing care has to assist them to present their self.[9] The caregiver does this by shaping social situations, preparing dress and appearance, drawing out personal stories, and downplaying inappropriate behaviors. These efforts need to respect that we don't have one but in fact three selves: past, present, and future. To treat homelooseness, the present, past, and future selves each need a home that is safe, social, and engaged.

In a short documentary about the Lantern, one of the construction workers who built the place expressed this quite elegantly. "As people move into this, they will feel like they are at home. They'll be able to go to the salon. They'll be able to go to the theater and watch a movie and being able to live life like they should be able to live life."[10]

It takes the wisdom of a person whose career is building homes and in turn communities to express what everyone—persons with dementia and persons without—needs. We need places where we can exercise our tastes and creativity to nurture the feeling of being at home.

In Australia, elections officials travel to long-term care facilities and set up a polling place for the residents to vote. Colleagues and I tested this in Vermont in the 2008 election.[11] The staff were elated. They explained how the residents felt valued and once again part of the community and the American political system (the staff also felt relieved of the challenge of how to properly assist a cognitively impaired person to vote).

In the Netherlands, day centers for adults with dementia are designed to cater to people's various tastes. For persons who enjoy the outdoors, there are centers set in woodsy areas with spaces to walk about. For persons who enjoy an urban life, there are centers decorated like a formal living room.

Entire cities and towns can become "dementia friendly."

In the city of Bruges, Belgium, for example, a sticker depicting a red handkerchief in the window of a shop signals that the shopkeepers are trained in how to communicate with older adults who show signs of memory problems. There and in other communities, persons with dementia and their caregivers attend "memory cafés" styled after the idea of a café as a place to linger, talk, and be entertained. There is one core rule. You present yourself simply as yourself, your name, not as either patient or caregiver.

HOMEBOUND

I have no doubt that by the close of the above section, some caregivers are quite frustrated, even angry. They're thinking: "Well, yes, that's all very fine. And what about *me*? What about my typical day?"

I entirely understand these sentiments.

As a person with dementia experiences more and more homelooseness, their caregiver needs to devote more time, task, and manipulation of the truth to maintain their relative's sense of feeling "at home." For the caregiver, these efforts create their own feeling of homelooseness, caused, paradoxically, by feeling homebound.

We've known this more publicly since the summer in 1980 when America first met an Alzheimer's disease caregiver. In her testimony to the first congressional hearing on Alzheimer's disease, Bobbie Glaze, one of the founding families of the Alzheimer's Association, told America how as her husband became more and more disabled, agitated, and withdrawn, they became impoverished. They moved multiple times, to smaller and simpler quarters. She told us she was alone. "I felt no sense of belonging."

Caregivers tell me how they have long given up taking trips, how they feel trapped in their home, trapped because they either must care for their loved one or, if their loved one lives somewhere else, such as the Lantern, they must continually check in on their relative (many also lack funds to travel). The experience, some say, is akin to social isolation during an epidemic.

Ten years later, Bobbie Glaze's friend and colleague Hilda Pridgeon testified at the 1990 congressional hearing *Alzheimer's: The Unmet Challenge for Research and Care* that "people are afraid. I'm afraid. They are afraid of what will happen to them if they get this disease. They are even more afraid of how their families will cope."

Even more afraid.

In the years to follow their testimonies, there has been progress to help families cope. The treatments I explained in part 3—caregiver training and education and adult day activity programs—can diminish this sense of being homebound. The creative care Basting and her colleagues have developed also helps.[12] Creating something together upends the bleak ideas of caregiving as mere time and task and dementia as a disease that robs a person of her humanity. For example, when a caregiver asks me how to respond when a patient asks after a dead relative, we talk about truth or deception and also a third way that sets aside memory as recall and instead embraces memory as meaning.

"Tell me about Mom. Tell me a story about her."

There needs to be a policy response to being homebound. We have to give families access to this care without the threat of fiscal ruin. Bill Walters—the husband of my patient who told me of his sadness over his wife's repeated inquiries about her long-deceased mother and father, her lack of interest in him or their children—was a proud, self-made businessman. Neither rich nor poor, he explained the fiscal situation this disease presented him.

It was, he said, "beyond belief."

Early on in her disease, his attorneys and accountants laid out three options. He could create an irrevocable trust that would shield their assets from ruin. This meant he'd surrender control of his finances to a trustee. "If I needed to buy a newspaper, I would have to ask them for the fifty cents." This was unacceptable. It would surrender too much of his self-determination and freedom, turning him into a kind of person with dementia, under the control of a caregiver. "I control my own destiny. I don't need to ask my trustee, whether it's an attorney or my kids, to buy a newspaper."

Or he could divorce her (adult children of course don't have this option, though some passively exercise it as they drift away). She would then be left an independent woman with her share of the divorce settlement to spend on her care. Once those funds ran out, she would become impoverished and thus qualify for Medicaid. That was morally unacceptable.

Mr. Walters chose the third option. The one most Americans take. "Pay until you can't pay anymore" and then, once impoverished, Medicaid steps in with its meager allocation of resources.

There were bills for home health aides, day care and respite care, and a live-in companion for when he was away at work. To have time to care for his wife, he turned away business, and therefore lost wages he might have earned. He was in a perverse race against time. The longer she lived, the more time and money he spent. The more he spent, the less was available to him in his own old age or available to his children and grandchildren. For ten years, he paid and paid and paid until the afternoon when, in the care of a hospice program, she died in their bedroom, surrounded by her family.

If he'd reached the precipice of near economic ruin—what policy makers call the poverty line—Medicaid would have stepped in to support her care. But long-term care supported by Medicaid is not mandated to pay for all who qualify for care. This explains why people who need care must wait on a list to receive Medicaid support for services such as help at home. This is a poison pill built into America's broken long-term care system.

And it is the vortex of the Alzheimer's crisis.

The solution isn't complex. Risks faced by millions of people with potentially catastrophic consequences are best solved with social insurance. Health insurance such as Medicare and the insurance purchased through the Affordable Care Act ensure that acute illness doesn't bankrupt us. We must do the same for persons with dementia and other chronic illnesses. They need social insurance to support their ability to live at home, wherever home may be and in whatever form it takes.

Sometimes these homes take on unusual arrangements.

LOVE STORIES

One more intervention is needed to keep people feeling at home, to treat homelooseness and being homebound. They say, we know we're at home if we're in a place where we feel our heart resides. But what if that heart is broken? How do you repair a broken heart that lives in a once great and happy home now riven by Alzheimer's disease?

At his wife's funeral, Mr. Walters made a startling announcement to the assembled mourners. "Today," he said, "I'm here to bury my wife who died of Alzheimer's disease. Last year, I was in this same church to bury my girlfriend, who died of cancer." For several years, as he cared for his wife in their home, he had another partner.

Not only caregivers but persons with dementia find new love. In 2007, America learned that John O'Connor, the husband of Justice Sandra Day O'Connor, the first woman to serve on the Supreme Court and a member of the Alzheimer's Study Group, was in a relationship with another woman.[13] John O'Connor had Alzheimer's disease. In 2005, Justice O'Connor retired from the court to take care of him. As his disabilities worsened, O'Connor had to break up their Phoenix, Arizona, home. She moved him to a new home. It was there that her husband of some sixty years met the other woman. She was a fellow resident at the Huger Mercy Living Center.

O'Connor's son Scott explained that his mother was thrilled. Her husband was finally relaxed and not complaining. He finally felt at home.

Mr. Walters's and Mr. O'Connor's relationships aren't unusual, though I cannot cite statistics. For spousal or partnered caregiver-patient dyads, this taking on of another partner is among the great unspoken facts of living with and caring for a person with dementia or of having dementia. I say "another partner" and not spouse because I've never encountered either a caregiver or a patient who divorced their spouse to then marry someone else. Instead, they maintain two quite different relationships.

This is the story of Ted, Ruth, and Beth.

The more intimate and certainly intensive care Ted Baker provided his wife, Ruth, such as helping her dress and bathe and use the toilet, the more he felt a stranger in their home. There was little coherent conversation, but sometimes Ruth was quite clear about what she wanted. She would insist he wasn't Ted, that he was some other man who'd replaced Ted.

"Leave! Get out!"

He learned from trial and error not to correct her to understand he was Ted, her husband. That was futile and painful for both of them. Instead, he obeyed her command. He'd leave the apartment, perhaps take a book, walk about, or just linger in the hall and, in time, return to the place that was less and less a home. There, he'd find Ruth calmed down.

When she insisted and yet again insisted "I want to go home!" he'd take her out, even to the bus stop, until, over time, she'd lose interest in trying to find the home that was nowhere to be found.

Both were suffering homelooseness.

Early in her disease, Ruth and Ted had moved to a continuing care retirement community because it promised a home until the end of their lives. For the healthy, there were apartments and two common dining rooms (one with waiters to serve and the other a more informal buffet). There was a gym, a swimming pool, a library, and a salon. A well-staffed nursing and rehabilitation unit offered care for those recovering from illness so that they could return to their private apartment. For a resident too disabled by dementia to live in his apartment, a memory unit provided small but comfortable rooms and common areas for meals and activities. The hall of this locked space was laid out in a rectangle to allow residents and their visitors to walk around and around.

This "continuing care retirement community" offered everything. Almost everything. It was up to the residents to make where they lived feel like home. There were staff at the community to assist with this. There were also the fellow residents.

One of them was Beth.

Beth was recently widowed (cancer). In earlier times, the two couples had been good friends. Beth helped Ted care for Ruth, staying with her so that he could tend to errands or an appointment. Each evening, Beth and Ted exchanged emails, back-and-forth messages about the day's events, ideas, and such. He described these exchanges as a lifeline that reminded him there was a real world outside his home.

I asked, "Why not a phone call?" And he explained plainly: "Ruth would hear."

This went on for years. Despite Ruth's outbursts, Ted perceived the pearl that was Ruth was still there, locked inside the shell created by the loss of her ability to communicate. In time though, the pearl dissolved.

After he moved Ruth to the community's memory unit, he visited her daily and he also visited Beth. In time, homes were rearranged. Ruth lived in the memory unit and Ted and Beth lived together a few floors above her in his apartment. They agreed to visit Ruth separately, never together.

When I recount the stories of John O'Connor or of Ted, Ruth, and Beth to people who haven't cared for a person with dementia or haven't been close to either a caregiver or a person with dementia, some are offended. They judge Ted's choices as morally wrong. They argue he committed the equivalent of an extramarital affair.

Some say Ted at least ought to have the courage to divorce Ruth. Ted told

me when a fellow resident asked him if he planned to divorce Ruth, he simply laughed. The idea was absurd.

Some say Mr. O'Connor should be separated from the woman. Each lacks
the capacity to engage in a relationship. Certainly matters of consent and exploitation must be addressed. Thoughtful long-term care facilities instruct
staff to assess and monitor relationships among residents to assure they're in
fact voluntary. The objection I'm reacting to is that of an adult child of one
of my patients who sternly reminds me that his mother and father's marital
vows (at least the Catholic vows) require devotion "in sickness and in health,
until death do us part."

A common counter to this severe objection is: "You don't understand. You
must walk in the shoes of a caregiver and a person with dementia." I would
further specify the path to understanding. You must ask: What is this sickness?

A caregiver who took a second partner explained the sickness. He was
caught in an existential dilemma. He was trying to do everything he possibly could to take care of his wife and at the same time live his life. He simply
had to make a choice. He had to pick the "least worst" of his options. Notably, several caregivers tell me they find solace in Viktor Frankl's book *Man's
Search for Meaning*. The neurologist, psychiatrist, and Holocaust survivor argues that life presents ghastly problems we cannot control, but we can control
how we think about the problem and so make meaning out of it.

Facts and figures of how many spousal caregivers choose a second partner are not available. I know many remain fiercely devoted to their spouse as
their only partner. This devotion is at least in part because the person living
with dementia recognizes them and, at least from time to time, engages in
meaningful communication.

I once cared for a woman whose husband kept her always at his side. He
told me how he'd ask her three questions: his name, hers, and, somewhat
oddly, I confess, her Social Security number. As long as she answered all
three correctly, he'd do whatever he could to keep her at home beside him.
For him, this was meaningful communication. The last time I met her at the
Memory Center, she looked at me and insisted to no one in particular: "Give
that boy a piece of cake."

Mr. Walters and his wife and partner; Sandra Day and John O'Connor and
the woman he met at the Huger Mercy Living Center; Ted, Ruth, and Beth;
the man who asked his wife the three questions—these are stories of love
with Alzheimer's disease, of people aging, growing apart but still together,
and trying as best they can to care for each other.

27

THE WORLDS WE END

For the end, for me as for cities,
Is total absence: what comes to be
Must go back into non-being.
    W. H. Auden, *Horae Canonicae*, "VI. Compline"

Io non mori' e non rimasi vivo.
(I did not die, and I did not remain alive.)
            —Dante, *Inferno*, canto 34

TILL DEATH DO you part.

Much of this book has been an effort to answer the essential question about the problem of living with Alzheimer's disease: "What's a good life when you're losing your ability to determine that life for yourself?"

But what about the end of that good life? What's the story of a good ending, and who determines that "goodness"?

The answers to these questions are quite unusual, unsettling, and incomplete. They bear little semblance to the answers for persons dying of other common diseases, the "diseases of the body," such as cancer or heart disease. For these people, death sometimes comes as the thief in the night who snatches away life. Other times, it is called in by means of "physician aid in dying" (or assisted suicide) to put an end to suffering. Whatever form it takes, when death does come, it is as definitive and certain as thunder. For persons living with Alzheimer's disease and for their caregivers, death is quite different. Easeful death lingers and takes its time.

AN EXISTENCE, NOT LIVING

Arthur Packel was, in August 2000, sixty-nine years old, married, and working as an attorney when I diagnosed him with mild-stage dementia caused by Alzheimer's disease. For one and a half decades, he and his wife, Renee, lived in every wing and room of the house of Alzheimer's.

In the last four years, when he needed someone to bathe, dress, and assist him with the toilet, and adult day care could no longer accommodate him, when conversations were a few fragmented words and he fled their apartment, she decided this home wasn't working. He was entirely homeloose. She moved him to a new home, to the "special care unit" of a nursing home.

In his first weeks there, he became increasingly disruptive and even physically aggressive. He'd walk uninvited into other residents' rooms. He struck out at residents and staff. Medications—antidepressants and antipsychotics—were started. He became sedated and unable to walk, and he was barely eating and drinking. At one of her visits, Mrs. Packel found him slumped in a chair, staring at the dull middle distance of linoleum.

"I called the doctor and said, 'I want him to die clearheaded! Take him off those medications.'" The doctor obeyed and so Mr. Packel began eating again.

She told me this story some five years later, as she and I sat in the living room of her small one-bedroom apartment. He'd died two months before. She recalled those days with bitter regret.

"I shouldn't have done that. I should have left him on the medications."

"Why?"

"Because he would have died. I just wanted him out of his misery. He was so healthy otherwise."

She described his life in the years to follow. "It was an existence. Not living."

Before I became an Alzheimer's doctor, when I practiced general geriatrics, death was often quite planned. Patients at the end stages of heart, lung, or kidney disease—many suffering in a maelstrom of these diseases—made a decision. Enough. Enough with visits to and from the hospital with its various units (intensive, cardiac, and step down) and floors. It's time to die. Hospice care was ordered. Sometimes in the hospital. Often at home.

Unleashed from medications and machines such as ventilators or dialysis, vital organs failed, and, as they did, we provided comfort with pills, patches, or drips of morphine. The patient went quickly back into nonbeing.

Often this happened when the patient was terminal, loosely defined as having six or fewer months of life remaining, but not always. Some patients who might have lived years more declined treatment. I made sure they understood the consequences of this decision, and if they did, I routinely respected it. I had an ethical obligation to respect their right to determine the course of their life and the timing of their death.

In the lives of persons with dementia, whether caused by Alzheimer's disease or other neurodegenerative brain diseases, these aren't the usual stories. Death is elusive and hard to plan. The problem begins with a simple fact. There is no lifesaving treatment, no dialysis for the brain to refuse.

There is, in a sense, a caesura, an interruption, between living with and dying of the disease, and this space is so vast and mysterious that physicians don't see either Alzheimer's disease or dementia as causes of death. They routinely don't list them as a cause of death on the death certificate they're required to complete, preferring instead to list causes such as pneumonia, sepsis, or complications of a hip fracture. The first time I recorded "Alzheimer's disease" as the cause of death, the nurse who stood beside me at the desk in the nursing home candidly volunteered: "I didn't know people died of Alzheimer's disease."

In 2014, researchers at Rush University made headlines with a report in the journal *Neurology* that Alzheimer's explained as many as half a million deaths.[1] This count was not the result of the disease killing more people but rather of discovering a different way to think about what it means to die of Alzheimer's disease.

They didn't discover a better way to persuade physicians to include Alzheimer's disease on death certificates. Instead, they'd calculated the number of people in whom Alzheimer's contributes to their risk of death. This method—called population attributable risk—is an appealing approach to rethinking death wherein multiple diseases are often at work. Each disease chips away at a person's life. Together, they ease him into nonbeing.

The problem for Mr. Packel and other persons living into the advanced stages of dementia is that the chipping away unfolds beyond anyone's control and at a mercilessly glacial pace. At our afternoon conversation, Mrs. Packel reminded me that seven years prior, I'd told her he had no more than five years of life remaining.

There seems only one way to pick up the pace. I asked Mrs. Packel if she considered it.

"You could have stopped feeding him?"

She shook her head no. "Eating was his joy. He opened up his mouth like a little bird," she explained. "Like a baby smacking his lips." On the occasion of the celebration of what would be his last birthday, his daughter fed him a half gallon of chocolate ice cream. One spoonful at a time.

I wondered what if, years before when Mr. Packel was first diagnosed, he commanded his wife and daughter in writing: "If my life is an existence, not living, then don't feed me?"

APPLESAUCE, NOT MASHED POTATOES

Maybe Margot Bentley sensed something was happening and she knew from her work as a nurse what life would be like if it got worse. She'd cared for persons like Arthur Packel. At sixty, the resident of British Columbia, Canada, decided to make plans. She wrote out how she should be cared for if, in the future, she developed dementia and could no longer direct her care.[2]

The document, commonly called a living will, instructed her daughters, Danielle and Katherine: "If at such time the situation should arise that there is no reasonable expectation of my recovery from extreme physical or mental disability, I direct that I be allowed to die and not be kept alive by artificial means or heroic measures." She detailed what she did and did not want them to do. She should not be given nourishment or liquids, and, if she was unable to recognize members of her family, "I ask that I be euthanized."

Eight years later, in 1999, she was diagnosed with dementia caused by Alzheimer's disease. Her mental and physical disabilities progressed slowly but relentlessly. Five years after her diagnosis, Danielle and Katherine decided home was impossible. They moved her to a nursing home.

Years passed. Speech vanished. She no longer recognized her daughters. She needed help to stand and required others to bathe, dress, groom, and feed her.

In 2011, twelve years after her diagnosis, Danielle and Katherine decided it was time. They'd said their goodbyes years before. Danielle hadn't seen her since 2009. Her mother wasn't dead, but she wasn't alive. It was time to honor Margot Bentley's living will to die. Her physician agreed. Oral feeding and hydration would cease and, as needed, comfort provided.

But then the daughters' plans were disrupted. By their mother. Margot Bentley changed her mind. She in fact wanted to eat. She wanted to keep on living. The staff at the Maplewood House announced they would of course therefore continue to feed her.

Her daughters insisted they cease.

The staff insisted otherwise. Ms. Bentley wanted to eat.

How did they know this?

A summary of events prepared by a social worker for one of several court hearings over the question of whether to honor Mrs. Bentley's living will or her current request to continue eating explained: "While Mrs. Bentley is completely unresponsive and totally dependent on health care providers, she does have one way of communicating—she often closes her mouth to main course foods but she opens it for sweet desserts."[3] She wanted to eat apple-sauce but closed her mouth to mashed potatoes. For the staff at Maplewood House, this meant she was able to decide whether to eat.

Her daughters disagreed. These behaviors were not evidence of her mind making a choice. They were a mere reflex, akin to an infant's rooting reflex when its lips are stroked or presented with a warm nipple. Feeding their mother was unconsented touching, a form of battery.

Intention or reflex? Care or battery?

As is typical in the care of persons living with advanced-stage dementia, the answer was a matter of interpretation. Mrs. Bentley no longer spoke. She couldn't nod or say yes to applesauce or shake her head or say no to mashed potatoes. Or blink once for this and twice for that. She could not telegraph her intentions.

Was she alive inside or merely displaying a neural reflex?

Applesauce not mashed potatoes. In the face of this evidence, the court decided that oral feeding must continue. To cease feeding was, in a sense, equivalent to disconnecting a person from dialysis who insists she wants to continue the lifesaving treatment.

The court also stated her best laid plans written when she was alive and well at sixty were in fact not plans. They were mere words on paper. Advance directives are used to plan medical care. Feeding someone, being fed, the court said, isn't medical care like cardiac resuscitation, a feeding tube inserted into her stomach, or chemotherapy. It is instead personal care. To assure this care would continue, her chart included an order. If her daughters came to move their mother from the nursing home, the police should be called.

In 2016, seventeen years after her diagnosis of dementia caused by Alzheimer's disease, five years after her daughters sought to honor her living will, Margot Bentley died.

It was a wrenching story. A private family matter became a headline-grabbing public drama played out in the pages of the *Vancouver Sun*. Her daughters said they were betraying their promise to their mother to honor her words. They refused to pay for their mother's care.

The staff caring for her likely suffered as well. They were being ordered to cease performing their vocation. Food—feeding—is among the essences of being and caring. Dying by cessation of eating and drinking is rough. The person has to exercise intense discipline, and the sensations of a dry mouth can be maddening. As the person becomes lethargic, caregivers who provide comfort by cleaning the dry mouth may witness a disturbing sight. The person is eager for water. Should more be given? So then withhold food but not water?

Variations on the sad story of Margot Bentley are all too common. They have a common theme. Once upon a time, years and years before dementia, the person wrote out how she ought to be cared for if, in some distant future, she developed dementia. Years pass and that same person, now disabled with dementia, is quite different, happy even.

When an infection or other medical event occurs, the person may agree to receive care he, years prior, declined. Or, if he is unable to understand the present problem or otherwise cannot communicate, family is asked to decide. Their instructions are a years-old living will.

Which person to listen to? Which person to care for? The past self who set forth a will for how to live in the future or the present self who is now living that future?

The essayist and journalist Judith Graham's account of deciding what was the right kind of care for her sister, Deborah, who had dementia (hers caused by frontal-lobar degeneration) shows how this is an ongoing, day-to-day moral struggle.[4] In her essay "My Sister Made Her End-of-Life Wishes Clear. Then Dementia Took Hold," Graham reflected on how Deborah changed in fundamental ways that were ethically significant.

"And I found myself wondering," she wrote, "whose wishes we should respect. My sister, as she had been? Or my sister, as she was now?"

Life with dementia was a life. She took pleasure in things. When, despite aides, home was no longer working, the family moved her to a new home at a memory unit. There, she enjoyed the staff, high-fiving them as she walked the halls. She danced with a male aide she seemed to like.

In time, like Margot Bentley, Deborah needed to be hand-fed and despite that, lost tens of pounds. Soon, swallowing became difficult. Nearly all patients with advanced-stage dementia develop these problems. Her family struggled with whether a feeding tube should be placed. To be sure, her sister's directive told them what to decide. Decline it. And yet, her sister was still a person who seemed to derive meaning from the presence of others.

"Her life had value," Judith reflected. To allow disability to erase that value was simply wrong.

They decided to exercise a kind of leeway over her prior wishes and listen to both selves: the one who wrote the living will and also the one who lived with dementia. Together, these selves guided them through the purgatory of finding goodness at the sorrowful end of Deborah's life. Deborah even contributed some lines to that text. Long after her capacity to meaningfully use language seemed gone, she wrote to Judith: "I don't want to be seen as disabled." For Graham, these paradoxically lucid words were an astonishing statement from a woman who was, by all others' accounts, profoundly disabled.

She was enrolled in hospice and, with family always at her side, they fed her liquid with a dropper and applesauce on a spoon. "We'd wait to hear a gulping swallowing sound. And then, after giving her time to rest, we'd try again."

The feeding tube was a side issue really. The care she received at the end of her life was neither an execution of the advance directive nor an overturning of it.

"We were honoring both the person she had been and the person she had become by making sure she didn't suffer unnecessarily. Every step of the way, we let her know her life had value. And when the hard times came, we didn't duck. We were fully present."

Renee Packel told me eating wasn't her husband's only pleasure. Music engaged him. So, too, his wife's hand. "I could hold his hand. Up to a month or two before he died, I could make him smile. That's why I hung on."

That is why she couldn't stop feeding him. He was, to some degree, still alive inside. Margot Bentley's children thought otherwise. They decided their mother was dead years before she died.

These stories of dying with dementia are not short stories but endless, sometimes gruesomely detailed chapters in a novel that seems to perpetually write itself. What makes the story particularly surreal is that we create the oddest of main characters. The person living with dementia is divided. Like fantasy writers, we imagine that they have one body but two selves—the "then self" and the "now self." That others, loving family and dedicated staff, must mediate among these selves only adds to the surreal tragedy.

The wisdom of Judith Graham's experience is the resolution of those two selves into one. She and her family rejected the dichotomy.

AMP, GENT, AND A FEEDING TUBE

Applesauce, mashed potatoes, liquids via a dropper.

Never mind the big-ticket medical decisions, the expensive machines, and whether to have a bed in one of a hospital's various units. Our focus ought to be on cleaning up the mess of the extraordinarily ordinary care we offer persons living with advanced dementia.

When I was a medical resident in training, a common admission to the wards was a very old, very frail person with advanced dementia, a fever, and pneumonia. These were typically cases of aspiration pneumonia caused, we reasoned, by the person's inability to coordinate a swallow. Our solution was "amp, gent, and a feeding tube," shorthand for two powerful antibiotics (ampicillin and gentamycin) and a consult to gastroenterology to place a feeding tube.

We came to learn that the antibiotics in fact weren't needed. Just oxygen until the inflammation abated. Sadly, the antibiotics caused devastating harms to the person and to society. The patients developed a horrible bacterial diarrhea that often reoccurred, a bacterium we spread about the hospital (this was in an age when we had such faith that antibiotics would rid us of all infections that we'd essentially stopped washing our hands). The bacteria became resistant to the once-powerful antibiotics.

The feeding tube was insidiously harmful. The patient was not allowed to eat by mouth for fear he might aspirate. Human contact faded—the dropper by dropper of liquids and spoonfuls of food were replaced by a slowly turning pump, set to infuse a plastic bag full of banana-colored formula. When the infusion was done, the device sounded to call staff back to the room. These feedings, researchers later discovered, did not extend the length of life.

If we did allow the person to eat by mouth, it was only after a tense negotiation with a speech pathologist. All liquids must be thickened. We reasoned that thin liquids, cool water, for example, would trickle into the lungs and sometimes we ordered sophisticated radiology studies to prove this. We argued that these thickened liquids wouldn't trickle into the lungs.

We called them honey-thickened liquids. We made them by adding a powder to the water or juice that turned the liquid into a kind of golden syrup. Or so it seemed. Colleagues once tried living off these for twelve hours. One recounted how he constantly felt thirst and bloating from the starchy material.

Amp, gent, and a feeding tube, honey-thickened liquids, all four bedrails up to keep the person from falling out of bed, sedating Benadryl for sleep, and wrist restraints for agitation. We did awful, iniquitous things.

And we still do. The particulars change, but the gruesome, confident indifference to care endures.

Just a few years ago, one Easter weekend when I was on call for the geriatrics practice, I took a call from a nurse to review the admission orders for a resident who had returned from hospital to the nursing home. At the close of her recitation of the list, she asked for one more medication, an "as needed" dose of Ativan, a sedative in the family of sedatives such as Valium and Xanax.

"Why?" I asked.

"In case she gets riled up. We like to have something to calm 'em down."

"Why not ask her why she's riled up?"

The nurse did *not* like that. "Do you *know* what it's like caring for these people?"

These people.

Even when we try to do the right thing and order hospice care, we seem to fail. The requirement that a person have a prognosis of six months or less of life results commonly in the patient being "not qualified." Neither alive nor dead.

That's ordinary medical care. What about personal care?

Mrs. Packel recounted how the staff would come up behind her husband and grab him by his thin shoulders to boost him up in the chair he was slumped into. He'd become agitated and yell.

"Why," she begged, "don't you face him and ask if you could lift him up?"

These matters of personal care seem so ordinary, so quotidian, but they are essential. What we fear is the care we receive. Being called sweetie in baby talk tones, dressed in sports clothing and pull-up sweat pants, listening to other people's televisions, and, for the afternoon activity, attending fake weddings performed by staff turned amateur actors. Being fed speciously named "honey-thickened liquids" or delegating all feeding to a machine.

This is what we fear. Threats not to our life but to our dignity. Absent dignity, what of life remains? We'd just as well pass into nonbeing.

But when does that happen?

MIDNIGHT AWAKENINGS

After Amyvid was approved by the FDA, after aducanumab made the front cover of *Nature*, after the A4 Study began enrolling subjects, I perceived the beginnings of a change in my practice as a physician. I began to be visited by women and just a few men who came alone. They opened their visit not with a complaint of memory problems but with a name.

"Ginnie Wolf."

I knew Ginnie Wolf. She was my patient. She had MCI and positive Alzheimer's biomarkers. She regularly used online brain games both to exercise and monitor her cognition. She began to struggle with the games. Her scores dropped. She also noted she could no longer follow the plot of a novel or plan and host a dinner party. It was time to execute her plan.

She said goodbye to her family and ended her life with a bottle of pills. A few months before her death, she told me, "I want to get this right. I want to live well up to the point I'm not living. I'm hoping there will be a time when I simply just know." She was insistent not to live with dementia.

Others spoke of Alice Howland, the protagonist in Lisa Genova's novel *Still Alice*, a third-person account of a Harvard professor of psychology's life as a person diagnosed with Alzheimer's disease at fifty years of age (Howland's disease is caused by one of the uncommon genetic mutations). Alice sets up what might be called the Butterfly plan, a five-question daily self-assessment of her cognition ("Where is your office?" for example) that if she fails, directs her to "Butterfly," a file on her computer with instructions on how to end her life. When she does set off her own alarm, she's too functionally impaired to follow her instructions.

These women wanted "the Alzheimer's test." They wanted an amyloid PET scan. Each explained a similar plan. A "not elevated" result would be a relief, and an "elevated" result would be a call to action. They would be even more vigilant in monitoring their cognitive and day-to-day functions. Some said that like Ginnie Wolf and Alice Howland, they had a plan to end their life before they could no longer do so themselves.

Once upon a time, Alzheimer's disease was a wild beast. It crept up, took hold of a person and then their family, and it never let them go. It was tireless. Efforts to tame it were futile. But now it is changing. It's becoming domesticated.

Biomarkers and MCI are allowing us to capture the disease when it's still young and seemingly harmless. Someday soon disease-slowing drugs will allow us to further tame it. Together, biomarkers and drugs will recast the natural history of the disease. They will redefine when we have it and, years later, when we are dying of it.

Robert Katzman foreshadowed this. The close of his 1976 essay that called America to action instructs us: "In focusing attention on the mortality associated with Alzheimer disease, our goal is not to prolong the lives of the severely demented persons, but rather to call attention to . . . a disease whose etiology must be determined, whose course must be aborted, and ultimately a disease to be prevented."

To be sure, a cure for each and every cause of dementia—amyloid, tau, TDP-43, vascular disease, inflammation, and a host of still-to-be-discovered others—could transform neurodegenerative diseases like Alzheimer's into polio, a problem of the past. Short of that spectacular but fantastical success, however, we shall have to confront morally difficult choices.

Imagine Ginnie Wolf was on aducanumab or some other drug like it, a drug that slowed but did not cure her disease. She'd be thoroughly scrutinized through the clear lens of the clinical gaze. The technologies monitoring her would keep me apprised on how she was functioning. I'd witness her slow decline. At regular visits to the Penn Memory Center, perhaps via telemedicine, she'd recount her troubles following the plot of a novel. I'd know that already of course as I'd have access to summaries of her use of her e-reader.

A robust ethic of respect for persons supports her right to interpret her disease experience, her illness, and decide: "Dr. Karlawish, this is only getting worse. The drug's not really working anymore. I want to stop treatment before I have dementia."

And so I would deprescribe the drug.

After that, after treatment has been stopped, what next? She's now back in the wild, back to nature, ready to return to nonbeing. What palliative care should I offer her when her death is not in six months but some six or more years? Physician aid in dying, available as of 2020 to residents of nine states and the District of Columbia, is not an option. Access to it, like hospice, requires a person to have a prognosis of six months.

What will be the terminal stage of Alzheimer's disease?

Stories about living with and dying of Alzheimer's disease will undoubtedly shape the contours of our answers to this question. We ought to reflect how the stories we share are typically about women, most of them white, middle class, and many quite successful in careers in academics and related professions. I respect their perspective. They fought to become a person in a culture that from their childhood onward told them what they could (wife, mother, maybe a teacher) and could not (medicine, engineering, the law) do. Alzheimer's disease is a disease of their hard-won autonomy.

And yet, we need stories with more diverse characters and cultures, where, for example, autonomy is understood as grounded and exercised in relationships.

We need to curate our language, both in word and image. A common term to describe a person like Margot Bentley is that she lives in a "vegetative state." The person is in a sense no longer an animal with a mind to which we owe moral respect but instead a mindless vegetable. In 2020, Biogen, the company that owns aducanumab, ran internet ads to promote their approach to studying their potential treatment for Alzheimer's disease. The image the company chose is frightening, perhaps even disgusting.

There is a woman, photographed from the shoulders up. She stares straight at you. Her mouth is fixed and expressionless as in a mug shot. A trickle of what looks to be white paint is pouring over her head, beginning to cover her face, obscuring her left eye and forehead. The text reads: "Even though she is just starting to forget important dates, Amyloid beta has been accumulating long before symptoms appeared."[5] Amyloid is coating her brain, turning her into a kind of living skull. Or, in a word, a zombie.

Stories of women caught in the cross hairs of outrageous public right-to-life versus death-with-dignity battles, words like "vegetable" and "vegetative," images of zombies—is this how we want to construct the ways we think and feel about living with Alzheimer's disease and dementia?

One morning at the Memory Center, the caregiver I was interviewing during a new patient visit for her father suddenly let forth a sob. It came like a fire alarm from a long-ago time and place. It was a memory of her grandfather. Years ago, he'd died of Alzheimer's disease.

Like Arthur Packel and Margot Bentley, he'd lived far into the disease, to the stage of being a "severely demented person" whose life Dr. Katzman wrote we do not want to prolong. She still visited him weekly, though at many of these visits, he spoke little. It seemed he didn't know who she was.

One day, he became quite ill. She explained, "We knew he was dying. He was on hospice in fact, but for some reason, he was sent to the hospital. We said, 'Nothing heroic, nothing extreme.'"

Something quite paradoxical happened.

The man who rarely spoke—who did not recognize his granddaughter, who was dying of dementia—took her hand and he looked at her. And then he spoke.

"He said he was happy I was there. He knew me. He spoke to me clearly. He expressed his happiness with seeing me there. It was not really long, just really clear. Like a miracle. He was himself again. Without a doubt, I just knew he knew who I was. It was very peaceful for both of us."

Three days later he died.

Before that day, she'd been mourning the loss of him for years, but then came this moment of lucidity. She told me it was a gift. He was still there. Still a person. Those weekly visits meant something to him.

This grandfather's words, Arthur Packel's hand, Deborah's note to her sister, Judith—"I don't want to be seen as disabled"—these are messages in a bottle. They are sent by people who are asking for our help to preserve their dignity and provide comfort. Our duty—caregivers, the health care system, government, society—is to do that, to be present from diagnosis to death.

In solitude, company.

ACKNOWLEDGMENTS

Writing is a most solitary act, but the creation of a book is a grand production that engages a host of persons. Here, I shall try to thank them all, though I'm certain I've neglected some.

I thank David McCormick and Emma Borges-Scott of McCormick Literary for their devotion to me and this book. Working with them—line by line, draft after draft—is a writer's pleasure. Daniela Rapp at Macmillan/St. Martin's Press is a dedicated editor and a fierce advocate. My thanks to the people at Macmillan/St. Martin's Press who shepherded this book through the various phases to bound book and to my copyeditor, Paula Cooper Hughes.

I've had the good fortune of a network of colleagues. Their willingness to listen, converse, read, and critique helped me create this book. The list is long. At the Penn Memory Center, I thank Terry Casey, Chris Clark, Felicia Greenfield, Kristin Harkins, Alison Lynn, and David Wolk. Elsewhere there are Jesse Ballenger, Maria Carrillo, Christine Cassel, Brad Dickerson, Joshua Grill, Allison Hoffman, Bryan James, Steve Joffe, Lara Keuck, Ken Langa, Jessica Langbaum, Emily Largent, David Lyreskog, Richard Milne, Andrew Peterson, Eric Reiman, Pamela Sankar, Lon Schneider, Reisa Sperling, Shana Stites, and Keith Wailoo. Elisa Petrini and Edwin Parker are master readers and editors. Great thanks to Peter Schankowitz and Anne Wright for urging me to always, always focus on the story.

Research for this book involved many interviews. Not all the candid and vivid stories I was told are explicitly quoted, but all are part of the book's warp and weft. I thank each of you who shared your stories. Great thanks to the Alzheimer's Association for access to your archives and for doing what you tirelessly do.

I have the great privilege of being a professor at the University of Pennsylvania, or what we affectionately call Penn. This academic home is quite unique. Truly, it is a nurturing "one university" that fosters a collegial competition of ideas and all kinds of inspiring collaborations. For several years,

I taught a class on Alzheimer's disease in the master's in public health program. The bright students' questions and ideas helped me polish points and clarify the themes and messages. I thank them.

Two other institutions deserve special thanks: the Greenwall Foundation and the Robert Wood Johnson Foundation. Both awarded me fellowships that supported work that led to this book. Both also invested in creating communities of scholars who engaged, inspired, and supported my sometimes wild ideas.

I am grateful to *Forbes.com*, *STATNews*, the *Philadelphia Inquirer*, and the *New York Times* for publishing my essays on aging and Alzheimer's disease that were the trial runs at the many ideas and themes that came together to form this book.

Finally, I thank my patients and their caregivers. Thank you for your courage to share your intimate and emotionally awesome stories of living with Alzheimer's disease and the other diseases that cause dementia. They are my foundational texts. Several years ago, Renee Packel was sharing her story with my class at Penn—I'd heard it many times before, nothing new—and yet I caught myself about to sob. I decided I need to make sense of this emotion.

And so I wrote this book.

NOTES

INTRODUCTION: THE DISEASE OF THE CENTURY

1 Lewis Thomas, "The Problem of Dementia," in *Late Night Thoughts on Listening to Mahler's Ninth Symphony* (New York: Viking Press, 1983): 120–26.
2 Robert Katzman, "The Prevalence and Malignancy of Alzheimer Disease: A Major Killer," *Archives of Neurology* 33, no. 4 (April 1, 1976): 217–18, https://doi.org/10.1001/archneur.1976.00500040001001.
3 Alzheimer's Study Group, *A National Alzheimer's Strategic Plan: The Report of the Alzheimer's Study Group* (Alzheimer's Association, March 24, 2009), https://www.alz.org/documents/national/report_asg_alzplan.pdf.

PART 1: ALZHEIMER'S UNBOUND

1. A PECULIAR DISEASE OF THE CEREBRAL CORTEX

1 G. McKhann et al., "Clinical Diagnosis of Alzheimer's Disease: Report of the NINCDS-ADRDA Work Group Under the Auspices of Department of Health and Human Services Task Force on Alzheimer's Disease," *Neurology* 34, no. 7 (July 1984): 939–44, https://doi.org/10.1212/wnl.34.7.939.
2 Being autonomous is often understood as making decisions, or "decision making." This requires a suite of cognitive abilities and also political conditions, as, for example, described by the philosopher Leslie Francis: "being able to value, being able to reason, being able to resist impulses, being able to imagine an ordered life, being able to order one's life, being able to put one's plans into practice, being able to participate in moral deliberation of an idealized kind, and being politically free." L. P. Francis, "Understanding Autonomy in Light of Intellectual Disability," in *Disability and Disadvantage* (Oxford, New York: Oxford University Press, 2011): 200–215. Other accounts of autonomy recognize that a person is embedded in relationships with other supportive persons (as well as supportive technologies). Catriona Mackenzie and Natalie Stoljar, *Relational Autonomy: Feminist Perspectives on Autonomy, Agency, and the Social Self* (New York: Oxford University Press, 2000). Part 4 explores these "relational" ideas of autonomy by examining the roles of technology such as robots, trusted others, repairing "homelooseness," and how persons living with dementia and their caregivers can co-create.

3   Arthur Kleinman, *The Soul of Care: The Moral Education of a Husband and a Doctor* (New York: Viking, 2019).

4   Arthur Kleinman, "Caregiving as Moral Experience," *Lancet* 380, no. 9853 (November 3, 2012): 1550–51, https://doi.org/10.1016/s0140-6736(12)61870-4.

5   H. A. Kiyak, L. Teri, and S. Borson, "Physical and Functional Health Assessment in Normal Aging and in Alzheimer's Disease: Self-Reports vs. Family Reports," *Gerontologist* 34, no. 3 (June 1994): 324–30, https://doi.org/10.1093/geront/34.3.324.

6   Martin Pinquart and Silvia Sörensen, "Differences Between Caregivers and Noncaregivers in Psychological Health and Physical Health: A Meta-Analysis," *Psychology and Aging* 18, no. 2 (June 2003): 250–67, https://doi.org/10.1037/0882-7974.18.2.250.

7   Nancy L. Mace and Peter V. Rabins, *The 36-Hour Day: A Family Guide to Caring for Persons with Alzheimer's Disease, Related Dementing Illnesses, and Memory Loss in Later Life* (Baltimore: Johns Hopkins University Press, 1981).

8   Esther M. Friedman et al., "US Prevalence and Predictors of Informal Caregiving for Dementia," *Health Affairs* 34, no. 10 (October 1, 2015): 1637–41, https://doi.org/10.1377/hlthaff.2015.0510.

9   *31-1011 Home Health Aides*, US Bureau of Labor Statistics, March 29, 2019, https://www.bls.gov/oes/current/oes311011.htm.

10 Michael D. Hurd et al., "Monetary Costs of Dementia in the United States," *New England Journal of Medicine* 368, no. 14 (April 4, 2013): 1326–34, https://doi.org/10.1056/NEJMsa1204629.

11 Norma B. Coe, Meghan M. Skira, and Eric B. Larson, "A Comprehensive Measure of the Costs of Caring for a Parent: Differences According to Functional Status," *Journal of the American Geriatrics Society* 66, no. 10 (October 2018): 2003–8, https://doi.org/10.1111/jgs.15552.

12 Meghan M. Skira, "Dynamic Wage and Employment Effects of Elder Parent Care," *International Economic Review* 56, no. 1 (January 23, 2015): 63–93, https://doi.org/10.1111/iere.12095.

13 John. M Glionna, "Only in Las Vegas: Alzheimer's Clinic Doubles as Party Venue," *STAT*, April 12, 2016, https://www.statnews.com/2016/04/12/alzheimers-brain-health-las-vegas/.

14 Lawrence K. Altman, "Reagan's Twilight—A Special Report: A President Fades into a World Apart," *New York Times*, October 5, 1997, https://www.nytimes.com/1997/10/05/us/reagan-s-twilight-a-special-report-a-president-fades-into-a-world-apart.html.

15 In the essay "The Living Dead? The Construction of People with Alzheimer's Disease as Zombies," the political scientist Susan Behuniak shows the pervasive use of the zombie trope to explain the disease, even in the titles of well-intended academic and popular writings, which employ phrases such as "coping with a living death," "death before death," and "death in slow motion." The word "zombie" isn't explicit, but it's there. This trope evokes feelings of disgust that, in turn, strip dignity and cause a politics of fear that marginalizes and dehumanizes persons living with Alzheimer's disease. Susan M. Behuniak, "The Living Dead? The Construction of People with Alzheimer's Disease as Zombies," *Ageing and Society* 31, no. 1 (January 2011): 70–92, https://doi.org/10.1017/S0144686X10000693.

2. NO ONE SAYS NO TO LEN KURLAND

1   Robert Ivnik, personal interview by Jason Karlawish, September 16, 2018.

2   Ronald Petersen, personal interview by Jason Karlawish, October 25, 2018.

3   Walter A. Rocca et al., "History of the Rochester Epidemiology Project: Half a Century of Medical Records Linkage in a US Population," *Mayo Clinic Proceedings* 87, no. 12 (December 2012): 1202–13, https://doi.org/10.1016/j.mayocp.2012.08.012.

3. ACCURATE BUT NOT PRESUMPTUOUS

1   Glenn Smith, personal interview by Jason Karlawish, August 29, 2018.
2   R. C. Petersen, G. E. Smith, et al., "Mild Cognitive Impairment: Clinical Characterization and Outcome," *Archives of Neurology* 56, no. 3 (March 1999): 303–8, https://doi.org/10.1001/archneur.56.3.303.
3   Ronald C. Petersen et al., "Prevalence of Mild Cognitive Impairment Is Higher in Men. The Mayo Clinic Study of Aging," *Neurology* 75, no. 10 (September 7, 2010): 889–97. https://doi.org/10.1212/WNL.0b13e3181f11d85.
4   John Lucas, personal interview by Jason Karlawish, September 25, 2018.
5   John C. Morris et al., "Mild Cognitive Impairment Represents Early-Stage Alzheimer Disease," *Archives of Neurology* 58, no. 3 (March 1, 2001): 397–405, https://doi.org/10.1001/archneur.58.3.397.

4. THE OLYMPICS OF PHARMACOKINETICS

1   Alois Alzheimer, "Über Eine Eigenartige Erkrankung der Hirnrinde" [On a peculiar disease of the brain cortex], *Allgemeine Zeitschrift für Psychiatrie und Psychisch-Gerichtliche Medizin* 64 (1907): 146–48. Trans. L. Jarvik and H. Greenson, "About a Peculiar Disease of the Cerebral Cortex," *Alzheimer's Disease and Associated Disorders* (1987), 7–8.
2   George G. Glenner and Caine W. Wong, Polypeptide marker for Alzheimer's disease and its use for diagnosis, 4666829, filed May 15, 1985, and issued May 19, 1987, http://www.freepatentsonline.com/4666829.html.
3   Chet Mathis, personal interview by Jason Karlawish, October 23, 2018.
4   Bill Klunk, personal interview by Jason Karlawish, July 26, 2018.
5   Laura Helmuth, "Long-Awaited Technique Spots Alzheimer's Toxin," *Science* 297, no. 5582 (August 2, 2002): 752–53, https://doi.org/10.1126/science.297.5582.752b.

5. THE REPUBLIC OF ALZHEIMER'S DISEASE

1   Laura Helmuth, "Long-Awaited Technique Spots Alzheimer's Toxin," *Science* 297, no. 5582 (August 2, 2002): 752–53, https://doi.org/10.1126/science.297.5582.752b.
2   Mike Weiner, personal interview by Jason Karlawish, July 22, 2018.
3   Ronald C. Petersen, Rosebud O. Roberts, et al., "Mild Cognitive Impairment: Ten Years Later," *Archives of Neurology* 66, no. 12 (December 2009): 1447–55, https://doi.org/10.1001/archneurol.2009.266.

6. A YOUNG MAN IN A HURRY

1   Daniel Skovronsky, personal interview by Jason Karlawish, September 4, 2018.
2   William E. Klunk et al., "Imaging Brain Amyloid in Alzheimer's Disease with Pittsburgh compound-B," *Annals of Neurology* 55, no. 3 (March 2004): 306–19, https://doi.org/10.1002/ana.20009.

3 Larry Goldstein et al., Department of Health and Human Services, United States Food and Drug Administration Center for Evaluation and Research. *Transcript of Peripheral and Central Nervous System Drugs Advisory Committee Meeting* (Washington, DC: October 23, 2008).

7. HOW DO YOU CAST A BROKEN BRAIN?

1 Christopher M. Clark et al., "Use of Florbetapir-PET for Imaging Beta-Amyloid Pathology," *JAMA* 305, no. 3 (January 19, 2011): 275–83, https://doi.org/10.1001/jama.2010.2008.
2 Eli Lilly and Company, "FDA Approves Amyvid (Florbetapir F 18 Injection) for Use in Patients Being Evaluated for Alzheimer's Disease and Other Causes of Cognitive Decline," PR Newswire, April 9, 2012, https://www.prnewswire.com/news-releases/fda-approves-amyvid-florbetapir-f-18-injection-for-use-in-patients-being-evaluated-for-alzheimers-disease-and-other-causes-of-cognitive-decline-146638165.html.
3 Larry Goldstein et al., Department of Health and Human Services, United States Food and Drug Administration Center for Evaluation and Research. *Transcript of Peripheral and Central Nervous System Drugs Advisory Committee Meeting* (Washington, DC: October 23, 2008).
4 Alzheimer's Association, "2013 Alzheimer's Disease Facts and Figures," *Alzheimer's and Dementia: The Journal of the Alzheimer's Association* 9, no. 2 (March 2013): 208–45, https://doi.org/10.1016/j.jalz.2013.02.003.
5 US Department of Health and Human Services, Centers for Disease Control and Prevention, "Promoting Brain Health: Be a Champion! Make a Difference Today!," February 2011, https://www.cdc.gov/aging/pdf/cognitive_impairment/cogImp_genAud_final.pdf.
6 Cliff Jack, personal interview by Jason Karlawish, August 30, 2018.
7 Maria Ellis et al., "Medicare Evidence Development and Coverage Advisory Committee" (Baltimore, MD, January 30, 2013).
8 Gina Kolata, "For Alzheimer's, Detection Advances Outpace Treatment Options," *New York Times*, November 15, 2012, https://www.nytimes.com/2012/11/16/health/for-alzheimers-detection-advances-outpace-treatment-options.html.
9 Louis Jacques et al., "Proposed Decision Memo for Beta Amyloid Positron Emission Tomography in Dementia and Neurodegenerative Disease (CAG-00431N)," September 27, 2013, https://www.cms.gov/medicare-coverage-database/details/nca-decision-memo.aspx?NCAId=265.
10 Alzheimer's Association, "2015 Alzheimer's Disease Facts and Figures," *Alzheimer's and Dementia* 11, no. 3 (March 1, 2015): 332–84, https://doi.org/10.1016/j.jalz.2015.02.003.

PART 2: THE BIRTH OF ALZHEIMER'S DISEASE

8. THE OLD WOMAN IN THE TOWER

1 Jesse F. Ballenger, "The Stereotype of Senility in Late-Nineteenth-Century America." In: *Self, Senility, and Alzheimer's Disease in Modern America: A History* (Baltimore: Johns Hopkins University Press, 2006): 11–35.

9. ALOIS ALZHEIMER: AN UNWITTING REVOLUTIONARY

1   These and other details of Alois Alzheimer's life are from Konrad Maurer and Ulrike Maurer, *Alzheimer: The Life of a Physician and the Career of a Disease*, trans. Neil Levi and Alistair Burns (New York: Columbia University Press, 2003).
2   Alzheimer, "Über Eine Eigenartige Erkrankung der Hirnrinde" [On a peculiar disease of the brain cortex]. *Allgemeine Zeitschrift für Psychiatrie und Psychisch-Gerichtliche Medizin* 64 (1907): 146–48. Trans. L. Jarvik and H. Greenson, "About a Peculiar Disease of the Cerebral Cortex," *Alzheimer's Disease and Associated Disorders* (1987): 7–8.
3   Alois Alzheimer, "Über Eigenartige Krankheitsfälle des Späteren Alters," *Zeitschrift für die Gesamte Neurologie und Psychiatrie* 4, no. 1 (December 1, 1911): 356–85, https://doi.org/10.1007/BF02866241. Trans. Hans Förstl and Raymond Levy, "On Certain Peculiar Diseases of Old Age," *History of Psychiatry* 2, no. 5 (March 1991): 71–73, doi:10.1177/0957154X9100200505.
4   Lara Keuck, "Diagnosing Alzheimer's Disease in Kraepelin's Clinic, 1909–1912," *History of the Human Sciences* 31, no. 2 (April 1, 2018): 42–64, https://doi.org/10.1177/0952695118758879.
5   Kraepelin as quoted in Maurer and Maurer, *Alzheimer*.

10. OBLIVION, OR WAR AND MADNESS

1   Wilfred Owen, *Wilfred Owen: Selected Letters*, ed. John Bell, 2nd ed. (Oxford, New York: Oxford University Press, 1998).
2   Adam Fergusson, *When Money Dies: The Nightmare of the Weimar Hyper-Inflation* (Melbourne, London: Scribe, 2011).
3   Andrew Scull, *Madness in Civilization: A Cultural History of Insanity, from the Bible to Freud, from the Madhouse to Modern Medicine*, reprint ed. (Princeton, NJ: Princeton University Press, 2016).
4   Emil Kraepelin, "Psychiatric observations on contemporary issues," *History of Psychiatry*, 3, no. 10 (1992): 253–256, https://doi.org/10.1177/0957154X9200301007.
5   Katja Guenther, *Localization and Its Discontents* (Chicago: University of Chicago Press, 2015), https://www.press.uchicago.edu/ucp/books/book/chicago/L/bo21163259.html.
6   Katie Maslow, personal interview by Jason Karlawish, January 22, 2019.

11. THE ESSAY HEARD ROUND THE WORLD

1   National Institute on Aging, "NOT-AG-18-053: Notice to Specify High-Priority Research Topic for PAR-19-070 and PAR-19-071," December 17, 2018, https://grants.nih.gov/grants/guide/notice-files/NOT-AG-18-053.html.
2   Robert Katzman, "The Prevalence and Malignancy of Alzheimer Disease: A Major Killer," *Archives of Neurology* 33, no. 4 (April 1, 1976): 217–18, https://doi.org/10.1001/archneur.1976.00500040001001.

3   Robert Butler, *Why Survive?: Being Old in America* (Baltimore: Johns Hopkins University Press, 2003).
4   R. D. Adams et al., "Symptomatic Occult Hydrocephalus with 'Normal' Cerebrospinal-Fluid Pressure: A Treatable Syndrome," *New England Journal of Medicine* 273 (July 15, 1965): 117–26, https://doi.org/10.1056/NEJM196507152730301.
5   Robert Katzman and Katherine Bick, *Alzheimer Disease: The Changing View* (San Diego: Academic Press, 2000).
6   Daniel Katzman, personal interview by Jason Karlawish, January 12, 2019.
7   Marjorie J. Spruill, *Divided We Stand: The Battle over Women's Rights and Family Values That Polarized American Politics* (New York: Bloomsbury USA, 2017).
8   Jesse F. Ballenger, *Self, Senility, and Alzheimer's Disease in Modern America: A History* (Baltimore: Johns Hopkins University Press, 2006).

12. A SELF-HELP GROUP FOR THE SELF-MADE MAN

1   Robert Katzman and Katherine Bick, *Alzheimer Disease: The Changing View* (San Diego: Academic Press, 2000).
2   Katzman and Bick, *Alzheimer Disease*, 340.
3   Michael Taylor, "Early Alzheimer's Crusader Anne Bashkiroff Dies," *SFGate*, November 23, 2008, https://www.sfgate.com/bayarea/article/Early-Alzheimer-s-crusader-Anne-Bashkiroff-dies-3183733.php.
4   Ryan Pridgeon, personal interview by Jason Karlawish, February 23, 2019.
5   Katzman and Bick, *Alzheimer Disease*, 316.
6   Jerome Stone, *The Self-Help Movement: Forming a National Organization* (Chicago: Alzheimer's Disease and Related Disorders Association, 1982).
7   Lonnie Wollin, personal interview by Jason Karlawish, February 22, 2019.

13. A CRISIS IN THE FAMILY

1   Minutes of the Board of Directors of the Alzheimer's Association, October 18, 1985, Archives of Alzheimer's Association.
2   US Congress, Office of Technology Assessment, *Losing a Million Minds: Confronting the Tragedy of Alzheimer's Disease and Other Dementias. Congressional Summary* (Washington, DC: US Congress, Office of Technology Assessment, April 1987), https://eric.ed.gov/?id=ED298420.
3   US Congress, Office of Technology Assessment, *Confused Minds, Burdened Families: Finding Help for People with Alzheimer's and Other Dementias*, OTA-13A-403 (Washington, DC: US Government Printing Office, 1990), https://catalog.hathitrust.org/Record/007415141.
4   US Congress, *Alzheimer's: The Unmet Challenge for Research and Care: Joint Hearing Before the Select Committee on Aging, House of Representatives, and the Subcommittee on Aging of the Committee on Labor and Human Resources, U.S. Senate, One Hundred First Congress, Second Session, April 3, 1990*, SCOA Comm. Pub. No. 101–783, Select Committee on Aging, House of Representatives, and the Subcommittee on Aging of the Committee on Labor and Human Resources, US Senate (1990).
5   Stephen McConnell to Public Policy Committee, "Congressional Action on Behalf of AD Patients/Families," memorandum, November 2, 1990.

6   Shelia Norman-Culp, "Alzheimer's Widow Reaches Out to Others," *Jacksonville Journal Courier*, August 31, 1989.
7   Robert Katzman and Katherine Bick, *Alzheimer Disease: The Changing View* (San Diego: Academic Press, 2000): 321–36.

14. THE LAST CASUALTIES OF THE COLD WAR

1   Steve McConnell, personal interview by Jason Karlawish, February 5, 2019.
2   Ronald Reagan, State of the Union Address, Washington, DC, January 26, 1982, https://millercenter.org/the-presidency/presidential-speeches/january-26-1982-state-union-address.
3   "News Conference: The Ronald Reagan Presidential Foundation and Institute," accessed April 13, 2020, https://www.reaganfoundation.org/ronald-reagan/reagan-quotes-speeches/news-conference-1/.
4   Reagan, State of the Union Address, 1982.
5   Julie Kosterlitz, "Anguish and Opportunity," *National Journal*, April 28, 1990.
6   *Ronald Reagan: Medicare Will Bring a Socialist Dictatorship*, accessed March 27, 2020, https://www.youtube.com/watch?v=Bejdhs3jGyw.
7   United States Code, Title 42—The Public Health and Welfare, Chapter 7—Social Security, Subchapter XVIII—Health Insurance for Aged and Disabled (2011): 42, https://www.govinfo.gov/content/pkg/USCODE-2011-title42/html/USCODE-2011-title42-chap7-subchapXVIII.htm.
8   Louis Friedfeld, "Geriatrics, Medicine, and Rehabilitation," *JAMA* 175, no. 7 (February 18, 1961): 595–98, https://doi.org/10.1001/jama.1961.03040070053012.
9   Michael M. Dacso, "Maintenance of Functional Capacity," *JAMA* 175, no. 7 (February 18, 1961): 592–94, https://doi.org/10.1001/jama.1961.03040070050011.
10 Marjorie J. Spruill, *Divided We Stand: The Battle over Women's Rights and Family Values That Polarized American Politics* (New York: Bloomsbury USA, 2017).
11 Minutes of the Board of Directors of the Alzheimer's Association, January 22, 1995, Archives of Alzheimer's Association.
12 Jonathan Oberlander, "The Political Life of Medicare," in *The Political Life of Medicare* (Chicago and London: University of Chicago Press, 2003): 62–63.
13 Julie Kosterlitz, "Anguish and Opportunity."
14 Denis A. Evans et al., "Prevalence of Alzheimer's Disease in a Community Population of Older Persons: Higher Than Previously Reported," *JAMA* 262, no. 18 (November 10, 1989): 2551–56, https://doi.org/10.1001/jama.1989.03430180093036.
15 Institute of Medicine (US) Committee to Study the AIDS Research Program of the National Institutes of Health, *The AIDS Research Program of the National Institutes of Health* (Washington, DC: National Academies Press, 1991), https://www.ncbi.nlm.nih.gov/books/NBK234085.
16 "What Is Alzheimer's Disease?," National Institute on Aging, accessed March 21, 2019, https://www.nia.nih.gov/health/what-alzheimers-disease.l.

15. HOPE IN A PILL

1   US Congress, *Impact of Alzheimer's Disease on the Nation's Elderly: Joint Hearing Before the Subcommittee on Aging of the Committee on Labor and Human Resources, United*

States Senate, and the Subcommittee on Labor, Health, Education, and Welfare of the Committee on Appropriations, House of Representatives, Ninety-Sixth Congress, Second Session, on to Analyze the Impact of Alzheimer's Disease and Other Dimentias [sic] of Aging on Our Society, July 15, 1980 (Washington, DC: US Government Printing Office, 1980).

2   William Koopmans Summers et al., "Oral Tetrahydroaminoacridine in Long-Term Treatment of Senile Dementia, Alzheimer Type," New England Journal of Medicine 315, no. 20 (November 13, 1986): 1241–45, https://doi.org/10.1056/NEJM198611133152001.

3   Philippe Bardonnaud, Pascal Dervieux, and Vanessa Descouraux, "Alzheimer: Les petits intérêts dans les grands," accessed March 23, 2019, https://www.franceinter.fr/emissions/interception/interception-11-janvier-2015.

4   "RFA-AG-17-005: Alzheimer's Clinical Trials Consortium (ACTC) (U24)," Department of Health and Human Services, July 25, 2016, https://grants.nih.gov/grants/guide/rfa-files/RFA-AG-17-005.html.

5   Jason Karlawish, "The Search for a Coherent Language: The Science and Politics of Drug Testing and Approval," in Ethics, Law, and Aging Review (New York: Springer, 2002): 39–56.

6   Sebastian Walsh, Elizabeth King, and Carol Brayne, "France Removes State Funding for Dementia Drugs," BMJ 367 (December 30, 2019), https://doi.org/10.1136/bmj.l6930.

7   Arnold S. Relman, "Tacrine as a Treatment for Alzheimer's Dementia—Editor's Note," New England Journal of Medicine 324, no. 5 (January 31, 1991): 349, https://doi.org/10.1056/NEJM199101313240525.

8   Barbara G. Vickrey et al., "The Effect of a Disease Management Intervention on Quality and Outcomes of Dementia Care: A Randomized, Controlled Trial," Annals of Internal Medicine 145, no. 10 (November 21, 2006): 713–26, https://doi.org/10.7326/0003-4819-145-10-200611210-00004.

9   Steven H. Belle et al., "Enhancing the Quality of Life of Dementia Caregivers from Different Ethnic or Racial Groups: A Randomized, Controlled Trial," Annals of Internal Medicine 145, no. 10 (November 21, 2006): 727–38, https://doi.org/10.7326/0003-4819-145-10-200611210-00005.

10   Kenneth E. Covinsky and C. Bree Johnston, "Envisioning Better Approaches for Dementia Care," Annals of Internal Medicine 145, no. 10 (November 21, 2006): 780, https://doi.org/10.7326/0003-4819-145-10-200611210-00011.

PART 3: LIVING WELL IN THE HOUSE OF ALZHEIMER'S

16. THE EXTRAORDINARY ORDINARY

1   Steven H. Zarit et al., "Effects of Adult Day Care on Daily Stress of Caregivers: A Within-Person Approach," Journals of Gerontology Series B: Psychological Sciences and Social Sciences 66B, no. 5 (September 2011): 538–46, https://doi.org/10.1093/geronb/gbr030.

2   Pam Barton, personal interview by Jason Karlawish, April 16, 2019.

3   Felicia R. Lee, "Surprise Grants Transforming 23 More Lives," New York Times, October 1, 2012, https://www.nytimes.com/2012/10/02/arts/macarthur-fellows-named-for-2012.html.

17. A CORRECTION

1   Keith A. Johnson et al., "Update on Appropriate Use Criteria for Amyloid PET Imaging: Dementia Experts, Mild Cognitive Impairment, and Education," *Journal of Nuclear Medicine: Official Publication, Society of Nuclear Medicine* 54, no. 7 (July 2013): 1011–13, https://doi.org/10.2967/jnumed.113.127068.
2   Margaret A. Noel, personal interview by Jason Karlawish, April 17, 2019.

18. DISCERNMENT

1   Rebecca Mitchell et al., "Hip Fracture and the Influence of Dementia on Health Outcomes and Access to Hospital-Based Rehabilitation for Older Individuals," *Disability and Rehabilitation* 38, no. 23 (2016): 2286–95, https://doi.org/10.3109/09638288.2015.1 123306.
2   Danielle S. Abraham et al., "Residual Disability, Mortality, and Nursing Home Placement After Hip Fracture over 2 Decades," *Archives of Physical Medicine and Rehabilitation* 100, no. 5 (2019): 874–82, https://doi.org/10.1016/j.apmr.2018.10.008.
3   Sharon Inouye, personal interview by Jason Karlawish, May 18, 2019.
4   S. K. Inouye et al., "A Predictive Model for Delirium in Hospitalized Elderly Medical Patients Based on Admission Characteristics," *Annals of Internal Medicine* 119, no. 6 (September 15, 1993): 474–81, https://doi.org/10.7326/0003-4819-119-6-199309150-00005.
5   Sharon K. Inouye and Peter A. Charpentier, "Precipitating Factors for Delirium in Hospitalized Elderly Persons: Predictive Model and Interrelationship with Baseline Vulnerability," *JAMA* 275, no. 11 (March 20, 1996): 852–57, https://doi.org/10.1001/jama.1996.03530350034031.
6   Sharon K. Inouye et al., "A Multicomponent Intervention to Prevent Delirium in Hospitalized Older Patients," *New England Journal of Medicine* 340, no. 9 (March 4, 1999): 669–76, https://doi.org/10.1056/NEJM199903043400901.
7   John W. Rowe, "Geriatrics, Prevention, and the Remodeling of Medicare," *New England Journal of Medicine* 340, no. 9 (March 4, 1999): 720–21, https://doi.org/10.1056/NEJM199903043400908.
8   Associated Press, "Study Suggests Common Sense Steps Alleviated Confusion Condition," March 4, 1999.
9   Robert McCann, personal interview by Jason Karlawish, April 30, 2019.
10 Daniel Mendelson, personal interview by Jason Karlawish, April 17, 2019.
11 Susan M. Friedman et al., "Impact of a Comanaged Geriatric Fracture Center on Short-Term Hip Fracture Outcomes," *Archives of Internal Medicine* 169, no. 18 (October 12, 2009): 1712–17, https://doi.org/10.1001/archinternmed.2009.321.

19. SOME THINGS TO WATCH OVER US

1   Jeffrey Kaye, personal interview by Jason Karlawish, May 21, 2019.
2   Jeffrey Kaye et al., "Methodology for Establishing a Community-Wide Life Laboratory for Capturing Unobtrusive and Continuous Remote Activity and Health Data," *Journal of Visualized Experiments*, no. 137 (July 27, 2018), https://doi.org/10.3791/56942.

3   H. H. Dodge et al., "In-Home Walking Speeds and Variability Trajectories Associated with Mild Cognitive Impairment," *Neurology* 78, no. 24 (June 12, 2012): 1946–52, https://doi.org/10.1212/WNL.0b013e318259e1de.

4   Tamara L. Hayes et al., "Medication Adherence in Healthy Elders: Small Cognitive Changes Make a Big Difference," *Journal of Aging and Health* 21, no. 4 (June 2009): 567–80, https://doi.org/10.1177/0898264309332836.

5   Jeffrey Kaye et al., "Unobtrusive Measurement of Daily Computer Use to Detect Mild Cognitive Impairment," *Alzheimer's and Dementia* 10, no. 1 (January 2014): 10–17, https://doi.org/10.1016/j.jalz.2013.01.011.

6   Adriana Seelye et al., "Computer Mouse Movement Patterns: A Potential Marker of Mild Cognitive Impairment," *Alzheimer's and Dementia: Diagnosis, Assessment and Disease Monitoring* 1, no. 4 (October 19, 2015): 472–80, https://doi.org/10.1016/j.dadm.2015.09.006.

7   Robert Katzman, "The Prevalence and Malignancy of Alzheimer Disease: A Major Killer," *Archives of Neurology* 33, no. 4 (April 1, 1976): 217–18.

20. NOT (LEGALLY) DEAD YET

1   C. E. Wells, "The Symptoms and Behavioral Manifestations of Dementia," *Contemporary Neurology Series* 9 (1971): 1–11.

2   Ellen Bouchard Ryan, Mary Lee Hummert, and Linda H. Boich, "Communication Predicaments of Aging: Patronizing Behavior Toward Older Adults," *Journal of Language and Social Psychology* 14 (March 1995): 144–46.

3   Fred Bayles et al., *Guardians of the Elderly: An Ailing System*, Associated Press, Special Report, September 19, 1987.

4   Bayles et al., *Guardians of the Elderly.*

5   Paul Appelbaum, personal interview by Jason Karlawish, May 15, 2019.

6   Charlie Sabatino, personal interview by Jason Karlawish, May 21, 2019.

7   L. H. Roth, A. Meisel, and C. W. Lidz, "Tests of Competency to Consent to Treatment," *American Journal of Psychiatry* 134, no. 3 (March 1977): 279–84, https://doi.org/10.1176/ajp.134.3.279.

8   Thomas Grisso and Paul S. Appelbaum, *Assessing Competence to Consent to Treatment: A Guide for Physicians and Other Health Professionals* (Oxford, New York: Oxford University Press, 1998).

9   Jason Karlawish et al., "The Ability of Persons with Alzheimer Disease (AD) to Make a Decision About Taking an AD Treatment," *Neurology* 64, no. 9 (May 10, 2005): 1514–19, https://doi.org/10.1212/01.WNL.0000160000.01742.9D.

10 Jason Karlawish, David J. Casarett, and Bryan D. James, "Alzheimer's Disease Patients' and Caregivers' Capacity, Competency, and Reasons to Enroll in an Early-Phase Alzheimer's Disease Clinical Trial," *Journal of the American Geriatrics Society* 50, no. 12 (December 2002): 2019–24, https://doi.org/10.1046/j.1532-5415.2002.50615.x.

11 Scott Y. H. Kim et al., "Preservation of the Capacity to Appoint a Proxy Decision Maker: Implications for Dementia Research," *Archives of General Psychiatry* 68, no. 2 (February 2011): 214–20, https://doi.org/10.1001/archgenpsychiatry.2010.191.

12 James M. Lai et al., "Everyday Decision-Making Ability in Older Persons with Cognitive Impairment," *American Journal of Geriatric Psychiatry: Official Journal of the American Association for Geriatric Psychiatry* 16, no. 8 (August 2008): 693–96, https://doi.org/10.1097/JGP.0b013e31816c7b54.

21. TARGETING AMYLOID

1   Jeff Sevigny et al., "The Antibody Aducanumab Reduces Aβ Plaques in Alzheimer's Disease," *Nature* 537, no. 7618 (September 2016): 50–56, https://doi.org/10.1038/nature19323.

2   Eric M. Reiman, "Attack on Amyloid-β Protein," *Nature* 537, no. 7618 (September 2016): 36–37, https://doi.org/10.1038/537036a.

3   D. Schenk et al., "Immunization with Amyloid-Beta Attenuates Alzheimer-Disease-Like Pathology in the PDAPP Mouse," *Nature* 400, no. 6740 (July 8, 1999): 173–77, https://doi.org/10.1038/22124.

4   *NewsHour with Jim Lehrer* (Washington, DC: NewsHour Productions, 1999), http://americanarchive.org/catalog/cpb-aacip_507-xd0qr4pk9k.

5   Lary Walker, "Dale Schenk, 59, Pioneer of Alzheimer's Immunotherapy," ALZFORUM, news article comment, October 5, 2016, https://www.alzforum.org/news/community-news/dale-schenk-59-pioneer-alzheimers-immunotherapy.

6   Minutes of the board of directors of the Alzheimer's Association, December 4, 1979, Archives of Alzheimer's Association.

22. HOPE IN A PLAN

1   Alzheimer's Study Group, "The Way Forward: An Update from the Alzheimer's Study Group," Special Committee on Aging, United States Senate (2009), https://www.aging.senate.gov/hearings/the-way-forward-an-update-from-the-alzheimers-study-group.

2   Alzheimer's Study Group, *A National Alzheimer's Strategic Plan: The Report of the Alzheimer's Study Group* (Alzheimer's Association, March 24, 2009), https://www.alz.org/documents/national/report_asg_alzplan.pdf.

3   "Alzheimer's Breakthrough Act," Alzheimer's Association, July 23, 2009, https://www.alz.org/national/documents/statements_breakthroughact.pdf.

4   Trish Vradenburg, "The Times They Are A-Changing," *US Against Alzheimer's: We Can Stop It by 2020* (blog), April 13, 2011, https://web.archive.org/web/20120310034437/http:/www.usagainstalzheimers.org/blog/view/the_times_they_are_a_changing/.

5   George Vradenburg, personal interview by Jason Karlawish, July 14, 2019.

6   "George and Trish Vradenburg's New Take on Alzheimer's Fight: More Speed, Fewer Galas," Reliable Source, *Washington Post*, April 9, 2012, https://www.washingtonpost.com/blogs/reliable-source/post/george-and-trish-vradenburgs-new-take-on-alzheimers-fight-more-speed-fewer-galas/2012/04/08/gIQAbMud4S_blog.html.

7   Robert Egge, personal interview by Jason Karlawish, July 15, 2019.

8   Consolidated and Further Continuing Appropriations Act 2015, Pub. L. No. 113–235, 113th Congress.

9   Tom Fagan and Gabrielle Stroebel, "Lilliputian Effect Size Fells Phase 3 Trial of Solanezumab, Leaving Its Future Uncertain," ALZFORUM: Networking for a Cure, November 23, 2016, https://www.alzforum.org/news/research-news/lilliputian-effect-size-fells-phase-3-trial-solanezumab-leaving-its-future.

10 "Biogen Plans Regulatory Filing for Aducanumab in Alzheimer's Disease Based on New Analysis of Larger Dataset from Phase 3 Studies," Biogen, October 22, 2019, https://investors.biogen.com/news-releases/news-release-details/biogen-plans-regulatory-filing-aducanumab-alzheimers-disease.

11 Sharon Begley, "The Maddening Saga of How an Alzheimer's 'Cabal' Thwarted Progress Toward a Cure," *STAT*, June 25, 2019, https://www.statnews.com/2019/06/25/alzheimers-cabal-thwarted-progress-toward-cure/.

12 Cynthia Helzel, "Making a Difference," Argentum, August 25, 2017, https://www.argentum.org/magazine-articles/making-a-difference/.

PART 4: A HUMANITARIAN PROBLEM

23. SOMETHING *MUST* BE WORKING

1 Ron Brookmeyer et al., "Forecasting the Prevalence of Preclinical and Clinical Alzheimer's Disease in the United States," *Alzheimer's and Dementia* 14, no. 2 (February 1, 2018): 121–29, https://doi.org/10.1016/j.jalz.2017.10.009.

2 Gill Livingston et al., "Dementia Prevention, Intervention, and Care," *Lancet* 390, no. 10113 (December 16, 2017): 2673–2734, https://doi.org/10.1016/S0140-6736(17)31363-6.

3 Thomas R. Dawber, Gilcin F. Meadors, and Felix E. Moore, "Epidemiological Approaches to Heart Disease: The Framingham Study," *American Journal of Public Health and the Nation's Health* 41, no. 3 (March 1, 1951): 279–86, https://doi.org/10.2105/AJPH.41.3.279.

4 Claudia L. Satizabal et al., "Incidence of Dementia over Three Decades in the Framingham Heart Study," *New England Journal of Medicine* 374, no. 6 (February 11, 2016): 523–32, https://doi.org/10.1056/NEJMoa1504327.

5 Fiona E. Matthews et al., "A Two-Decade Comparison of Prevalence of Dementia in Individuals Aged 65 Years and Older from Three Geographical Areas of England: Results of the Cognitive Function and Ageing Study I and II," *Lancet* 382, no. 9902 (October 26, 2013): 1405–12, https://doi.org/10.1016/S0140-6736(13)61570-6.

6 Pam Belluck, "Education May Cut Dementia Risk, Study Finds," *New York Times*, February 10, 2016, https://www.nytimes.com/2016/02/11/health/education-may-cut-dementia-risk-study-finds.html.

7 E. A. Maguire et al., "Navigation-Related Structural Change in the Hippocampi of Taxi Drivers," *Proceedings of the National Academy of Sciences* 97, no. 8 (April 11, 2000): 4398–403, https://doi.org/10.1073/pnas.070039597.

8 Eleanor A. Maguire, Katherine Woollett, and Hugo J. Spiers, "London Taxi Drivers and Bus Drivers: A Structural MRI and Neuropsychological Analysis," *Hippocampus* 16, no. 12 (2006): 1091–101, https://doi.org/10.1002/hipo.20233.

9 Lisa Barnes, personal interview by Jason Karlawish, September 5, 2018.

10 Megan Zuelsdorff et al., "Stressful Life Events and Racial Disparities in Cognition Among Middle-Aged and Older Adults," *Journal of Alzheimer's Disease* 73, no. 2 (January 1, 2020): 671–82, https://doi.org/10.3233/JAD-190439.

11 Bruce S. McEwen, "Plasticity of the Hippocampus: Adaptation to Chronic Stress and Allostatic Load," *Annals of the New York Academy of Sciences* 933, no. 1 (2001): 265–77, https://doi.org/10.1111/j.1749-6632.2001.tb05830.x.

24. EXISTENTIAL DREAD

1 Kristin Harkins et al., "Development of a Process to Disclose Amyloid Imaging Results to Cognitively Normal Older Adult Research Participants," *Alzheimer's Research and Therapy* 7, no. 1 (2015): 26, https://doi.org/10.1186/s13195-015-0112-7.

2   Emily A. Largent et al., "Cognitively Unimpaired Adults' Reactions to Disclosure of Amyloid PET Scan Results," *PLOS ONE* 15, no. 2 (February 13, 2020): https://doi.org/10.1371/journal.pone.0229137.

25. CARING FOR EACH OTHER

1   Kirk R. Daffner, "Reflections of a Dementia Specialist: I Want to Stop Working Before I Embarrass Myself," *Washington Post*, accessed March 25, 2020, https://www.washingtonpost.com/national/health-science/reflections-of-a-dementia-specialist-i-want-to-stop-working-before-i-embarrass-myself/2018/04/13/adb08158-3111-11e8-8abc-22a366b72f2d_story.html.
2   "Whealthcare," Whealthcare, accessed March 27, 2020, http://www.whealthcare.org.
3   Jilenne Gunther and Robert Neill, "Snapshots: Banks Empowering Customers and Fighting Exploitation," AARP (February 2016), https://www.aarp.org/content/dam/aarp/ppi/2016-02/Snapshots-Banks-Empowering-Customers-and-Fighting-Exploitation-Brochure.pdf.
4   "PARO Therapeutic Robot," accessed March 25, 2020, http://www.parorobots.com/.
5   "A Korean Team Develops Dementia-Caring Robot, Marking Emergency Call Automatically," *China Daily*, October 27, 2016, http://www.chinadaily.com.cn/regional/2016-10/27/content_27195065.htm.
6   Dennis Thompson, "Robots May Soon Become Alzheimer's Caregivers," WebMD, June 28, 2018, https://www.webmd.com/alzheimers/news/20180628/robots-may-soon-become-alzheimers-caregivers#1.
7   Lawrence K. Altman, "Reagan's Twilight—A Special Report: A President Fades into a World Apart," *New York Times*, October 5, 1997, https://www.nytimes.com/1997/10/05/us/reagan-s-twilight-a-special-report-a-president-fades-into-a-world-apart.html.

26. THE WORLDS WE CREATE

1   Jean Makesh, personal interview by Jason Karlawish, October 15, 2019.
2   Matthew Butler, *Ground Breaking Biophilic Assisted Living and Memory Care, Only One in the World*, 2019, https://www.youtube.com/watch?time_continue =1&v=IKl-jUt642-g&feature=emb_logo.
3   "TOWN SQUARE: The George G. Glenner Alzheimer's Family Centers, Inc.," accessed April 13, 2020, https://glenner.org/town-square/.
4   Sumathi Reddy, "To Help Alzheimer's Patients, a Care Center Re-Creates the 1950s," *Wall Street Journal*, September 18, 2018, https://www.wsj.com/articles/to-help-alzheimers-patients-a-care-center-recreates-the-1950s-1537278209.
5   Christopher A. Thurber, Edward Walton, and American Academy of Pediatrics Council on School Health, "Preventing and Treating Homesickness," *Pediatrics* 119, no. 1 (January 2007): 192–201, https://doi.org/10.1542/peds.2006-2781.
6   Richard Schulz et al., "End-of-Life Care and the Effects of Bereavement on Family Caregivers of Persons with Dementia," *New England Journal of Medicine* 349, no. 20 (November 13, 2003): 1936–42, https://doi.org/10.1056/NEJMsa035373.
7   Ira Glass, "Give the People What They Want," *This American Life*, accessed March 17, 2020, https://www.thisamericanlife.org/216/give-the-people-what-they-want.
8   Anne Basting, personal interview by Jason Karlawish, November 14, 2019.

9   I credit this idea of "assisted presentations of self" to Anders Næss, Eivind Grip Fjær, and Mia Vabø, "The Assisted Presentations of Self in Nursing Home Life," *Social Science and Medicine* 150 (February 1, 2016): 153–59, https://doi.org/10.1016/j.socscimed.2015.12.027.

10 Butler, *Ground Breaking Biophilic Assisted Living and Memory Care, Only One in the World*.

11 Jason Karlawish et al., "Bringing the Vote to Residents of Long-Term Care Facilities: A Study of the Benefits and Challenges of Mobile Polling," *Election Law Journal: Rules, Politics, and Policy* 10, no. 1 (March 1, 2011): 5–14, https://doi.org/10.1089/elj.2010.0065.

12 Anne Basting, *Creative Care: A Revolutionary Approach to Dementia and Elder Care* (New York: HarperOne, 2020).

13 Joan Biskupic, "A New Page in O'Connors' Love Story," ABC News, February 19, 2009, https://abcnews.go.com/TheLaw/Politics/story?id=3858553&page=1.

27. THE WORLDS WE END

1   Bryan D. James et al., "Contribution of Alzheimer Disease to Mortality in the United States," *Neurology* 82, no. 12 (March 25, 2014): 1045–50, https://doi.org/10.1212/WNL.0000000000000240.

2   Katherine Hammond, "Kept Alive: The Enduring Tragedy of Margot Bentley," *Narrative Inquiry in Bioethics* 6, no. 2 (October 3, 2016): 80–82, https://doi.org/10.1353/nib.2016.0023.

3   Pamela Fayerman, "Patient's Family Sues B.C. as Nursing Home Keeps Her Alive Against Her Wishes," August 7, 2013, http://www.vancouversun.com/health/patient+family+sues+nursing+home+keeps+alive+against+wishes/8756167/story.html.

4   Judith Graham, "My Sister Made Her End-of-Life Wishes Clear. Then Dementia Took Hold," *STAT*, September 16, 2016, https://www.statnews.com/2016/09/16/dementia-last-wishes/.

5   "Identify Alzheimer's Disease Earlier, Brought to You by Biogen," US Healthcare Professionals Website, Biogen, accessed January 26, 2020, https://www.identifyalz.com/?cid=smc-li-dse-hp-alzdsasite-112018.

GLOSSARY

A4 Study   Anti-Amyloid Treatment in Asymptomatic Alzheimer's Study

AARP   American Association for Retired Persons

ADAS   Alzheimer's Disease Assessment Scale

ADNI   Alzheimer's Disease Neuroimaging Initiative

ADPR   Alzheimer's Disease Patient Registry

AMA   American Medical Association

ARIA   Amyloid Related Imaging Abnormalities. There are two subtypes: ARIA-E to signify edema and effusions, and ARIA-H to signify microscopic hemorrhage.

CNN   Cable News Network

ERA   Equal Rights Amendment

FDA   Food and Drug Administration

HELP   Hospital Elder Life Program

JAMA   *Journal of the American Medical Association*

MCI   mild cognitive impairment

MEDCAC   Medicare Evidence Development and Coverage Advisory Committee

NIA   National Institute on Aging

NIH   National Institutes of Health

OHSU   Oregon Health and Science University

PDAPP   Platelet-derived amyloid precursor protein, the name given to a transgenic mouse model of Alzheimer's disease

PET   positron-emission tomography

PiB   Pittsburgh compound B

SELECTED BIBLIOGRAPHY

Alzheimer, Alois. 1911. "Über Eigenartige Krankheitsfälle des Späteren Alters." *Zeitschrift für die Gesamte Neurologie und Psychiatrie* 4 (1): 356–85. https://doi. org/10.1007/BF02866241. Translated by Hans Förstl and Raymond Levy. "On Certain Peculiar Diseases of Old Age." *History of Psychiatry* 2, no. 5 (March 1991): 71–73. doi:10.1177/0957154X9100200505.

Alzheimer's Study Group, *A National Alzheimer's Strategic Plan: The Report of the Alzheimer's Study Group.* Alzheimer's Association, March 24, 2009. https://www.alz.org/ documents/national/report_asg_alzplan.pdf.

Agich, George J. *Autonomy and Long-Term Care.* New York: Oxford University Press, 1993.

Ballenger, Jesse F. *Self, Senility, and Alzheimer's Disease in Modern America: A History.* Baltimore: Johns Hopkins University Press, 2006.

Basting, Anne. *Creative Care: A Revolutionary Approach to Dementia and Elder Care.* New York: HarperOne, 2020.

Bayles, Fred, Scott McCartney, Lisa Levitt Ryckman, Sharon Cohen, Strat Douthat, George Esper, and Tamara Jones. *Guardians of the Elderly: An Ailing System.* Associated Press: Special Report, September 19, 1987.

Behuniak, Susan M. "The Living Dead? The Construction of People with Alzheimer's Disease as Zombies." *Ageing and Society* 31, no. 1 (January 2011): 70–92. https://doi. org/10.1017/S0144686X10000693.

Belle, Steven H., Louis Burgio, Robert Burns, David Coon, Sara J. Czaja, Dolores Gallagher-Thompson, Laura N. Gitlin, et al. "Enhancing the Quality of Life of Dementia Caregivers from Different Ethnic or Racial Groups: A Randomized, Controlled Trial." *Annals of Internal Medicine* 145, no. 10 (November 21, 2006): 727–38. https:// doi.org/10.7326/0003-4819-145-10-200611210-00005.

Bessel, Richard. *Germany After the First World War.* Oxford: Clarendon Press, 1993.

Boris, Eileen, and Jennifer Klein. *Caring for America: Home Health Workers in the Shadow of the Welfare State.* New York: Oxford University Press, 2012.

Butler, Robert. *Why Survive?: Being Old in America.* Baltimore: Johns Hopkins University Press, 2003.

Clark, Christopher M., Julie A. Schneider, Barry J. Bedell, Thomas G. Beach, Warren B. Bilker, Mark A. Mintun, Michael J. Pontecorvo, et al. "Use of Florbetapir-PET for Imaging Beta-Amyloid Pathology." *JAMA* 305, no. 3 (January 19, 2011): 275–83. https://doi. org/10.1001/jama.2010.2008.

Coe, Norma B., Meghan M. Skira, and Eric B. Larson. "A Comprehensive Measure of the Costs of Caring for a Parent: Differences According to Functional Status." *Journal of the American Geriatrics Society* 66, no. 10 (October 2018): 2003–8. https://doi.org/10.1111/ jgs.15552.

Congress of the US, Washington, DC, Office of Technology Assessment. *Losing a Million Minds: Confronting the Tragedy of Alzheimer's Disease and Other Dementias*. Congressional Summary. Washington, DC: US Congress, Office of Technology Assessment, April 1987. https://eric.ed.gov/?id=ED298420.

Degler, Carl N. *At Odds: Women and the Family in America from the Revolution to the Present*. New York: Oxford University Press, 1981.

"Department of Health and Human Services United States Food and Drug Administration Center for Evaluation and Research. Transcript of Peripheral and Central Nervous System Drugs Advisory Committee Meeting." Department of Health and Human Services, United States Food and Drug Administration, October 23, 2008.

Evans, D. A., H. H. Funkenstein, M. S. Albert, P. A. Scherr, N. R. Cook, M. J. Chown, L. E. Hebert, C. H. Hennekens, and J. O. Taylor. "Prevalence of Alzheimer's Disease in a Community Population of Older Persons. Higher Than Previously Reported." *JAMA* 262, no. 18 (November 10, 1989): 2551–56.

Fee, Elizabeth, and Daniel M. Fox, eds. *AIDS: The Burden of History*. Berkeley: University of California Press, 1988. https://publishing.cdlib.org/ucpressebooks/view?docId=ft7t1nb59n&chunk.id=d0e5789&toc.depth=1&toc.id=d0e5789&brand=ucpress.

Fergusson, Adam. *When Money Dies: The Nightmare of the Weimar Hyper-Inflation*. Scribe, 2011.

Francis, L. P. "Understanding Autonomy in Light of Intellectual Disability." In *Disability and Disadvantage*, 200–215. Oxford, New York: Oxford University Press, 2011.

Friedman, Esther M., Regina A. Shih, Kenneth M. Langa, and Michael D. Hurd. "US Prevalence and Predictors of Informal Caregiving for Dementia." *Health Affairs* 34, no. 10 (October 1, 2015): 1637–41. https://doi.org/10.1377/hlthaff.2015.0510.

Friedman, Susan M., Daniel A. Mendelson, Karilee W. Bingham, and Stephen L. Kates. "Impact of a Comanaged Geriatric Fracture Center on Short-Term Hip Fracture Outcomes." *Archives of Internal Medicine* 169, no. 18 (October 12, 2009): 1712–17. https://doi.org/10.1001/archinternmed.2009.321.

Grisso, Thomas, and Paul S. Appelbaum. *Assessing Competence to Consent to Treatment: A Guide for Physicians and Other Health Professionals*. Oxford, New York: Oxford University Press, 1998.

Guenther, Katja. *Localization and Its Discontents*. Chicago: University of Chicago Press, 2015. https://www.press.uchicago.edu/ucp/books/book/chicago/L/bo21163259.html.

Harkins, Kristin, Pamela Sankar, Reisa Sperling, Joshua D. Grill, Robert C. Green, Keith A. Johnson, Megan Healy, and Jason Karlawish. "Development of a Process to Disclose Amyloid Imaging Results to Cognitively Normal Older Adult Research Participants." *Alzheimer's Research and Therapy* 7, no. 1 (May 26, 2015): 26. https://doi.org/10.1186/s13195-015-0112-7.

Hurd, Michael D., Paco Martorell, Adeline Delavande, Kathleen J. Mullen, and Kenneth M. Langa. "Monetary Costs of Dementia in the United States." *New England Journal of Medicine* 368, no. 14 (April 4, 2013): 1326–34. https://doi.org/10.1056/NEJMsa1204629.

Inouye, S. K., S. T. Bogardus, P. A. Charpentier, L. Leo-Summers, D. Acampora, T. R. Holford, and L. M. Cooney. "A Multicomponent Intervention to Prevent Delirium in Hospitalized Older Patients." *New England Journal of Medicine* 340, no. 9 (March 4, 1999): 669–76. https://doi.org/10.1056/NEJM199903043400901.

Institute of Medicine (US) Committee to Study the AIDS Research Program of the National Institutes of Health. *The AIDS Research Program of the National Institutes of Health*. Washington, DC: National Academies Press, 1991. https://www.ncbi.nlm.nih.gov/books/NBK234085.

Jack, Clifford R., David S. Knopman, William J. Jagust, Leslie M. Shaw, Paul S. Aisen, Michael W. Weiner, Ronald C. Petersen, and John Q. Trojanowski. "Hypothetical Model of Dynamic Biomarkers of the Alzheimer's Pathological Cascade." *Lancet Neurology* 9, no. 1 (January 1, 2010): 119–28. https://doi.org/10.1016/S1474-4422(09)70299-6.

Jack, Clifford R., David S. Knopman, William J. Jagust, Ronald C. Petersen, Michael W. Weiner, Paul S. Aisen, Leslie M. Shaw, et al. "Tracking Pathophysiological Processes in Alzheimer's Disease: An Updated Hypothetical Model of Dynamic Biomarkers." *Lancet Neurology* 12, no. 2 (February 1, 2013): 207–16. https://doi.org/10.1016/S1474-4422(12)70291-0.

James, Bryan D., Sue E. Leurgans, Liesi E. Hebert, Paul A. Scherr, Kristine Yaffe, and David A. Bennett. "Contribution of Alzheimer Disease to Mortality in the United States." *Neurology* 82, no. 12 (March 25, 2014): 1045–50. https://doi.org/10.1212/WNL.0000000000000240.

Johnson, K. A., S. Minoshima, N. I. Bohnen, K. J. Donohoe, N. L. Foster, P. Herscovitch, J. H. Karlawish, et al. "Appropriate Use Criteria for Amyloid PET: A Report of the Amyloid Imaging Task Force, the Society of Nuclear Medicine and Molecular Imaging, and the Alzheimer's Association." *Journal of Nuclear Medicine* 54, no. 3 (March 1, 2013): 476–90. https://doi.org/10.2967/jnumed.113.120618.

Kasper, Judith D., Vicki A. Freedman, Brenda C. Spillman, and Jennifer L. Wolff. "The Disproportionate Impact of Dementia on Family and Unpaid Caregiving to Older Adults." *Health Affairs* 34, no. 10 (October 1, 2015): 1642–49. https://doi.org/10.1377/hlthaff.2015.0536.

Katzman, Robert, and Katherine Bick. *Alzheimer Disease: The Changing View.* San Diego: Academic Press, 2000.

Katzman, Robert. "The Prevalence and Malignancy of Alzheimer Disease: A Major Killer." *Archives of Neurology* 33, no. 4 (April 1, 1976): 217–18. https://doi.org/10.1001/archneur.1976.00500040001001.

Kaye, Jeffrey, Christina Reynolds, Molly Bowman, Nicole Sharma, Thomas Riley, Ona Golonka, Jonathan Lee, et al. "Methodology for Establishing a Community-Wide Life Laboratory for Capturing Unobtrusive and Continuous Remote Activity and Health Data." *Journal of Visualized Experiments: JoVE*, no. 137 (July 27, 2018). https://doi.org/10.3791/56942.

Keuck, Lara. "Diagnosing Alzheimer's Disease in Kraepelin's Clinic, 1909–1912." *History of the Human Sciences* 31, no. 2 (April 1, 2018): 42–64. https://doi.org/10.1177/0952695118758879.

Khachaturian, Zaven S., and Ara S. Khachaturian. "Prevent Alzheimer's Disease by 2020: A National Strategic Goal." *Alzheimer's and Dementia: The Journal of the Alzheimer's Association* 5, no. 2 (March 1, 2009): 81–84. https://doi.org/10.1016/j.jalz.2009.01.022.

Khachaturian, Zaven S., Ronald C. Petersen, Serge Gauthier, Neil Buckholtz, Jodey P. Corey-Bloom, Bill Evans, Howard Fillit, et al. "A Roadmap for the Prevention of Dementia: The Inaugural Leon Thal Symposium." *Alzheimer's and Dementia: The Journal of the Alzheimer's Association* 4, no. 3 (May 1, 2008): 156–63. https://doi.org/10.1016/j.jalz.2008.03.005.

Kiyak, H. A., L. Teri, and S. Borson. "Physical and Functional Health Assessment in Normal Aging and in Alzheimer's Disease: Self-Reports vs. Family Reports." *Gerontologist* 34, no. 3 (June 1994): 324–30. https://doi.org/10.1093/geront/34.3.324.

Kleinman, Arthur. *The Soul of Care: The Moral Education of a Husband and a Doctor.* New York: Penguin, 2019.

Klunk, William E., Henry Engler, Agneta Nordberg, Yanming Wang, Gunnar Blomqvist,

Daniel P. Holt, Mats Bergström, et al. "Imaging Brain Amyloid in Alzheimer's Disease with Pittsburgh Compound-B." *Annals of Neurology* 55, no. 3 (March 2004): 306–19. https://doi.org/10.1002/ana.20009.

Largent, Emily A., Kristin Harkins, Christopher H. van Dyck, Sara Hachey, Pamela Sankar, and Jason Karlawish. "Cognitively Unimpaired Adults' Reactions to Disclosure of Amyloid PET Scan Results." *PLOS ONE* 15, no. 2 (February 13, 2020): e0229137. https://doi.org/10.1371/journal.pone.0229137.

Lieberman, Morton A., and Leonard D. Borman. *Self-Help Groups for Coping with Crisis: Origins, Members, Processes, and Impact.* San Francisco: Jossey-Bass, 1979.

Livingston, Gill, Andrew Sommerlad, Vasiliki Orgeta, Sergi G. Costafreda, Jonathan Huntley, David Ames, Clive Ballard, et al. "Dementia Prevention, Intervention, and Care." *Lancet* 390, no. 10113 (December 16, 2017): 2673–2734. https://doi.org/10.1016/S0140-6736(17)31363-6.

Lock, Margaret. *The Alzheimer Conundrum: Entanglements of Dementia and Aging.* Princeton, NJ: Princeton University Press, 2013.

Mace, Nancy L., and Peter V. Rabins. *The 36-Hour Day: A Family Guide to Caring for Persons with Alzheimer's Disease, Related Dementing Illnesses, and Memory Loss in Later Life.* Baltimore: Johns Hopkins University Press, 1981.

Mackenzie, Catriona, and Natalie Stoljar. *Relational Autonomy: Feminist Perspectives on Autonomy, Agency, and the Social Self.* New York: Oxford University Press, 2000.

Maguire, E. A., D. G. Gadian, I. S. Johnsrude, C. D. Good, J. Ashburner, R. S. Frackowiak, and C. D. Frith. "Navigation-Related Structural Change in the Hippocampi of Taxi Drivers." *Proceedings of the National Academy of Sciences* 97, no. 8 (April 11, 2000): 4398–403. https://doi.org/10.1073/pnas.070039597.

Maurer, Konrad, and Ulrike Maurer. *Alzheimer: The Life of a Physician and the Career of a Disease.* Translated by Neil Levi and Alistair Burns. New York: Columbia University Press, 2003.

McKhann, G., D. Drachman, M. Folstein, R. Katzman, D. Price, and E. M. Stadlan. "Clinical Diagnosis of Alzheimer's Disease: Report of the NINCDS-ADRDA Work Group Under the Auspices of Department of Health and Human Services Task Force on Alzheimer's Disease." *Neurology* 34, no. 7 (July 1984): 939–44. https://doi.org/10.1212/wnl.34.7.939.

Næss, Anders, Eivind Grip Fjær, and Mia Vabø. "The Assisted Presentations of Self in Nursing Home Life." *Social Science and Medicine* 150 (February 1, 2016): 153–59. https://doi.org/10.1016/j.socscimed.2015.12.027.

Oberlander, Jonathan. "The Political Life of Medicare." In *The Political Life of Medicare*, 62–63. Chicago, London: University of Chicago Press, 2003.

Petersen, R. C., G. E. Smith, S. C. Waring, R. J. Ivnik, E. G. Tangalos, and E. Kokmen. "Mild Cognitive Impairment: Clinical Characterization and Outcome." *Archives of Neurology* 56, no. 3 (March 1999): 303–8. https://doi.org/10.1001/archneur.56.3.303.

Pinquart, Martin, and Silvia Sörensen. "Differences Between Caregivers and Noncaregivers in Psychological Health and Physical Health: A Meta-Analysis." *Psychology and Aging* 18, no. 2 (June 2003): 250–67. https://doi.org/10.1037/0882-7974.18.2.250.

Qiu, Chengxuan, Eva von Strauss, Lars Bäckman, Bengt Winblad, and Laura Fratiglioni. "Twenty-Year Changes in Dementia Occurrence Suggest Decreasing Incidence in Central Stockholm, Sweden." *Neurology* 80, no. 20 (May 14, 2013): 1888–94. https://doi.org/10.1212/WNL.0b013e318292a2f9.

Reiman, Eric M. "Attack on Amyloid-β Protein." *Nature* 537, no. 7618 (September 2016): 36–37. https://doi.org/10.1038/537036a.

Rocca, Walter A., Barbara P. Yawn, Jennifer L. St. Sauver, Brandon R. Grossardt, and L. Joseph Melton. "History of the Rochester Epidemiology Project: Half a Century of Medical Records Linkage in a US Population." *Mayo Clinic Proceedings* 87, no. 12 (December 2012): 1202–13. https://doi.org/10.1016/j.mayocp.2012.08.012.

Ronald Reagan—Medicare Will Bring a Socialist Dictatorship. Accessed March 27, 2020. https://www.youtube.com/watch?v=Bejdhs3jGyw.

Ronald Reagan Presidential Library. "Physician's Explanation of Ronald Reagan's Alzheimer's Diagnosis." Accessed June 13, 2019. https://www.reaganlibrary.gov/sreference/physician-s-explanation-of-ronald-reagan-s-alzheimer-s-diagnosis.

Rosenberg, Charles E., and Janet Lynne Golden, eds. *Framing Disease: Studies in Cultural History.* New Brunswick, NJ: Rutgers University Press, 1992.

Roth, L. H., A. Meisel, and C. W. Lidz. "Tests of Competency to Consent to Treatment." *American Journal of Psychiatry* 134, no. 3 (March 1977): 279–84. https://doi.org/10.1176/ajp.134.3.279.

Satizabal, Claudia L., Alexa S. Beiser, Vincent Chouraki, Geneviève Chêne, Carole Dufouil, and Sudha Seshadri. "Incidence of Dementia over Three Decades in the Framingham Heart Study." *New England Journal of Medicine* 374, no. 6 (February 11, 2016): 523–32. https://doi.org/10.1056/NEJMoa1504327.

Schenk, D., R. Barbour, W. Dunn, G. Gordon, H. Grajeda, T. Guido, K. Hu, et al. "Immunization with Amyloid-Beta Attenuates Alzheimer-Disease-Like Pathology in the PDAPP Mouse." *Nature* 400, no. 6740 (July 8, 1999): 173–77. https://doi.org/10.1038/22124.

Schulz, Richard, Aaron B. Mendelsohn, William E. Haley, Diane Mahoney, Rebecca S. Allen, Song Zhang, Larry Thompson, Steven H. Belle, and Resources for Enhancing Alzheimer's Caregiver Health Investigators. "End-of-Life Care and the Effects of Bereavement on Family Caregivers of Persons with Dementia." *New England Journal of Medicine* 349, no. 20 (November 13, 2003): 1936–42. https://doi.org/10.1056/NEJMsa035373.

Scull, Andrew. *Madness in Civilization: A Cultural History of Insanity, from the Bible to Freud, from the Madhouse to Modern Medicine.* Repr. ed. Princeton, NJ: Princeton University Press, 2016.

Sevigny, Jeff, Ping Chiao, Thierry Bussière, Paul H. Weinreb, Leslie Williams, Marcel Maier, Robert Dunstan, et al. "The Antibody Aducanumab Reduces Aβ Plaques in Alzheimer's Disease." *Nature* 537, no. 7618 (September 2016): 50–56. https://doi.org/10.1038/nature19323.

Spruill, Marjorie J. *Divided We Stand: The Battle over Women's Rights and Family Values That Polarized American Politics.* New York: Bloomsbury USA, 2017.

Stites, Shana D., Jonathan D. Rubright, and Jason Karlawish. "What Features of Stigma Do the Public Most Commonly Attribute to Alzheimer's Disease Dementia? Results of a Survey of the U.S. General Public." *Alzheimer's and Dementia* 14, no. 7 (July 1, 2018): 925–32. https://doi.org/10.1016/j.jalz.2018.01.006.

Summers, W. K., L. V. Majovski, G. M. Marsh, K. Tachiki, and A. Kling. "Oral Tetrahydroaminoacridine in Long-Term Treatment of Senile Dementia, Alzheimer Type." *New England Journal of Medicine* 315, no. 20 (November 13, 1986): 1241–45. https://doi.org/10.1056/NEJM198611133152001.

Thomas, Lewis. "The Problem of Dementia." In *Late Night Thoughts on Listening to Mahler's Ninth Symphony,* 121. New York: Viking Press, 1983.

United States Congress, Office of Technology Assessment. *Confused Minds, Burdened Families: Finding Help for People with Alzheimer's and Other Dementias,* OTA-13A-403. Washington, DC: US Government Printing Office, 1990. https://catalog.hathitrust.org/Record/007415141.

United States Congress, Senate Committee on Labor and Human Resources, Subcommittee on Aging. *Impact of Alzheimer's Disease on the Nation's Elderly: Joint Hearing Before the Subcommittee on Aging of the Committee on Labor and Human Resources, United States Senate, and the Subcommittee on Labor, Health, Education, and Welfare of the Committee on Appropriations, House of Representatives, Ninety-Sixth Congress, Second Session, on to Analyze the Impact of Alzheimer's Disease and Other Dimentias [i.e., Dementias] of Aging on Our Society.* Washington, DC: US Government Printing Office, 1980.

United States Congress. *Alzheimer's: The Unmet Challenge for Research and Care.* Joint Hearing Before the Select Committee on Aging, House of Representatives, and the Subcommittee on Aging of the Committee on Labor and Human Resources, US Senate, 101st Cong., 2d Sess., April 3, 1990, SCOA Comm. Pub. No. 101–783.

Vickrey, Barbara G., Brian S. Mittman, Karen I. Connor, Marjorie L. Pearson, Richard D. Della Penna, Theodore G. Ganiats, Robert W. Demonte, et al. "The Effect of a Disease Management Intervention on Quality and Outcomes of Dementia Care: A Randomized, Controlled Trial." *Annals of Internal Medicine* 145, no. 10 (November 21, 2006): 713–26. https://doi.org/10.7326/0003-4819-145-10-200611210-00004.

Zarit, Steven H., Kyungmin Kim, Elia E. Femia, David M. Almeida, Jyoti Savla, and Peter C. M. Molenaar. "Effects of Adult Day Care on Daily Stress of Caregivers: A Within-Person Approach." *Journals of Gerontology Series B: Psychological Sciences and Social Sciences* 66B, no. 5 (September 2011): 538–46. https://doi.org/10.1093/geronb/gbr030.

INDEX

ABOUT THE AUTHOR

Jason Karlawish is a physician and writer. He researches and writes about issues at the intersections of bioethics, aging, and the neurosciences. He is the author of the novel *Open Wound: The Tragic Obsession of Dr. William Beaumont* and his essays have appeared in *The New York Times*, *The Washington Post*, *Forbes*, and the *Philadelphia Inquirer*. He is a Professor of Medicine, Medical Ethics and Health Policy, and Neurology at the University of Pennsylvania and Co-Director of the Penn Memory Center, where he cares for patients. He lives in Philadelphia. To learn more, visit www.jasonkarlawish.com.

616.8311 KARLAWISH
Karlawish, Jason,
The problem of Alzheimer's :
R2005855560 PTREE

Fulton County Library System